BIOLOGY OF THE IMMUNE RESPONSE

Biology of the Immune Response

Peter Abramoff, Ph.D.
Professor and Chairman
Department of Biology
Marquette University

Mariano F. La Via, M.D.
Professor of Pathology
The Bowman Gray School of Medicine
Wake Forest University

McGraw-Hill Book Company
New York   St. Louis   San Francisco   Düsseldorf   London   Mexico   Panama
Sydney   Toronto

Biology of the Immune Response

Library of Congress Catalog Card Number 79–102446
00135

1 2 3 4 5 6 7 8 9 0   MAMM   7 9 8 7 6 5 4 3 2 1 0

This book was set in Electra by Monotype Composition Company, Inc., and printed on perma-nent paper and bound by The Maple Press Company. The designer was Merrill Haber; the drawings were done by B. Handelman Associates, Inc. The editors were James R. Young and Sally Mobley. Stuart Levine supervised the production.

Preface

In this age of the "information explosion" we can hardly cope with the thousands of printed pages that come our way each day. It might seem ironic, in this context, that we chose to add yet another book to the massive amount of "informational" matter being produced.

We undertook the writing of this book, together with eleven contributing authors, to fill what to us appeared to be a gap in the immunological literature: a presentation of the biological aspects of immunological phenomena. The past 10 years have witnessed a tremendous growth in research dealing with immunobiological phenomena, both at the basic level and in the clinical areas. The elucidation of cell types involved in antibody production and of their kinetics and interactions is one example. The recent successful transplantations of organs and tissues have added much more information to our understanding of the homograft reaction and have also generated many more unsolved problems. The basic scientist and clinician have interdigitated their efforts in this area as well as in the search for an explanation for the puzzle of "autoimmune" phenomena.

This tremendous burst of activity has created the need for better communication at all investigative levels. This need prompted us to produce a well-organized and integrated textbook which would serve as a medium to accomplish this end. We have made every possible effort to see that this book would be an organic textbook and not a series of disjointed papers on various aspects of immunobiology. We have tried to provide core information, clearly and in a well-integrated fashion, with abundant, up-to-date references for those who want to expand their reading on a subject of interest to them. We hope that our efforts will benefit both the student of immunology and of medicine and the professional man who has been left behind by the "information explosion" and who needs to "catch up". If this hope is fulfilled, we will feel that our efforts have not been in vain.

It takes many hours of hard work to bring a book to the reader; the authors cannot, however, take full credit for all this work. Without the invaluable help of many of our close collaborators, students, and friends, this task would have been impossible.

We would like to mention particularly our faithful secretaries, Mrs. Jerry Comm, Mrs. Emily Cook, and Miss Marilyn Mutzenbauer, for their inexhaustible energy and enthusiasm in typing and retyping the manuscript, checking references, editing our grammar and syntax, and correcting page and galley proofs. Mr. John McIntyre, Dr. Damodar Vakil, and Mrs. Nancy Brien also assisted in various phases of manuscript preparation.

Finally, we owe a special debt of gratitude to Dr. Robert Good and Mrs. Joanne Finstad-Good for their generous assistance in providing abundant illustrative material from their files. Dr. Good in a way shares with us the responsibility of bringing this book to the reader as he provided stimulation and encouragement to us from the birth of the idea to the final manuscript.

PETER ABRAMOFF

MARIANO F. LA VIA

List of Contributors

Nancy K. Brien, M.Sc.
Marquette University

Edward A. Chaperon, Ph.D.
Creighton University Medical School

Henry N. Claman, M.D.
University of Colorado Medical Center

Richard S. Farr, M.D.
National Jewish Hospital and Research Center

William S. Hammond, M.D.
University of Colorado Medical Center

Kimishige Ishizaka, M.D.
Children's Asthma Research Institute

Phyllis D. Kind, Ph.D.
University of Colorado Medical Center

Percy Minden, M.D.
National Jewish Hospital and Research Center

George C. Saunders, V.M.D.
University of Colorado Medical Center

David W. Talmage, M.D.
University of Colorado Medical Center

Darcy B. Wilson, Ph.D.
University of Pennsylvania School of Medicine

Contents

9
Immunoenhancement 260
Phyllis D. Kind

10
Immunosuppression 272
Edward A. Chaperon

11
Theories of Antibody Formation 304
David W. Talmage

13
Immunologic Protection
William S. Hammond

14
Immunologic Injury
Kimishige Ishizaka / Phyllis D. Kind

BIOLOGY OF THE IMMUNE RESPONSE

1
Nature of Immunity

Thucydides reported in his writings that during the plague in Athens it was observed that those who had recovered would not catch the disease a second time, even though they were ministering to the sick. Voltaire, in his letters, related that in China there was a very widely practiced custom of inhaling powder prepared from the scabs of smallpox lesions, since the inhalation of these powders would protect from the disease. Because of the common occurrence of smallpox, the exposure of healthy individuals to diseased ones and even inoculation with human smallpox was practiced in European countries and was shown to have a protective effect. After the demonstration by Jenner in the eighteenth century that inoculation of cowpox material would protect from smallpox, this practice became quite common. It was Pasteur, however, who placed immunology on a scientific basis through his studies on microbes and development of methods to induce immunity. The term *vaccination*, introduced by Pasteur in honor of Jenner's use of vaccinial pox, has been used traditionally to indicate methods of inoculation with a number of antigens which confer immunity against disease.

Immunology is concerned with the general field of resistance to infectious diseases, both naturally existing or artificially induced, by introduction of antigens. It has developed explosively during the last few years, and the tremendous growth is immediately apparent upon perusal of the current literature. This growing interest in understanding the mechanisms of acquired as well as natural immunity has captured the attention of biologists from various scientific fields. Biochemists, clinicians, microbiologists, pathologists, and biophysicists have found fruitful areas to explore with their specialized techniques. This has led to a clearer understanding of the mechanism of acquired immunity, the nature of antigens and antibodies, the participation of antibodies in the pathogenesis of disease, and the phylogenetic and ontogenetic development of immunological responsiveness. It has also led to great advances in the field of human organ transplantation for the treatment of chronic disabling diseases.

The entry into the field of so many investigators has created a need for subdivision of this vastly growing discipline. The work dealing primarily with the nature of antigens, the chemical and physical properties of the immunoglobulins, and antigen-antibody reactions has been classified under the heading of *immunochemistry*. The term *immunobiology* has been used to designate the studies on the more biological aspects of immunology, such as the mechanism of antibody production at the cellular and subcellular level, the participation of various lymphoid cells in the production of antibodies, the biological manifestations of immunity, and participation of antibodies in the pathogenesis of disease. Other areas, such as immunohematology, clinical immunology, etc., comprise specialized fields of study of particular entities.

Immunochemistry is quite old as a discipline, since the study of the chemistry of antigens and antibodies, of their interaction, and of the chemical basis of immunity dates back to the early 1900s. It was Landsteiner (1) who first investigated the possibility of creating chemically defined artificial antigens in the hope of gaining a better understanding of how antibodies might be induced and how they may interact with antigens. His pioneering work, showing that antibodies would be formed in response to artificially prepared antigens, led to the discarding of the "side-chain" theory, which had been proposed by Ehrlich (2–4). This theory stated that the outside of the cell had a number of "side chains" (haptophore groups) which were capable of combining with and neutralizing toxins, foreign proteins, nutritional materials, etc. Groups which combined with noxious materials were shed, and this in turn led to the production of more haptophore groups, which accumulated in the serum. Thus antigen was needed only to bind haptophore groups so that overproduction would result and antibody would increase. The observations of Landsteiner (1) that artificial antigens could be prepared, which had never been seen by the cell, made it appear that the theory postulated by Ehrlich could not be used to explain the infinite number of patterns necessary for recognition of all possible artificial antigens. A new theory resulted from Landsteiner's observations, postulating that the process of antibody production was initiated by the introduction in the cell of a substance which was previously unknown (antigen) and which acted as a "template" for the de novo synthesis of a protein capable of reacting with it (antibody). This hypothesis, which was advanced independently by Breinl and Haurowitz (5), by Alexander (6), and by Mudd (7), was attractive and, in its original form or in some variation of it, dominated the thinking of immunologists for many years (8). Chapter 11 summarizes some of the theoretical aspects of these observations and reviews the historical development of theories of antibody production.

The work of Landsteiner was very important in initiating a series of investigations into the whole problem of antigen and antibody chemistry and of the mechanism of antigen-antibody reactions. In subsequent years, attempts to quantitate the antibody response and antigen-antibody reactions were made. Heidelberger and Kendall (9) can be credited with establishing the beginnings of the quantitative measurement of antibodies by the technique of the quantitative precipitation test (see Chap. 14). The recent history of immunochemistry is linked to experiments which have led to the characterization of immunoglobulins and the elucidation of their primary, tertiary, and quaternary structure and to a more complete understanding of some of the events involved in the reactions of antigens and antibodies. The same progress has been made in studying complement and understanding how complement participates in antigen-antibody reactions (see Chaps. 3 and 14).

Immunobiology has also progressed rapidly, achieving greater understanding of the phenomena occurring at the organ, tissue, cellular, and subcellular level during immune response, of the development of immune responses during phylogeny and ontogeny, of the participation of antibodies, and in the pathogenesis of disease.

TYPES OF IMMUNITY

It is clear that the acquired immunity, which is brought about by the introduction of foreign materials into the organism, is not the only way in which the organism protects itself against foreign materials. There is a natural immune state which can be demonstrated in individuals who

TABLE 1-1
A Summary of Types of Immunity

I. Innate immunity
  A. Nonsusceptibility ("genetic" immunity)
  B. Natural immunity
II. Specific acquired immunity
  A. Active
    1. Naturally acquired
    2. Artificially acquired
  B. Passive
    1. Naturally acquired
    2. Artificially acquired
  C. Adoptive

---

have never had any contact with an antigen. The types of immunity are outlined in Table 1-1.

Innate Immunity

Nonspecific, or *innate, immunity* can cover the range from complete nonsusceptibility to a certain disease all the way to a resistance so low that every person exposed to the disease will contract it. The best known examples of this immunity are diseases such as typhoid fever or measles. *Constitutional,* or *"genetic," immunity* is the capacity which a normal organism possesses to remain relatively unharmed by agents which are harmful and are present in its environment. It is brought about by physiologic and anatomic features associated with the species and does not depend upon antibodies which can be detected by the ordinary methods that we possess today. It is inherited in the same fashion as any other characteristic of the species. This type of immunity has been poorly understood. It should be pointed out, for example, that causes where natural antibodies cannot be demonstrated are not necessarily to be included within the sphere of genetic immunity. It is possible that with more refined measurement methods, antibody may eventually be found in some of these cases. The concept of nonsusceptibility is borne out, however, by the occurrence of infections in some species but not in others. Man, for example, will not be infected by a large number of animal pathogens (distemper, hog cholera, cattle plague, etc.). On the other hand, many human diseases, such as cholera, dysentery, measles, syphilis, or mumps, do not affect lower animals. Cold-blooded animals are nonsusceptible to tetanus toxin, perhaps because some physiologic factors (body temperature, diet, etc.) contribute to this nonsusceptibility. Therefore, nonsusceptibility can depend upon the following characteristics of an organism: (1) a barrier to the penetration of an organism at the level of the skin or integuments; (2) inhibition of the growth and reproduction of microorganisms after penetration in the tissues; (3) inactivation of toxins liberated by microorganisms.

The skin and the mucous membranes are physical barriers because of their lack of permeability to most microorganisms. The surface of the skin also exerts some bactericidal action, perhaps due to secretions such as fatty acids or sebaceous gland products. On mucosal surfaces, the mucous films which are present in the respiratory and genital canals have definite bactericidal and virucidal properties, some of which cannot be attributed to the presence of antibodies, although some are dependent on antibody-containing secretions. The gastrointestinal tract provides active epithelial protection and also a host of bactericidal enzymes in saliva, mucus, and the gastric juices.

The tissues and body fluids also contain bactericidal substances. Lysozyme is an example of a bactericidal enzyme which is found in the tissues and the body fluids of several animal species (10). Egg albumin is quite rich in lysozyme. This is a mucolytic enzyme which is capable of splitting sugar from the amino polysaccharides of the bacterial membrane so that the cellular contents are lost and the bacterial integrity destroyed. Other substances which have been implicated in natural defenses are some polypeptides with antibacterial activity (11). These may be related to beta lysine, a humoral bactericidal agent which has bactericidal action against aerobic spore-forming bacilli (11). It appears to be a complex system of enzymes which are very effective bactericidal agents. The properdin system can also be regarded as a bactericidal system in serum. Properdin itself is inactive, but in combination with certain components of complement and in the presence of magnesium, it will cause bacteriolysis (12). While it appears that, unlike antibodies, properdin is nonspecific, it might be that it is an antibody to certain components of the bacterial cell wall. Interferon is an antiviral substance which has been shown to be present in normal body fluids and to be very active in the destruction of viral particles (13).

The physiologic barriers which are effective in protection are many. Body temperature is effective in combating infection, and changes in it will inhibit organisms which would otherwise grow well in animal tissue. The chicken, which is normally resistant to anthrax, becomes susceptible if its body temperature is lowered. Lizards, which are usually resistant to anthrax, become susceptible if their body temperature is raised to that of mammals. In some cases tissue metabolites, which are necessary for microbial multiplication, may fail to be provided and multiplication will fail.

It is also possible that changes in metabolic activities of cells, which are invaded by microbial organisms, will lead to an environment which is not optimal for multiplication. On the other hand, changes in a different direction with abundance of necessary metabolites may lead to more active multiplication. Oxygen tension is another important factor controlling bacterial infection, since the availability of oxygen is essential for facultative aerobes. If the oxygen tension is low, aerobic microorganisms will not multiply. Conversely, for anaerobic microorganisms such as *Clostridium perfringens*, the lowered oxygen tension will lead to considerable multiplication and invasion with pathogenic effects being manifested.

Phagocytosis is another very important mechanism of protection (14). The system of phagocytic cells, which is present in the body and which is part of the lymphoreticular system and of the hematopoietic system, consists primarily of two types of phagocytic cells: the circulating phagocytic cells of the blood (polymorphonuclear leukocytes) and the so-called macrophages, which are connective tissue–bound, but will circulate upon demand. Macrophages are found in very close relationship to the vascular endothelia and reticulum of the lymphoid organs, the liver, and the lung. Another system of phagocytic cells is present in the central nervous system and is comprised of the so-called microglial cells.

The phagocytes present an initial barrier to any attack by foreign microorganisms or, in general, to any foreign matter that is presented to the organism. They have a highly developed system of digestive vacuoles which have the capacity of removing and digesting most foreign materials. The usual sequence of events is initiated when the phagocytic cell comes in contact with foreign matter and engulfs it by a series of membrane changes which lead to the production of a cytoplasmic vacuole containing the phagocytosed particle (15). A protolysosome, which originated in the Golgi region, will then approach the phagocytic vacuole and fuse with it, discharging its enzymatic contents into the vacuole so as to digest the particle. When digestion is completed, the terminal lysosome is left in the cell as a darkly staining body. The mechanism by which phagocytic cells are attracted to bacteria and to other inert particulate matter is not very clear, but it is apparent that such a chemotropism operates in natural defenses. It is known that some components of complement are needed for chemotropism of polymorphonuclear leukocytes (16). Phagocytosis is the most active contributing factor to native resistance. This mechanism is very effective because the phagocytic cells are spread throughout the body and can be mobilized very readily.

Another line of defense, which is usually exercised by the organism, particularly in higher animals, is inflammation. This response is primarily manifested in a series of vascular phenomena leading to vasodilatation with leakage of phagocytic cells and of plasma constitutents into the tissues. The polymorphonuclear leukocytes exercise their phagocytic capacity, and this is facilitated by the formation of fibrin, which traps bacteria. In addition, bactericidal factors in the plasma will be beneficial in aiding the process of defense. The repair, which follows inflammatory phenomena, is also mediated through some of these factors.

Natural Immunity

In animals that have not been immunized and have not been infected with the disease to which they are immune, natural immunity may be present. It is probably brought about by substances which cross-react with the infectious agent involved or with some of its by-products. There are substances which bind to erythrocytes of other species or even to those of different individuals of the same species. These substances, which are very much like antibodies in their behavior, are called *normal*, or *natural*, *antibodies*. For instance, in the globulin fraction separated from pooled normal human plasma, one finds isohemagglutinin, which is an antibody directed to the erythrocytes of other individuals in the human species (17). Other antibodies are present too, such as diphtheria antitoxin and antibody to dysentery bacilli, to herpes virus, to the toxin of streptococcus, and to typhoid H and O antigens. Natural antibodies to cholera, typhoid, and dysentery have been observed in the horse and to pneumonia and dysentery in rabbits. Natural antibodies directed to foreign erythrocytes are found in the blood of various animal species, such as swine, which possess antibodies for the red cells of sheep, goats, rabbits, and humans. Rabbits have antibodies to guinea pig, horse, sheep, and human erythrocytes. Human sera contain natural antibodies for rabbit, sheep, ox, horse, pigeon, and guinea pig erythrocytes.

The origin of natural antibodies of this type is not certain. They are present in the blood of newborn animals, generally decrease in the neonatal period, and eventually return to moderate levels which are maintained throughout adulthood. For instance, one will find very high titers of pneumococcal antibodies in young adults, and it is interesting to note that pneumococcal pneumonia is lowest during this time. What constitutes natural antibodies is a difficult question to answer. Some of these antibodies are probably induced in response to a subclinical attack by an infectious agent. It is possible that a small dose was introduced, and the infection which followed was latent or subclinical with production of some antibody. That this may indeed be the case has been proven in at least some cases of normal antidiphtheria and antitoxin antibodies. The possibility exists that in some instances the production of antibody has occurred in response to organisms which entered by abnormal routes. For instance, gastrointestinal absorption of antigen in some cases may account for the production of antibodies which might be considered normal, since this is not a usual route of antigen absorption. It is also possible that some of the natural antibodies are produced in response to organisms related to the one against which they are directed. Another possibility is that they are directed to unrelated organisms which contain an antigen common to one contained in the organism with which they react. For instance, the anti-sheep hemolysins found in rabbits that have not been immunized with sheep erythrocytes may be produced as a consequence of the introduction of bacteria which contain antigens that cross-react with sheep erythrocytes. On the other hand, the presence of antigens which are related to sheep erythrocytes in the food which the rabbit eats may also lead to the production of natural antibodies. Not all natural antibodies can be accounted for in this manner. Some appear to be present as a physiological component of the individual's serum proteins. Some are found in all serum proteins. Some are found in all individuals of a species, but not in individuals of another species, even though these latter could have had the same opportunity to come in contact with the antigen which might be considered as the stimulus for the production of these antibodies if they had been produced by antigenic stimulation. It was suggested by Landsteiner (1) that most of the normal hemagglutinins and hemolysins which are directed to the blood of foreign species are of spontaneous origin. This idea is supported by the lower degree of specificity that is exhibited by these antibodies, which are sometimes poorly absorbed by the cells toward which they are directed. Some of the activity of these antibodies may perhaps be due to properdin.

Another group of natural antibodies comprises the agglutinins (isoagglutinins) of the human blood groups (17). Formation of these isohemagglutinins is definitely under genetic control. These antibodies, which appear after birth, react with the red blood cells of other human individuals. They reach peak concentration by ten years of age and slowly decrease thereafter. The genetic origin of hemagglutinins is easily demonstrated, but the role of heredity in natural immunity to disease is difficult to prove. Some of the normal antibodies found in the blood of several animals have a high degree of specificity, and this is not surprising, if they are the result of some antigenic stimulation which is not readily apparent. Others, on the other hand, are only specific to a lesser degree up to the point that they may react with a number of different antigens. These may be real natural antibodies which are not present as a result of unknown or undetected antigenic stimulation.

Acquired Immunity

The immunity which is acquired by introduction of an immunogenic substance depends on the ability of the animal to produce antibodies to some of its components in response to the immunogen. Thus, infection is not the only way in which immunity can be acquired or the antibody-producing mechanism can be stimulated. Immunity can be conferred by purified antigenic substances which are only part of the original antigen and can be transmitted artificially. Active immunity usually develops following a natural or artificial stimulation of the antibody-producing mechanism. By *natural stimulation* is meant the type of stimulation which is imparted by contracting a disease and recovering from it, for example. This will usually result in a long-lasting immunity to another attack of the same disease. This immunity also occurs in the case of subclinical or undetected infections. Many people who carry antibodies against a certain disease have almost certainly had the disease in a subclinical form. Before immunity can be developed by actual immunization, some time has to elapse. This is due to the tissue reactions necessary for the production of antibodies (see Chaps. 5, 6, and 7). Because of this time lag, active immunization is used only as a preventive measure. Immunizing at the time the disease is contracted would in most cases not leave enough time for the production of antibodies to protect against the disease before it develops to a harmful degree.

Another type of immunity is the *artificial immunity* in which antibody-producing mechanisms are stimulated artificially by introduction into the body of microorganisms or some of their component products which cause disease. Nearly all pathogenic agents produce fatal disease only when a susceptible individual receives a sufficiently large dose, usually by certain routes. Smaller doses, or organisms introduced by a route other than the normal one, may cause short illness and at times no illness at all, with only local inflammation. Sublethal doses of virulent microorganisms are not considered sufficiently safe for human immunization, and attenuated organisms are employed. The virulence of the organisms may be reduced by such treatments as aging of the cultures, exposing them to high temperatures, various passages in tissue culture, growing them in an unnatural host, etc.

The preferred method of stimulating active immunity against many diseases is to employ killed microorganisms. Many methods can be employed to kill the microorganisms and the most commonly used are merthiolate, acetone, formaldehyde, phenol, and heat. These preparations of killed bacteria are known as vaccines and are commonly used in protection from human disease. In the case of toxins, treatment with formaldehyde will convert most of these to antigenic toxoids which are nontoxic. These are so harmless that large doses may be administered with no risk of tissue damage or of producing death. They are commonly employed and may be used in conjunction with adjuvants.

Since most antigens will produce some degree of active immunization, it would be reasonable to protect by immunization against all known infectious diseases. This is not done for many practical reasons. It is clear that although immunization is of great importance in the prevention and control of certain diseases, not all diseases are amenable to prevention in this manner. In many cases, the causative agent is not known or not available in sufficient quantities or too toxic to be administered. Sometimes, antigenicity is lost when the infectious agent is cultured in artificial media and the antigen produces antibodies which are not protective.

Passive Immunity

This type of immunity is achieved by transfer of antibodies that have been made in another individual. It usually lasts only a short while, since these antibodies are catabolized like normal globulins and disappear after a short period of time.

Naturally Acquired

During the first months of an animal's life, many diseases are not contracted which would ordinarily affect the animal. This can be attributed to antibodies which have been transferred from the mother to the infant. Such transferral can be achieved either by transplacental passage or by the colostrum (first milk of the mother) shortly after birth. Antibody passage through the placenta has been demonstrated in several animals. In others, where the placental and fetal circulatory systems are separated by more than one layer of cells, the passage of antibodies occurs with the administration of colostrum in the first few days of life. The antibodies that are administered with colostrum are absorbed through the gastrointestinal tract of the newborn. The immunity which has been passed in this fashion is lost rapidly, and then acquired immunity is conferred by the animal's own immunologic mechanisms. The existence of naturally acquired passive immunity is very important, since this mechanism protects newborn animals during the period when their own immune capacities have not developed.

Artificially Acquired

The injection of antibody containing sera from artificially immunized animals or from humans that have experienced a disease and have recovered has been practiced quite extensively in the treatment of some diseases of humans and animals. It was common practice, before the introduction of sulfanilamides and of antibiotics, in the treatment of diseases such as pneumonia for which no good active immunologic response could be obtained before the disease had developed too far. The use of specific antibodies has in more recent years given way to the administration of pooled normal gamma globulin from human subjects as a means of boosting natural immunity. The usefulness of passively administered antibody has been limited by a number of factors. In the first place, the duration of immunity is short and depends on the amount of antibody injected and its life in the circulation of the host. Secondly, the antiserum has to be given very shortly after exposure to the disease and will not be helpful after the disease has developed fully and damage has been done. Thirdly, antiserum or gamma globulin has to be given in as large amounts as possible, since the rate of loss is high. Finally, when one uses an antiserum from another animal, there is also danger of producing a serum sickness which may in some cases be lethal or at least lead to severe side reactions. (See Chap. 14 for a more detailed discussion of serum sickness.)

Adoptive Immunity

Adoptive immunity is the type of passively acquired immunity which is transferred from one animal to another by lymphocytes which are immunologically active. This can be considered as somewhat intermediate between active and passive immunity. It is passive in the sense that the immunity is not produced in the host and is not the outcome of its own active response to immunization. It is active in the sense that it is based on the presence of actively functioning cells which have been exposed to antigenic stimulus and are now growing and functioning in a host after having been transferred from a donor. It is apparent that because the cells are functioning, a secondary response can be elicited in the host that has been adoptively immunized, while this could not be done by passive immunity conferred by antiserum.

Summary

It is clear then that the mechanisms leading to an acquired immune response are only some of the ways in which protection from disease can be achieved. A system of natural resistance or natural immunity to various infectious agents and foreign substances exists. This has been developed very rapidly throughout phylogenesis and is most important in those species which do not exhibit a true immune response as found in higher vertebrates. The tremendous progress of our knowledge in immunology has made us aware of these mechanisms by which protection is achieved. The understanding, which has been gained recently, of genetic factors controlling antibody response and the development of naturally acquired immunologic responses, as well as the studies on the immunochemical parameters of defense responses, have contributed greatly to a better understanding of some of these phenomena. There remains a lot to be learned, particularly in the areas of antigenic stimulation and of the way in which this leads to the immune response. Although the ground which has been covered is quite extensive, what lies ahead is still of tremendous proportions and challenges the imagination of the investigator. The ultimate goal of immunology is the control of disease before it becomes manifest, namely, prevention or prophylaxis. It is apparent that this is a worthwhile objective and that further work and understanding of immunologic phenomena will bring us closer to it.

REFERENCES

1. Landsteiner, K.: "The Specificity of Serological Reactions," Harvard University Press, Cambridge, Mass., 1945.
2. Ehrlich, P.: "Das Sauerstoff—Bedürfniss des Organismus," Hirschwald, Berlin, 1885.
3. Ehrlich, P.: *Proc. Roy. Soc. (Biol.)*, **66**:424, 1900.
4. Ehrlich, P.: "Gesammelte Arbeiten über Immunitätsforschung," Hirschwald, Berlin, 1904.
5. Breinl, F., and Haurowitz, F.: *Z. Physiol. Chem.*, **192**:45, 1930.
6. Alexander, J.: *Protoplasma*, **14**:296, 1931.
7. Mudd, S.: *J. Immunol.*, **23**:423, 1932.
8. Haurowitz, F.: in A. M. Pappenheimer, Jr. (ed.), "The Nature and Significance of the Antibody Response," Columbia University Press, New York, 1953.
9. Heidelberger, M., and Kendall, F. E.: *J. Exp. Med.*, **50**:809, 1929.
10. Perutz, M. F.: *Proc. Roy. Soc. (Biol.)*, **167**:348, 1967.
11. Donaldson, D. M., Jensen, R. S., Jensen, B. M., and Matheson, A.: *J. Bacteriol.* **88**:1049, 1964.
12. Pillemer, L., Blum, L., Lepow, I. H., Ross, O. A., Todd, E. W., and Wardlaw, A. C.: *Science*, **120**:279, 1954.
13. Wolstenholme, G. E. W., and O'Connor, C. M. (eds.): "Interferon," Ciba Foundation Symposium, Little, Brown and Company, Boston, 1967.
14. Hirsch, J. G.: *Ann. Rev. Microbiol.*, **19**:339, 1965.
15. Gordon, G. B., Miller, L. R., and Bensch, K. G.: *J. Cell Biol.*, **25**:41, 1965.
16. Ward, P. A., Cochrane, C. G., and Müller-Eberhard, H. J.: *J. Exp. Med.*, **122**:327, 1965.
17. Race, R. R., and Sanger, R.: "Blood Groups in Man," 4th ed., Blackwell, Oxford, 1962.

2
Antigens and Antigenicity

TYPES OF ANTIGENS

The generally accepted definition of an antigen is functional in that an antigen is generally considered to be a substance which, when introduced into an organism, will elicit an immunological response. Secondly, this substance must react with the antibody that is produced in some demonstrable way. More recently a number of investigators have chosen to restrict the term *antigenicity* to those characteristics of a molecule which deal with its capacity to interact with antibodies and have adopted the term *immunogenicity* to refer to those characteristics of molecules (immunogens) which elicit the production of specific antibodies.

The term *antigenic* is relative, since the response is frequently a property of the route of injection, method of preparation of the antigen, or the individual animal or species used. For example, saline preparations of pneumococcal polysaccharides, when injected by certain routes (intracutaneously and subcutaneously) into human beings or mice, will elicit significant levels of antibody formation. On the other hand, these same preparations, when injected by other routes in human beings or mice or when administered to other species such as the rabbit, will not induce antibody formation. Finally, it is also probable that certain molecules have been considered to be nonimmunogenic largely on the basis of an inability to demonstrate a visible in vitro interaction of antigen and antibody. As our techniques for detection of antigen-antibody reactions become more sophisticated, it is possible that a number of substances previously considered to be nonantigenic will be shown to be antigenic.

Most of the reactions which measure the interaction of antigen with antibody can best be demonstrated by using the serum of the organism undergoing the reaction and are manifested in a number of visible reactions depending upon the type of antigen used. For example, when the serum of an animal which has been injected with a soluble antigen such as bovine serum albumin (BSA) is mixed with a suitable proportion of BSA, a precipitate consisting of complexes of the antigen and antibody is formed. This is termed a *precipitin reaction* and the antibody is termed a *precipitin*. When an antiserum prepared by injecting such particulate antigens as bacteria or erythrocytes is added to a suspension of the antigen, dissolution or lysis of the bacteria or red blood cells is observed. Antibodies producing this type of reaction are called *lysins*, and depending upon whether their action is directed toward bacteria or red blood cells, they are termed *bacteriolysins* or *hemolysins*, respectively. This particular reaction requires the presence of a thermolabile factor called *complement*, which is found in fresh normal serum of a variety of animals and is particularly active in guinea pig serum. The reaction of antigen and antibody with complement is called *complement fixation*. Further details regarding antigen-antibody reactions will be discussed in Chap. 12.

In addition to those antigenic molecules which stimulate antibody formation and can be demonstrated to interact visibly with such antibodies there are a number of substances which, although they react with antibodies, have not been shown to produce antibodies when injected into animals. Landsteiner (1) proposed the term *hapten* to describe substances that react with antibody in vitro but do not elicit the production of antibodies when injected into an organism. Haptens can be divided into two types depending upon whether they combine with antibody molecules to form an insoluble antigen-antibody complex which then precipitates out of solution (*complex haptens*), or whether they combine and do not form a visible reaction (*simple haptens*).

Complex haptens include such substances as alcoholic extracts of guinea pig kidney, which do not produce antibodies in a rabbit but nevertheless can be shown to react with antibodies produced by injection of rabbits with saline extracts of guinea pig kidney.

Simple haptens include such natural small molecules as the extracts of pollen called allergens, polynucleotides, certain steroids, and such simple chemical compounds as picryl chloride and formaldehyde which can produce sensitization when injected, applied to the skin, or inhaled. Such substances are not in themselves antigenic but readily form complexes with proteins of the skin or with plasma proteins to form artificial antigens in the host.

Since simple haptens do not produce a visible antigen-antibody reaction following their interaction with antibody, an indirect method must be used to demonstrate their activity. Landsteiner (2) attached various artificial haptens such as arsanilic acid and p-aminobenzoic acid to various protein molecules and then produced antibodies against such protein-hapten complexes in rabbits. He found that rabbit antisera against such conjugated antigens containing simple haptens were often specific for the hapten used and readily formed visible precipitates with the protein-hapten complex. However, he found that no visible reaction occurred if the antisera were mixed with the hapten alone, instead of with the hapten-protein complex. On the other hand, antisera first treated with hapten did not give a visible precipitin reaction when later reacted with the protein-hapten complex, thus indicating that the hapten had indeed reacted with the antibody in such a way as to prevent the precipitation by antibody of the conjugated antigen. This type of reaction is called an inhibition reaction.

Historically, Landsteiner's classic demonstration (3) that an organic molecule of low molecular weight, e.g., arsanilic acid, functions as a hapten when it is linked covalently to a protein carrier, opened up a new avenue for the study of antigenicity, antibody structure, and the mechanisms of antibody formation. The fact that antibodies can be produced against hapten-carrier complexes has led to the consensus that the carrier enables the hapten to be taken up by immunologically competent cells, thus permitting it to participate in the induction of antibody specific for the hapten.

FACTORS DETERMINING IMMUNOGENICITY

Considerable experimental evidence has accumulated in recent years regarding the specific chemical characteristics of antigenic molecules and the properties which determine the extent of their antigenicity. As previously stated the antigenic characterization of any substance depends upon our ability to demonstrate its capacity to induce antibody formation. It is sometimes difficult to determine whether the antigenic substance is antigenic per se or whether it first forms a complex with the test animal's own molecules to form an essentially foreign complex which then becomes antigenic in the host. Furthermore, most of our immunological tests are relatively insensitive when dealing with an antigen or antibody in small amounts, and thus some molecules are not detected as being antigenic. Finally, immune reactions involving such biological tests as anaphylaxis and skin sensitivity are generally found to be far more sensitive than most of our present in vitro tests of antigen-antibody reactions. Such assays must be used cautiously for studies of antigenicity since even a small amount of a powerful antigenic contaminant will confer an apparent antigenicity to nonantigenic substances.

However, in spite of these difficulties there are some generalizations which can be stated regarding the factors that determine antigenicity.

1. It has been clearly established that there is a certain minimal molecular weight below which substances are not in themselves antigenic. Furthermore, it can generally be stated that the larger the molecular weight, the more antigenic a molecule will be. The smallest known antigenic molecule is the pancreatic hormone glucagon with a molecular weight of about 3800. Other small molecules that are antigenic are ribonuclease (mol. wt about 15,000), a phenylisocyanate of clupeine (mol. wt about 5000), and a variety of synthetic polypeptides with molecular weights as low as 4000 (4). On the other hand, histones (mol. wt about 10,000), protamines, gelatin, lysozyme, cytochromes, and a number of other small molecules are nonantigenic. However, some apparently nonantigenic small molecules can be demonstrated to be antigenic by mixing them with adjuvants which tend to enhance antibody production against these molecules (5). For example, insulin with a mol. wt of about 6000 will fairly regularly induce antibody formation if injected with adjuvants (see Chap. 9 for a more detailed discussion of adjuvants). Some normally nonantigenic small molecules can be made antigenic by attaching them to latex carrier particles to produce a complex which is then taken up by immunocompetent cells (6). For example, the human gastric-acid–stimulatory hormone, gastrin, has a mol. wt of about 2200 and has been shown to be nonantigenic. However, antibodies to gastrin have been produced in chickens after injection of gastrin which has been attached to polymethylmethacrylate latex particles (7).

2. According to Haurowitz (8) size alone does not seem to be enough to make a molecule antigenic. He suggests that a rigid structure of the determinant groups is a prerequisite for antigenicity. For example, sulfonated polystyrene, which is a large molecular polymer made up of a single repeating unit, is nonantigenic. It is also for this reason that gelatin has not been generally considered to be antigenic. Gelatin, a derived protein resulting from the partial hydrolysis of collagen, is poorly antigenic because it is a denatured protein containing large amounts of glycine, no tryptophan or cystine, and very little histidine or tyrosine. Therefore, free rotation occurs around the longitudinal axis, and thus the molecule has no fixed configuration. Gelatin is also easily digested and rapidly excreted in the urine. However, several investigators (9,10) have demonstrated that attachment of L-tyrosine, L-tryptophan, or L-phenylalanine converted gelatin into a relatively powerful antigen. As little as 2 percent tyrosine residues sufficed to enhance strongly the antigenicity of gelatin (11). On the other hand, the attachment of DL-alanine, L-glutamic acid, L-lysine, L-serine, or L-proline did not convert gelatin into a more antigenic substance. Thus it appears that the addition of aromatic groups has enhanced the antigenicity of gelatin by increasing its rigidity or nonflexibility. Haurowitz (12) believes that the highly specific action of the aromatic diazo compounds is due to the rigidity of the benzene rings, while the inability of long-chain fatty acids to act as determinant groups is due to the fact that the paraffin chains are easily distorted, and their shape constantly alters.

3. It is also generally accepted that in order to be immunogenic, molecules must be foreign to an organism, and the more foreign, the more immunogenic will the molecule be. It has long been recognized that an organism does not ordinarily produce antibodies against the myriad kinds and types of molecules produced by its own body. Ehrlich (13) called this principle "horror autotoxicus," which states that an animal will never produce antibodies to any substance normally found in his own circulation. Burnet and Fenner (14) based their discussions of the mechanism of antibody formation on this ability of the antibody-producing mechanism to distinguish "self" from "not self."

It has also been demonstrated that molecules fulfilling similar functions in different species are structurally quite similar and thus are generally found to be poorly immunogenic in a wide range of taxonomically unrelated organisms. For example, insulin apparently fulfills basically the same function in all higher animals, and when examined chemically is also found to vary little from one species to the next. The same is true of hemoglobin and thyroglobulin, which are poorly immunogenic among the mammalian species. Furthermore, Goodman (15) has demonstrated that proteins which arise early in vertebrate ontogeny are less immunogenic within closely related species than those proteins which appear late in development. For example, Boyden (16) has reported systematic serologic studies which demonstrate that there is a higher degree of correspondence for the serum albumins of closely related mammalian species than for the serum globulins.

Under certain specialized circumstances an organism will produce antibodies against certain of its own body constituents. The process whereby an antigenic component of the body's own tissues calls forth the production of antibody or results in specific sensitization to this antigen is called *autoimmunization* or *autosensitization*. (See Chap. 14 for further discussion of autoimmunity.)

4. It has also been suggested that an immunogen must be soluble to induce antibody formation. This is not strictly true and is probably based on the fact that a number of highly antigenic materials are soluble proteins. However, bacteria, red blood cells, and other cells (particulate antigens) are powerfully antigenic. It may be that such insoluble antigens are broken down into various soluble antigenic components. It has been suggested that macrophages "process" antigenic materials by reducing them to immunogenic fragments which are combined with macrophage ribonucleic acid (RNA) (17). Such complexes may serve to enhance the cellular uptake of the antigenic fragment by antibody-forming cells. It is not known whether a macrophage-processing step, that is, the linkage of an antigenic fragment to the antigen-carrier RNA, is a necessary step for the production of antibody to all antigens. However, in the case of the high-molecular-weight antigens studied to date, it seems clear that antigen processing takes place. A more detailed discussion of the role of macrophage and "immunogenic RNA" is found in Chaps. 5 and 7.

5. Antigen metabolism may regulate antibody formation by controlling the amount of antigen left intact and capable of stimulating antibody formation. For example, Felton (18) observed that whereas the injection of 0.5 μg of pneumococcal polysaccharide would immunize a mouse, the injection of larger doses (0.5 to 5.0 mg) not only did not immunize, but rendered the animal impossible to immunize to the type-specific pneumococcus for many months. Felton et al. (19) called this phenomenon *immunological paralysis*. It appears that antigens such as D-polypeptides (20) and pneumococcal polysaccharides are poorly degraded, and thus the concentration of the intact antigens is high enough to induce immunologic paralysis. Good antigens are rapidly degraded, so that over a wide range of doses, optimal amounts of antigen are available to stimulate antibody formation (21). Thus there appears to be a balance between stimulation and paralysis for every antigen, and this balance is under genetic control (22). Gill et al. (23) have postulated that a poor antigen induces paralysis easily, whereas a good antigen stimulates antibody formation under a wide variety of conditions.

IMMUNOGENICITY OF VARIOUS MOLECULES

Proteins

Most known proteins have been tested for immunogenicity at one time or another and, except for only a few, have been found to be immunogenic. The best-known immunogens are the proteins with molecular weights of 40,000 or more. Albumins with molecular weights of 40,000 to 60,000 and gamma globulins (mol. wt in excess of 6,000,000) and tobacco mosaic virus (mol. wt about 40,000,000 or more) are among the most powerful antigens known to date.

Polysaccharides

Polysaccharides are immunologically important components of most cells. Many are not immunogenic but may dominate the specificity of proteins with which they are combined. The ability of a few polysaccharides to induce antibody formation has been well established. However, the study of the immunogenicity of polysaccharides is always tempered by the possibility that a given polysaccharide may contain traces of a protein and thus one should always be suspicious of an immunogenic polysaccharide which contains nitrogen unless it can be accounted for.

One type of polysaccharide which has been shown to induce antibody formation is a nitrogen-free polysaccharide of many parasitic helminths as well as that of mollusks. These polysaccharides are similar to glycogen but have the power of inducing precipitin production in rabbits and sensitized guinea pigs.

Bacterial Polysaccharides

The most extensively studied polysaccharides are those isolated from microorganisms. Dochez and Avery (24) discovered the presence of a polysaccharide in the capsule of virulent pneumococci which precipitated with antipneumococcal serum. Zinsser and Parker (25) found antigenic polysaccharides in staphylococci, pneumococci, and in influenza, typhoid, and tubercle bacilli. Precise information concerning the antigenic properties of such polysaccharides began with their isolation by Avery and Heidelberger (26) from pneumococcal capsules. For some years it was believed that these substances were haptens capable only of reacting with antibody induced by the capsule of the bacterial cell. Pappenheimer (27) obtained polysaccharides without drastic chemical manipulation and was able to obtain antibody production to them when injected intracutaneously or subcutaneously into human beings or mice. There are two possible reasons why antibodies to such polysaccharides are not produced in rabbits: (1) antigenicity of the polysaccharide may depend on its adsorption to tissue protein (and this does not occur); (2) tissue enzymes may be present in the rabbit which inactivate pneumococcal polysaccharides.

Humans and mice are the only two animals in which the isolated, purified polysaccharides have definitely been shown to be immunogenic. The optimal amount in mice was found to be 0.5 μg, whereas 50 μg is a sufficient dose for the average human being, injected subcutaneously or intracutaneously. Consequently, it is obvious that these polysaccharides, in the right animal, are among the most powerful antigens known.

Dextran, a large molecular weight polysaccharide synthesized from sucrose by the bacterium *Leuconostoc mesenteroides*, is apparently non-immunogenic for rabbits and guinea pigs but is immunogenic for man (28,29). Purified blood group A and B substances are fair immunogens in man but not in rabbits.

The polysaccharides which are present in the capsule of virulent (smooth-type) pneumococci are referred to as soluble specific substances (SSS) and are specific for each type of pneumococcus. In fact, SSS is the basis of type specificity in the pneumococci, since as far as is known all types of pneumococci contain the same proteins and the differences between the various types seem to reside solely in the differences of these capsular polysaccharides. All pneumococci also contain true protein antigens in their cells and they can survive the loss of the capsule and then grow as R (rough) forms, whereas the capsulated pneumococci grow in colonies of the S (smooth) form. At present there are more than 70 serologic types, which are designated by Roman numerals (30). Immune sera are available representing each type. If encapsulated pneumococci are mixed with a type-specific antiserum, swelling of the capsules occurs. This is spoken of as a *quellung* (German for swelling) *reaction*. The quellung method of serological typing or grouping is applicable to the study of many other species of encapsulated organisms. If deprived of their capsules such organisms are immunologically indistinguishable and avirulent (in the case of pathogens). Similar series of capsular types are found in influenza bacilli (*Haemophilus influenzae*; types A, B, C, D, E), in meningococci (*Neisseria meningitidis*; types I, II, II alpha), in beta-type hemolytic streptococci, and many others (31).

Many of the different types of type-specific polysaccharides can be differentiated not only serologically, but also chemically. The type III pneumococcal polysaccharide is a polymer of cellobiuronic acid which consists of alternate residues of glucose and glucuronic acid united by glucosidic linkage (32). It has been suggested that there are perhaps 180 cellobiuronic acid molecules so linked to make up a polysaccharide of minimum molecular weight 62,000. The type VIII polysaccharide is also composed of cellobiuronic units and has a molecular weight of 140,000. The polysaccharide antigen of type I pneumococci contains galacturonic acid, galactose, fucose, and glucosamine; that of type II contains rhamnose, glucose, and glucuronic acid (33). The group A streptococcal carbohydrate is composed of only two monosaccharide constituents, rhamnose and N-acetylglucosamine, in a ratio of approximately 2:1 (31).

Many gram-negative bacteria contain in their cell walls complex antigens composed of carbohydrate, lipid, and a protein or polypeptide-like material called *lipoglycoproteins*. These complex molecules which are very toxic are called endotoxins. *Shigellae, Salmonellae,* and other pathogenic bacteria contain such endotoxins. The endotoxins produce fever and also inflammation in the site of local application and cause many of the pathological symptoms such as scarlet fever, typhoid, gonorrhea, and other diseases. It is not clear whether only the lipid or also the carbohydrate portion of the endotoxins is responsible for their toxicity.

The best investigated of the endotoxins are those of *Salmonella* bacilli. The species of *Salmonella* have been shown to contain in their cells a somatic antigen, called O-antigen, and another antigen, called H-antigen, in their flagella. The O-antigens are type specific and have been used to serologically differentiate more than 20 types of *Salmonella* which are designated by Arabic numerals. These antigens, which are lipopolysaccharides, are extracted from the bacteria by treatment with trichloracetic acid or with water and phenol (34).

Blood Group Substances

Landsteiner (3) in 1900 discovered that the serum of most individuals contains substances which agglutinate and hemolyze the red blood cells of many other individuals. Such agglutination reactions can be used to differentiate four major groups of human red blood cells which have been designated as A, B, AB, and O. The basis for determining the four blood groups is the presence of naturally occurring antigens and antibodies. The factors that determine the antigens and antibodies are inherited, the antigen appearing in the offspring only if present in at least one parent. The two antigens that were discovered by Landsteiner are called A and B, and they are found on the surface of the erythrocytes (red blood cells). The antibodies, found in the serum, are known as anti-A and anti-B antibodies. The antigens determining the four blood groups are the result of the expression of three allelic genes—O, A, and B, the latter two apparently being dominant to O. The genotypes AA and AO and genotypes BB and BO cannot be distinguished serologically and are classified as phenotypes A and B, respectively. Thus only four phenotypes (A, B, AB, O) can be recognized, although six genotypes occur (OO, AO, AA, BO, BB, AB). Table 2-1 shows the distribution of these antigens and antibodies in the four blood group phenotypes.

Cells containing antigen A are agglutinated by anti-A antibody; cells containing antigen B are agglutinated by anti-B antibody. The degree of agglutination may depend upon a factor such as the concentration of antibodies in the serum. When blood is given in a transfusion, the kind of agglutinogen of the donor and the kind of agglutinin of the recipient are all that matter. The reason for this is that the agglutinins of the donor are too diluted by the blood of the recipient for them to be effective in ag-

TABLE 2-1
The ABO Human Blood Groups

Phenotype	Genotype	Agglutinogen (Antigen found on surface of erythrocytes)	Agglutinin (Antibody found in serum)
O	OO	none	anti-A and anti-B
A	AA or AO	A	anti-B
B	BB or BO	B	anti-A
AB	AB	A and B	none

glutinating the recipient's agglutinogens. Blood transfusions can be safely made only when blood groups are compatible. Compatibility means that the recipient and donor in a transfusion belong to the same group and, furthermore, that any possibility of additional reactions has been eliminated by cross matching. Blood transfusions are often needed after severe hemorrhages and in certain diseases.

There are at least 12 different blood group systems besides the ABO system (35). The M and N series and the Rh blood groups have received the most attention in recent years. Each of these systems is determined by a separate locus, and most of these in turn show multiple alleles. The Rh blood group system was discovered in 1940 by Landsteiner and Weiner (36) by means of the serum injected with the blood of a rhesus monkey. The connection between the Rh blood groups and erythroblastosis fetalis was revealed by the work of Levine et al. (37). The presence of the Rh blood group substance in the embryo of an Rh-negative mother can elicit formation of antibodies in the mother. If these antibodies pass through the placenta into the fetus, they react with the fetal Rh-positive cells, causing anemia, jaundice, and a general edema. The anemic condition in turn causes the fetus to produce immature erythrocytes (erythroblasts) at a high rate, leading to the condition called *erythroblastosis fetalis,* or *hemolytic disease of the newborn.*

The blood group A and B substances are found not only in the erythrocytes but also in other tissue cells such as sperm, liver, muscle, spleen, kidney, and lung cells (35). They are also present in various body fluids of 75 to 80 percent of individuals, including saliva, seminal fluid, gastric juice, and sweat. These persons are known as "secretors." The capacity to secrete water-soluble blood group substances is inherited as a mendelian dominant character. Blood group substances in such fluids can be detected by a precipitin test with anti-A and anti-B typing sera or by an inhibition test as previously described.

The blood group substances have been characterized as being glyco-lipids which contain fatty acids, sphyngosine, and mucoproteins or muco-peptides which on hydrolysis yield amino acids and carbohydrates (38). The serologic specificity of the blood group substances is largely deter-mined by their carbohydrate moieties. They contain 22 to 25 percent of a peptide rich in serine, threonine, and proline. This peptide probably forms the backbone to which the oligosaccharide chains are attached (39). It has now been demonstrated that the carbohydrate portion of the human blood group substances A, B, and M contains galactose, N-acetylgalacto-samine, N-acetylglucosamine, and fucose (40,41).

Heterophile Substances

Some of the antigenic determinants of the blood group substances also occur in bacterial polysaccharides. Thus, the polysaccharides of the type XIV pneumococci will cross-react serologically with the human blood group A substance. Antigens of this type are called heterophile antigens (42). Forssman (43) in 1911 discovered that emulsions of guinea pig liver, kidney, adrenals, testis, and brain, when injected into rabbits, pro-duced high concentrations of antibodies capable of lysing sheep red blood cells in the presence of complement. Furthermore, these sheep red cell hemolysins could be removed by absorption of the antiserum with guinea pig kidney extract. The antigenic substance, which has also been found in the tissues of the horse, dog, cat, mouse, fowl, tortoise, and many other animals, has been designated the *Forssman antigen*, and the hemolysin is called the *Forssman antibody*. The Forssman antigens of different animal species possess a common determinant which appears to be a lipopoly-saccharide complex loosely bound to a protein (44). It appears that the antigenic specificity of the Forssman antigen is associated with the poly-saccharide moiety of the complex.

There are many heterophile systems, of which the Forssman antigen is only one (42). The terms *Forssman antigen* and *heterophile antigen* have erroneously been used synonymously. The term *Forssman antigen* should be limited to the antigen discovered by Forssman in guinea pig tissues, and *heterophile antigen* should be used to denote a broad group of antigens present in various plant and animal tissues which possess char-acteristics similar to those of the Forssman antigen. Other common heterophile antigens are the Paul-Bunnell and Buchbinder antigens. In the serum of patients suffering from infectious mononucleosis, Paul and Bunnell (45) discovered strong agglutinins for sheep erythrocytes. Buch-binder (46) found a heterophile antigen in bacteria of the hemorrhagic septicemia group and in the erythrocytes of a wide variety of birds. Rabbit antisera against these organisms were found to agglutinate and lyse sheep erythrocytes. Other heterophile antigens have been described, and many more probably exist. In general, red blood cells have been involved in all systems described to date.

Lipids

Although many reports have been made of the functional immunogenicity of lipids, there is no undisputed proof of any purified lipid being capable of eliciting an immune response. It appears that even the high-molecular-weight lipids, such as phospholipids (lecithin and cephalin), sterols (cholesterol and ergosterol), the sex hormones, and some of the sterols involved in tumor studies, will not function as immunogens when injected alone. However, the ability of such lipids to induce specific antibody formation when mixed with a foreign serum is fairly well established, but the underlying mechanism is not understood. Alcoholic extracts of animal tissues and organs which alone are nonimmunogenic may be capable of stimulating an immune response when mixed with foreign protein such as swine serum. This procedure has been called combined immunization. Landsteiner and Sims (47) have suggested that the lipid might form a loose union with the serum proteins. On the other hand, Sachs et al. (48) have suggested that the protein merely served as an "envelope" which enhanced entry of nonprotein substances into cells. Combined immunization has been used with extracts of brain, testis, and other organs.

It has been mentioned in preceding sections of this chapter that lipids form part of the endotoxins, the blood group substances, and the heterophile antigens. However, in each of these substances, the specific combining activity of the antibodies is directed against the carbohydrate moiety of the complex and not against the lipid. Heidelberger (49) believes that the lack of clearly defined immunogenicity in the lipids is explained by the lack of repetition of structural units in the molecule, so that no definite pattern is present to serve as an antigenic determinant.

Nucleic Acids

Before the late 1950s it was generally believed that nucleic acids were not antigenic and that nucleotides could not act as antigenic determinants. However, since that time considerable evidence has been accumulated which clearly suggests that under appropriate conditions nucleic acids may act as antigens (50,50a,51). The evidence to support this contention consists of the following: (1) a participation of nucleic acids in antigenic reactions involving DNA-rich complexes (52,53); (2) the serum of patients suffering from a disease known as lupus erythematosus (LE) was found to contain a factor specifically reactive with highly purified DNA (54,55); (3) antibodies capable of reacting with phage DNA possessing an unusual base were discovered (56); and (4) antisera against nucleic acid-rich ribosomes have been found to react with polyribonucleotides (57).

CHEMICAL NATURE OF ANTIGENICITY

Having defined the general characteristics which determine the immunogenicity of molecules, we will now examine those chemical structures which apparently must be present in a molecule to endow it with antigenic properties. Four lines of investigation have been used to study this parameter.

Degradation Studies

These studies have involved the selective removal or masking of suspected groupings through chemical modification so as to examine their involvement in determining the immunogenicity of molecules. If the capacity of the antigen or antibody to participate in the interaction remains unimpaired after the chemical modification, then the groupings may be presumed to be nonessential. However, if the modification results in a loss of activity, then that grouping may be essential for the immunogenicity of that particular molecule.

Maurer and Ram (58) conducted a series of studies to determine whether amino groups were essential to the antigenicity of bovine serum albumin (BSA). They modified the amino groups of BSA by three different procedures: deamination (removal of amino groups), acetylation, and guanidination (masking of amino groups by the addition of acetic anhydride and guanidine, respectively). Acetylated BSA, with 85 percent of its amino groups masked, was shown to have about 50 percent cross-reaction with antinative BSA, while guanidinated BSA, with 95 percent substitution, exhibited 100 percent cross-reaction. Furthermore, a deaminated derivative having only 10 percent of the original amino groups of BSA still showed a 40 percent cross-reaction with anti-BSA. These observations suggest that at least 90 percent of the amino groups of BSA have no major role in the antigenicity of BSA. They also concluded that the relative unimportance of the amino groups of BSA is applicable to other protein antigens, such as rabbit serum albumin (RSA), human serum albumin (HSA), and rabbit gamma globulin (RGG).

The carboxyl groups of BSA also do not seem to be essential for its antigenicity, since methylated BSA still combines with anti-BSA. On the other hand, acetylation (addition of acetyl groups with acetic anhydride to active hydrogens of HOH, C_2H_5OH, or NH_2H) of rabbit serum albumin makes this protein antigenic in rabbits.

Denaturation Studies

Almost all soluble proteins coagulate upon heating, particularly in slightly acidic solutions. This is a common, but not a necessary, sign of denaturation. The term *denaturation* is applied to the structural changes of protein which result in a concomitant loss of such biologic properties as enzyme, hormonal, or antigenic activity, with a drop in solubility and with general changes of chemical and physical properties. It is believed that denaturation results from the uncoiling or unfolding of polypeptide chains to give extended chains without gross intramolecular rearrangements involving covalent bond breakdown.

There are a number of substances with denaturing action, namely, acids, bases, organic solvents, salts of heavy metals, concentrated solutions of urea or guanidine, aromatic acids (e.g., salicylic acid), and detergents (e.g., dodecylsulfate). Protein antigens are not all equally susceptible to these substances or even to physical treatment like heat, light, radiation, or adsorption onto surfaces. Susceptibility itself depends to different degrees on pH, salt content, etc., of the protein solvent.

Acids and alkalis react with proteins to form acid and alkali metaproteins which have decreased antigenicities when compared with their native counterparts. Alkalis tend to be more active than acids in denaturing proteins.

Heating most proteins in solution soon destroys their ability to interact with antibodies produced against their undenatured counterparts. However, unless the proteins have been coagulated by heating, they are still antigenic and will induce the production of antibodies which, however, will have a different specificity than those directed against unheated protein.

Shaking protein solutions leads to the formation of insoluble strands or films of protein due to unfolding of the polypeptide chains at the air-water interface (foam). Such proteins also show changes in specificity without loss of antigenicity unless the treatment has been rather drastic.

In general it can be stated that denatured proteins lose most, or all, of their original antigenic specificity, and acquire new specificities instead. Furthermore, no denaturing agent has been found which will destroy the functional immunogenicity of proteins without destroying the whole molecule. The specificity may be changed but the immunogenicity is not altered (3,59).

Conjugation (Coupling Studies)

Conjugation of proteins with reactive chemical groups (haptens) has been shown to confer upon the foreign proteins the immunologic specificity of the haptens (3). Similarly, the conjugation of hapten groups with non-antigenic, homologous, or even autologous serum albumins render them antigenic with the specificity directed primarily toward the hapten (60). The 2,4 dinitrophenyl group (DNP), recognized as a strong antigenic hapten by several animal species, has been used extensively in such experiments. In similar studies, Sela and Arnon (61,62) conjugated amino acids to gelatin, which is itself a very weak antigen.

Sela and Arnon (61) produced several polypeptidyl derivatives of gelatin—polyalanyl, polyglutamyl, polylysyl, polycysteinyl, polytyrosyl, polytryptophanyl, and polyphenylalanyl gelatins. They also produced several copolymers of α-amino acids. It was shown that attachment of tyrosine (Tyr), tryptophan (Trp), or phenylalanine (Phe) peptides to gelatin converts it into a relatively powerful antigen. However, it has not been shown whether this enhancement results specifically from the aromatic character of the attached amino acids or if it is due to an increase in the rigidity of the molecule. Arnon and Sela (62) also produced three polytyrosyl gelatins differing in their tyrosine content, as well as a gelatin enriched with both tyrosine and glutamic acid which were tested for their immunogenicity in rabbits. It was found that the extent of the immunogenicity of gelatin depends on the amount of tyrosine attached. As little as 2 percent tyrosine was found to strongly enhance the immunogenicity of gelatin. The addition of alanine, glutamine, and lysine, on the other hand, did not enhance the immunogenicity of gelatin. Whereas the attachment of polar amino acid residues to gelatin caused almost no change in the extent of antigenicity, the enrichment of gelatin with dipeptides consisting of tyrosine and glutamic acid yielded an antigen that elicited more antibodies than a polytyrosyl gelatin with a similar tyrosine content. The antibodies to poly-Glu-Tyr-Gel were specific and the only substance that interacted with and precipitated with these antibodies was a copolymer of Glu and Tyr, thus indicating that all of the antigenic specificity lies in the dipeptide chains attached to gelatin.

Immunogenicity of Synthetic Polypeptides

Synthetic polypeptide antigens have been used extensively to define the chemical factors involved in immunogenicity and in the structure of antigenic sites. The results of these studies have been extensively reviewed recently (4,9).

Maurer et al. (4) have carried out a series of experiments to determine the immunogenicity of synthetic polymers of α-amino acids in guinea pigs, mice, rabbits, and human beings. No antibodies against polymers containing the single amino acids listed in Table 2-2 were obtained. Although some of the polymers tested were of low molecular weight, which could explain their nonimmunogenicity, others had large molecular weights but were still nonimmunogenic.

Maurer et al. (63) also synthesized copolymers of glutamic acid and lysine in varying ratios of the two AA as outlined in Table 2-3. Only the copolymer 6:4 Glu-Lys was found to be weakly immunogenic in the rabbit. Since this had a mol. wt of 38,000, it would appear that molecular weight, although an important factor, could not be the prime factor governing the immunogenicity of these copolymers. Perhaps more important than molecular weight is the molecular configuration which the polypeptide assumes. Employing adjuvant techniques, precipitable amounts of antibody could be produced in rabbits with the 6:4 copolymer of Glu-Lys. However, intramuscular injections of this copolymer in man produced no detectable antibody. On the other hand, in guinea pigs, copolymers of Glu-Lys of ratios 6:4, 7:3, or 5:5 were all found to be antigenic (64). The responses to immunization with the copolymers in adjuvant were much better than when the material was incorporated in saline alone. However, at no time did 100 percent of the guinea pigs react even after repeated injections of the copolymer in adjuvants.

Pinchuck and Maurer (65) have found that neither Swiss strains nor a number of inbred strains of mice could respond to copolymers of only two amino acids ($G_{60}L_{40}$, $G_{60}A_{40}$, $G_{90}T_{10}$). Upon introduction of as little as 4 percent of a third amino acid (tyrosine, phenylalanine, lysine), good immune responses were obtained, regardless of the nature of the third amino acid. Furthermore, the level of the immune response to a series of Glu-Lys-Ala polymers increased with increasing alanine content of the polymer.

TABLE 2-2
Polymers of Single Amino Acids

Polymer	Molecular weight
Polyalanine (Ala)	3,500
Polyglutamic acid (Glu)	6,400
Polyglutamic acid	80,000
Polyaspartic acid (Asp)	4,000
Polylysine (Lys)	18,000
Polyproline (Pro)	50,000
Polyhydroxyproline (HPro)	7,000

TABLE 2-3
Immunogenicity of Copolymers

Copolymers	Mole ratios	Molecular weight	Immunogenicity (rabbits)
Glu-Lys	6:4	38,000	Weakly immunogenic
Glu-Lys	5:5	39,000	Nonimmunogenic
Glu-Lys	7:3	110,000	Nonimmunogenic

SOURCE: From Maurer et al. (63) with permission.

Maurer et al. (66) studied the immunogenicity of a series of copolymers consisting of two and three α-amino acids as outlined in Table 2-4. From these studies it can be concluded that, in contrast to the importance placed upon aromatic amino acids in enhancing immunogenicity, it would appear that their contribution, if any, is small. From the observation that GT is slightly immunogenic, whereas polyglutamic acid is not immunogenic at all, one could infer that tyrosine has enhanced the immunogenicity of poly-Glu. The same could be said about the immunogenicity of GLT and GLPhe as compared to GL, since it appears that the two former copolymers are better immunogens than GL. However, when the data on the immunogenicity of GA and GAT are compared, it seems that the introduction of tyrosine has not significantly enhanced the immunogenicity of GA. It is important to note that GA was an exceptionally good immunogen in 10 of 12 rabbits. In fact, it was almost as good as the GLA30. Furthermore, the introduction of tyrosine into polyglutamic acid did not enhance the immunogenicity as much as did the introduction of alanine (GA). GLA5 was a poor immunogen but was slightly better than GL. The introduction of more alanine in the polymer to produce GLA30 en-

TABLE 2-4
Synthetic Polymers Studied for Immunogenicity

Copolymer	Ratio of AA	Nomen-clature	Molec-ular weight	Percent reactors	Titer μg N/ml serum
Glu-Lys-Ala	57:38:5	GLA5	50,000	63.6	15
Glu-Lys-Ala	42:28:30	GLA30	62,000	100.0	95
Glu-Lys-Tyr	58:38:4	GLT	94,000	75.0	13
Glu-Tyr	90:10	GT	65,000	41.7	0.4
Glu-Ala	60:40	GA	33,000	83.3	80
Glu-Ala-Tyr	60:30:10	GAT	25,000	72.7	44
Glu-Lys-Phe	58:38:4	GLPhe	48,000	81.8	23
Glu-Lys-Ala-Tyr	36:24:35:5	GLAT	35,000		

SOURCE: Adapted from Maurer et al. (66) with permission.

hanced the immunogenicity considerably, possibly by increasing the number of GA residues.

Since polyglutamic acid, polylysine, and polyalanine have been found to be nonimmunogenic by themselves, it is reasonable to assume that much of the antigenic specificity is directed against multiples of two or three amino acids. This assumption is supported by the fact that attachment of glutamic acid to polyalanine did not enhance the antigenicity of the compound. Also, the addition of glutamic acid to a polymer consisting of polylysine as backbone with attached chains of alanine failed to show antigenicity.

Another factor governing immunogenicity is the "foreignness" of the molecules. With random linear copolymers, as one increases the number of different amino acids in the polymer and the percentage of each AA, the probability of producing random sequences which may be foreign to the host increases. This may explain why GLA30 is a better antigen than GLA5 not only in guinea pigs (67), but also in rabbits (68) and man (69).

More recently Gill et al. (23) have studied the influence of charge and optical isomerism on the immunogenicity of synthetic polypeptides. The effect of charge of the antigen on the amount of antibody elicited was examined with a series of glutamic acid–lysine and glutamic acid–lysine-tyrosine polymers. Completely charged homopolymers (poly-Lys or poly-Glu) or a modified copolymer (poly 59Glu-41Lys) did not elicit any antibody even though they had relatively large molecular weights (Table 2-5). Highly charged polymers (e.g., poly-96Lys-4Tyr) elicited small amounts of antibody whether or not they contained the aromatic acids tyrosine or phenylalanine. The best antigens fell in the range of +75 to −75 percent net charge density, and within this range there appeared to be no effect of charge on the amount of antibody produced. An antigen with no net charge elicited a comparable amount of antibody. Thus, charge is not a requirement of antigenicity, but excessively high charges can decrease or, under some conditions, abolish the ability to elicit antibody formation.

Gill et al. (23) also tested a wide variety of synthetic polypeptides composed of D-amino acids for their ability to elicit antibody formation when given by different immunization schedules. Whereas immunization with relatively large doses of antigens composed of L-amino acids (2 to 20 mg) elicits significant levels of antibody formation in rabbits, no such antibody levels could be produced with similar doses of D-polypeptides. On the other hand, low doses (0.3 to 0.6 mg) of D-polypeptides administered over a long period of time induced antibody formation to a wide variety of D-polypeptides. But there is no significant secondary response with D-polypeptides, and indeed there is eventual suppression (immune paralysis) of the antibody response upon repeated injection of antigen.

TABLE 2-5
Antibody Response to Synthetic Polypeptides of
Different Composition and Charge

Polymer	Molecular weight	Charge	µg AbN/ml Average antibody response	Animals responding
Poly-Glu	84,000	−100	0	0/8
Poly-97Glu-3Lys	125,000	−95	0	0/9
Poly-96Glu-4Tyr	114,000	−100	5	5/8
Poly-59Glu-41-Lys	100,000	−100	0	0/8
Poly-84Glu-10Lys-6Tyr	110,000	−75	56	13/14
Poly-96Lys-4Tyr	487,000	+100	16	4/10
Poly-Lys	324,000	+100	0	0/8
Poly-84Glu-10Lys-6Tyr	110,000	−75	56	13/14
Poly-62Glu-33-Lys-5Phe	63,000	−25	101	9/9
Poly-51Glu-33Lys-16Tyr	13,000	−25	135	15/15
Poly-42Glu-28Lys-30Ala	74,000	−15	97	15/15
Poly-49Glu-51Lys	63,000	0	22	9/9
Poly-36Glu-60Lys-4Tyr	—	+25	136	5/5
Poly-23Glu-71Lys-6Tyr	300,000	+50	150	14/14
Poly-11Glu-85Lys-4Tyr	148,000	+75	121	9/9

SOURCE: Adapted from Gill et al. (23) with permission.

Similar findings have been reported when mice are immunized with
D-polypeptides (70). These observations indicate that the D-polypeptides
behave immunologically like the pneumococcal polysaccharides in their
low degree of antigenicity, in the lack of a booster effect, and in the easy
induction of immunologic paralysis. The paralysis is probably due to the
prolonged tissue storage (20,21) of the D-polymers and their gradual release
over a long period of time. Thus, very small amounts of antigen must be
used over prolonged periods of time to induce antibody formation to
synthetic D-polypeptides.

These investigators were also able to elicit antibody formation to
charged D- and L-homopolymers (e.g., poly-Glu, poly-D-Glu, poly-Lys,
poly-D-Lys) with small amounts of antigen administered over long periods
of time. Thus the induction of antibody formation by D-polypeptides and
charged homopolymers indicates that all types of synthetic polypeptides
are immunogenic in rabbits under the proper dosage conditions.

Antigenicity of Coupled Synthetic Polypeptides

Kantor et al. (71) have studied the nature of immunogenicity by the
conjugation of an antigenic hapten with synthetic polypeptides. The
antigenicity of DNP (2,4 dinitrophenyl group) polylysine and a DNP

copolymer of lysine and glutamic acid was studied in guinea pigs and compared with the immune response shown by the same animals to the unconjugated polyamino acids. These two polymers were selected because polylysine is nonantigenic while Glu-Lys is immunogenic in some guinea pigs. Conjugation with DNP was introduced because this hapten, which conjugates easily with the free NH_2 group of lysine, is recognized by guinea pigs as an antigenic determinant when bound to nonantigenic guinea pig serum albumin.

It was found that three different size DNP polylysine polymers, when conjugated with varying numbers of DNP groups, proved to be immunogenic. The most extensive immunogenicity was obtained with the largest mol. wt polymer (182,000) as compared with those of mol. wt 62,000 or 3300. It was also found that only those animals responding to DNP-polylysine responded to the DNP Glu-Lys copolymer.

In summary, studies of systematically varied series of synthetic polypeptides have provided several generalizations about the chemical factors involved in immunogenicity. Polymers containing aromatic amino acids generally elicit more antibody than those not containing them. This is not an exclusive property, however, since the incorporation of alanine can enhance immunogenicity in some cases. Tyrosine and phenylalanine are equally effective in enhancing antibody formation, but there is no correlation between the amount of antibody elicited and the amount of amino acid in the polypeptide. The charge of the antigen plays essentially a restrictive role: completely charged and highly charged polypeptides are poor antigens. Finally, small doses of poor antigens stimulate antibody formation and larger doses generally induce immunologic paralysis.

REFERENCES

1. Landsteiner, K.: *Biochem. Z.*, **119**:294, 1921.
2. Landsteiner, K.: *Biochem. Z.*, **86**:343, 1917.
3. Landsteiner, K.: "The Specificity of Serological Reactions," rev. ed., Harvard University Press, Cambridge, Mass., 1945.
4. Maurer, P.: *Progr. Allergy*, **8**:1, 1964.
5. Freund, J.: *Annu. Rev. Microbiol.*, **1**:291, 1947.
6. Litwin, S. D., and Singer, J. M.: *J. Immunol.*, **95**:1147, 1965.
7. Stremple, J. F., Abramoff, P., van Oss, C. J., Wilson, S. D., and Ellison, E. D.: *Lancet*, II: 1180, 1967.
8. Haurowitz, F.: *Biol. Rev.*, **27**:247, 1952.
9. Sela, M.: *Advan. Immunol.*, **5**:29, 1966.
10. Haurowitz, F.: "Chemistry and Biology of Proteins," Academic Press, Inc., New York, 1950.

11. Arnon, R., and Sela, M.: *Biochem. J.*, **75**:103, 1960.
12. Haurowitz, F.: in "Serological Approaches to Studies of Protein Structure and Metabolism," Rutgers University Press, New Brunswick N.J., 1954.
13. Ehrlich, P.: "Das Sauerstoff—Bedürfniss des Organismus," Hirschwald, Berlin, 1885.
14. Burnet, F. M., and Fenner, F.: "The Production of Antibodies," 2d ed., Macmillan, Melbourne, 1949.
15. Goodman, M.: *Amer. Naturalist*, **94**:153, 1960.
16. Boyden, A. A.: in "Serological and Biochemical Comparisons of Proteins," Rutgers University Press, New Brunswick, N.J., 1958.
17. Gottlieb, A. A.: *J. Reticuloendothel. Soc.*, **5**:270, 1968.
18. Felton, L. D.: *J. Immunol.*, **61**:107, 1949.
19. Felton, L. D., Prescott, B., Kauffmann, G., and Ottinger, B.: *J. Immunol.*, **74**:205, 1955.
20. Carpenter, C. B., Gill, T. J., III, and Mann, L. T., Jr.: *J. Immunol.*, **98**:236, 1967.
21. Gill, T. J., III, Papermaster, D. S., and Mowbray, J. F.: *J. Immunol.*, **95**:794, 1965.
22. Sela, M.: *Advan. Immunol.*, **5**:29, 1966.
23. Gill, T. J., III, Kunz, H. W., and Papermaster, D. S.: *J. Biol. Chem.*, **242**:3308, 1967.
24. Dochez, A. R., and Avery, O. T.: *J. Exp. Med.*, **26**:477, 1917.
25. Zinsser, H., and Parker, J. T.: *J. Exp. Med.*, **37**:275, 1923.
26. Avery, O. T., and Heidelberger, M.: *J. Exp. Med.*, **38**:81, 1923.
27. Pappenheimer, A. M., Jr., and Enders, J. F.: *Proc. Soc. Exp. Biol. Med.*, **31**:37, 1933–34.
28. Kabat, E. A., and Berg, D.: *J. Immunol.*, **70**:514, 1953.
29. Allen, P. Z., and Kabat, E. A.: *J. Immunol.*, **80**:495, 1958.
30. White, B., Robinson, E. S., and Barnes, L. A., "The Biology of Pneumococcus," Commonwealth Fund, New York, 1938.
31. McCarty, M., and Morse, S. I.: *Advan. Immunol.*, **4**:249, 1964.
32. Heidelberger, M., Kabat, E. A., and Mayer, M.: *J. Exp. Med.*, **75**:35, 1942.
33. Aspinall, G. O.: *Annu. Rev. Biochem.*, **31**:79, 1962.
34. Lüderitz, O., Staub, A. M., and Westphal, O.: *Bacteriol. Rev.*, **30**:192, 1966.
35. Race, R. R., and Sanger, R.: "Blood Groups in Man," 4th ed., Blackwell, Oxford, 1962.
36. Landsteiner, K., and Wiener, A. S.: *Proc. Soc. Exp. Biol. Med.*, **43**:223, 1940.
37. Levine, P., Burnham, N. J. L., Englewood, N. J., Katzin, E. M., and Vogel, P.: *Amer. J. Obstet. Gynecol.*, **42**:925, 1941.
38. Koscielak, J.: *Biochem. Biophys. Acta*, **78**:313, 1963.
39. Pusztai, A., and Morgan, W. T. J.: *Biochem. J.*, **88**:546, 1963.
40. Morgan, W. T. J., and Watkins, W. M.: *Brit. Med. Bull.*, **15**:109, 1959.

41. Kabat, E. A.: "Blood Group Substances," Academic Press, Inc., New York, 1956.
42. Jenkin, C. R.: *Advan. Immunol.* **3**:351, 1963.
43. Forssman, J.: *Biochem. Z.*, **37**:78, 1911.
44. Goebel, W. F., Shedlovsky, T., Lavin, G. I., and Adams, M. H.: *J. Biol. Chem.*, **148**:1, 1943.
45. Paul, J. R., and Bunnell, W. W.: *Amer. J. Med. Sci.*, **183**:90, 1932.
46. Buchbinder, L.: *Arch. Pathol.*, **19**:841, 1935.
47. Landsteiner, K., and Sims, S.: *J. Exp. Med.*, **38**:127, 1923.
48. Sachs, H., Klopstock, A., and Weil, A. J.: *Deut. Med. Wochschr.*, **51**:589, 1925.
49. Heidelberger, M.: *J. Mt. Sinai Hosp.*, **9**:893, 1943.
50. Plescia, O. J., and Braun, W.: *Advan. Immunol.*, **6**:231, 1967.
50a. Levine, L., and Stollar, B. D.: *Progr. Allerg.*, **12**:161, 1968.
51. Plescia, O. J., and Braun, W. (eds.): "Nucleic Acids in Immunology," Springer-Verlag, New York, 1968.
52. Phillips, J. H., Braun, W., and Plescia, O. J.: *Nature (London)*, **181**:573, 1958.
53. Lawlis, J. F., Jr.: *Proc. Soc. Exp. Biol. Med.*, **98**:300, 1958.
54. Ceppellini, R., Polli, E., and Celada, F.: *Proc. Soc. Exp. Biol. Med.*, **96**:572, 1957.
55. Holman, H. R., and Kunkel, H. G.: *Science*, **126**:162, 1957.
56. Levine, L., Murakami, W. T., Van Vunakis, H., and Grossman, L.: *Proc. Nat. Acad. Sci. U.S.*, **46**:1038, 1960.
57. Barbu, E., and Panijel, J.: *Compt. Rend.*, **250**:1382, 1960.
58. Maurer, P. H., and Ram, J. S.: in "Serological and Biochemical Comparisons of Proteins," Rutgers University Press, New Brunswick, N.J., 1958.
59. Kabat, E. A., and Mayer, M. M.: "Experimental Immunochemistry," 2d ed., Charles C Thomas, Springfield, Ill., 1961.
60. Gell, P. G. H., and Benacerraf, B.: *J. Exp. Med.*, **113**:571, 1961.
61. Sela, M., and Arnon, R.: *Biochem. J.*, **75**:91, 1960.
62. Arnon, R., and Sela, M.: *Biochem. J.*, **75**:103, 1960.
63. Maurer, P. H., Subrahmanyam, D., Katchalski, E., and Blout, E. R.: *J. Immunol.*, **83**:193, 1959.
64. Maurer, P. H.: *J. Immunol.*, **90**:493, 1963.
65. Pinchuck, P., and Maurer, P. H.: *J. Exp. Med.*, **122**:665, 1965.
66. Maurer, P. H., Gerulat, B. F., and Pinchuck, P.: *J. Immunol.*, **90**:381, 1963.
67. Maurer, P. H., and Cashman, T.: *J. Immunol.*, **90**:393, 1963.
68. Maurer, P. H., Gerulat, B. F., and Pinchuck, P.: *J. Immunol.*, **90**:388, 1963.
69. Maurer, P. H., Gerulat, B. F., and Pinchuck, P.: *J. Exp. Med.*, **116**:521, 1962.
70. Janeway, C. A., and Sela, M.: *Immunology*, **13**:29, 1967.
71. Kantor, F. S., Ojeda, A., and Benacerraf, B.: *J. Exp. Med.*, **117**:55, 1963.

3
Structure and Function of Immunoglobulins

IMMUNOGLOBULIN FAMILY AND CLASSIFICATION

Immunoglobulin Classes

Antibodies in man and other animals are associated with a group of proteins called immunoglobulins. Tiselius and Kabat (1) first demonstrated that precipitating antibodies in hyperimmunized rabbit sera are associated with γ-globulin, which has the slowest mobility on free electrophoresis. In all species investigated, the main component of γ-globulin had a molecular weight of 150,000, and antibody in serum was usually found in the 7S γ-globulin fraction. As the methods for separation and identification of serum proteins advanced, however, it became apparent that the molecules having antibody activity were not restricted to this protein. Serum proteins with β mobility on electrophoresis were also found to have antibody activity. The molecular size of antibodies was also found to be heterogeneous. About 5 to 10 percent of human γ-globulin consisted of protein having a molecular weight of about 900,000 and was referred to as 19S γ-globulin. The fraction was identified by immunoelectrophoresis (2), indicating that the protein was antigenically distinct from 7S γ-globulin. The presence of antibody activity in 19S γ-globulin was demonstrated about 30 years ago (3). Furthermore, immunoelectrophoresis of human sera revealed a third type of γ-globulin which was antigenically related to but distinct from 7S and 19S γ-globulins (2). This protein, called β_{2A}- or γ_{1A}-globulin, is mainly of a molecular size similar to that of 7S γ-globulin but has a relatively high carbohydrate content.

Since the proteins having antibody activity are heterogeneous with respect to physicochemical properties and antigenic structure, the term *immunoglobulin* has been applied to the family of serum proteins containing antibody activity. By analogy with the nomenclature of the hemoglobins, the 7S-, 19S-, and γ_{1A}-globulins were referred to as IgG (γG), IgM (γM), and IgA (γA) respectively. Despite their diversity, the family of immunoglobulins have common properties. They all cross-react antigenically, indicating that common structures exist in the molecules, and all appear to be associated with antibody activity. Furthermore, all of the immunoglobulins are probably the product of the plasma cell series.

In certain diseases of the plasma cell series, such as multiple myeloma and Waldenström's macroglobulinemia, high concentrations of homogeneous proteins accumulate in the patient's serum. The myeloma proteins and Waldenström-type macroglobulin in the sera have structures similar to normal immunoglobulins and possess antigenic determinants specific for one of the normal immunoglobulins. Bence-Jones proteins excreted in the urine of some of these patients also react with antisera to normal immunoglobulin. Although the pathological proteins generally lack a recognizable antibody activity, the proteins are included in the immunoglobulin family. Since the myeloma proteins of a single patient are apparently the product of cells from a single clone, the proteins are homogeneous as compared with normal immunoglobulins. Therefore, structural studies of the pathological proteins have contributed significantly to the knowledge of normal immunoglobulins and antibodies. Indeed, Waldenström-type macroglobulin and γA myeloma proteins were described before IgM and IgA were detected in normal serum. Studies on an atypical myeloma protein, which was antigenically distinct from IgG, IgM, and IgA, led to the discovery of the fourth class of human immunoglobulin, IgD. Several investigators found low-molecular-weight immunoglobulin resembling Bence-Jones protein in the urine and plasma of normal persons.

Since the definition of immunoglobulin is based on immunologic properties, i.e., presence of antibody activity and of common antigenic determinants in the molecules rather than physicochemical properties of the proteins, the family of immunoglobulins is classified by their antigenic structure. As will be described later, it has been shown that immunoglobulins are composed of multiple polypeptide chains. The antigenic determinants responsible for cross-reactions among all immunoglobulin classes are present in polypeptide chains (light chains) common to the immunoglobulins, and the determinants characteristic for each immunoglobulin class exist in other types of polypeptide chains (heavy chains), which are different depending on the immunoglobulin class. Therefore, the antigenic structure of immunoglobulins is related to their chemical structure in portions of the molecules.

Classification of immunoglobulins is performed using antisera specific for one of the immunoglobulin classes. In rabbits immunized with human IgA, the antiserum reacts with human IgG, IgA, and IgM. However, the antibodies reacting with IgG and IgM can be removed by adding IgG and/or IgM. After absorption the supernatant reacts only with IgA. In a similar manner, an antiserum specific for the homologous immunoglobulin used for immunization can be prepared. Each of the antisera specific for one of the human IgG, IgA, or IgM gives a single precipitin band with normal serum indicating that normal human serum contains all of the three immunoglobulins. When myeloma proteins are tested by the antisera, most of the myeloma proteins give a precipitin band with either anti-IgG or anti-IgA indicating that the myeloma proteins have the antigenic determinants characteristic for either IgG or IgA. The pathological macroglobulin from Waldenström's macroglobulinemia reacts with anti-IgM serum but not with anti-IgG or anti-IgA antiserum. Thus, most of the pathological myeloma proteins could be classified into one of the IgG, IgA, or IgM classes.

Rowe and Fahey (4) found an atypical myeloma protein which did not react with any of the anti-IgG, anti-IgA, or anti-IgM serum. The antiserum against the myeloma protein, after absorption with G myeloma protein and with a serum from a case of hypogammaglobulinemia, gave a precipitin band with the myeloma protein but not with myeloma proteins of the three immunoglobulin classes. Furthermore, the antiserum gave a single precipitin band with most of the normal sera tested, and the specificity of the precipitin band was different from that of the precipitin bands formed with the known immunoglobulin classes, indicating that the counterpart of the myeloma protein exists in normal serum. Antigenic analysis of the protein revealed that it possesses characteristic antigenic determinants not shared by other immunoglobulin classes and determinants common to the other three immunoglobulins which are present in light chains.

Furthermore, structural studies showed that the basic structure of this protein is similar to that of other immunoglobulins. Although antibody activity had not been detected in this protein, it became clear that the protein represents a distinct immunoglobulin class and was designated as IgD (γD) (5).

The fifth human immunoglobulin class was found in studies on reaginic antibody. The antiserum specific for this protein was obtained by immunizing rabbits with a reagin-rich fraction from atopic patients' sera, followed by absorption with normal IgG, A, and D myeloma proteins. The antiserum did not react with any of the known immunoglobulin classes but gave a γ_1 precipitin band with a reagin-rich fraction. Furthermore, antibody activity was detected in the protein by radioimmunoelectrophoresis (6,7). This protein has light-chain antigenic determinants common to other immunoglobulin classes as well as determinants not shared by any of the four immunoglobulins (IgG, IgM, IgA, and IgD) (8). Recently a myeloma protein, antigenically related to this protein, was found (9). It thus became apparent that the globulin represents a fifth immunoglobulin class and has been officially designated IgE or γE. As will be described later, IgE is a carrier of reaginic activity in atopic patients' sera.

Type K and Type L Immunoglobulins

The normal and pathological immunoglobulins, such as myeloma proteins, Bence-Jones proteins, and Waldenström macroglobulins, have common antigenic determinants. However, cross-reactivity of pathological proteins with antisera to normal IgG is variable. On the basis of the cross-reactivity, myeloma proteins have been classified into three groups (10). Subsequently, the third group, having the least cross-reactivity, was found to be A myeloma protein (11) and the two groups belonged to G myeloma proteins. Similarly, Bence-Jones proteins were classified into two groups. The two groups of Bence-Jones proteins have mutually exclusive antigenic determinants (12). With antisera to normal human IgG in immunodiffusion, the normal IgG spurs over groups 1 and 2 myeloma proteins. Representative proteins of the two groups spur over each other, indicating the presence of different determinants in the proteins of each group. Mannik and Kunkel (13) found that the grouping of myeloma proteins is clearly demonstrated with antisera to Bence-Jones proteins. The antiserum to group 1 Bence-Jones protein reacted only with multiple myeloma proteins of group 1 but not with the proteins from group 2. Similarly, the antiserum to group 2 Bence-Jones proteins gave a reaction with myeloma proteins from group 2 but not with group 1 proteins. Furthermore, A myeloma proteins and the Waldenström-type macroglobulins were classified into two antigenic groups by the same antisera (13,14). The antigenic determinants responsible for this grouping are common to all immunoglobulins. These two groups are now called type K and type L. The Bence-Jones protein and the serum myeloma protein from the same myeloma patients belong to the same antigenic type. It was also found that normal immunoglobulins consist of the two major types of molecules. Approximately 60 percent of IgG-immunoglobulin carries K antigenic determinants and 30 percent of the molecule carries L antigenic determinants (15). The ratio of type K and type L IgG in normal serum corresponds to the frequency of these types in G myeloma proteins. The same two antigenic groups of molecules are present in normal γA, γM, γD, γE, and normal γL globulins found in plasma and urine.

Subclasses of Immunoglobulins

Studies on G myeloma proteins revealed that at least four subclasses of IgG can be distinguished by antigenic analysis. Grey and Kunkel (16) found three subclasses using rabbit and monkey antisera to individual myeloma proteins. After absorption of the antisera with heterologous myeloma proteins, they found that some myeloma proteins still gave a precipitin band with the absorbed serum. Terry and Fahey (17) also distinguished three subclasses using monkey antisera to normal human IgG. Some of the resulting monkey serum produced three precipitin bands with human serum or human IgG in immunoelectrophoresis, but did not react with any of the purified IgA, IgM, and IgD. Comparison of the findings of these investigators revealed that two of the three subclasses corresponded, but the third subclass was different from each of the others. Therefore, it is apparent that there are four subclasses of IgG. All of the IgG molecules in the four subclasses possess γG antigenic determinants, since immunization of rabbits with these proteins gives rise to anti-IgG antibody. In addition to the antigenic determinants, the IgG in each subclass has antigenic determinants not shared by any of the other subclasses. The subclasses were designated γG_1, γG_2, γG_3, and γG_4, which correspond to γ_{2b}, γ_{2a}, γ_{2c}, and γ_{2d} by Terry and Fahey (17) and We, Ne, Vi, and Ge by Grey and Kunkel (16). Frequency of G myeloma proteins belonging to the four subclasses approximately corresponds to the relative concentration of these proteins in normal serum. Among Caucasians, the frequency of γG_1 is 50 percent; γG_2, 24 percent; γG_3, 8 percent; and γG_4, 8 percent (18,19). Antibody activity against thyroglobulin was detected in γG_1, γG_2, and γG_3 subclasses by radioimmunoelectrophoresis in sera from patients with chronic thyroiditis.

Subclasses of IgA were reported by Kunkel and Prendergast (20) as

well as by Vaerman and Heremans (21). They found that some of the
A myeloma proteins were clearly identified as IgA with some anti-γA
serum but were difficult to type by another anti-γA antiserum. Further
studies showed that such γA-globulin is antigenically deficient. The latter
antiserum gave a faint band with the deficient A myeloma proteins, and
the antigenically complete IgA formed a spur over the faint precipitin
band. The antiserum specific for the complete type IgA was obtained
by absorption of the antiserum with the deficient-type protein. Among
the 32 myeloma proteins studied, Kunkel and Prendergast found 3 deficient proteins. Vaerman and Heremans found four deficient proteins in 58
myeloma proteins tested. The major component having complete antigenic determinants was called Le-type, and the deficient proteins were
called He-type. Both groups of investigators indicated that the larger part
of IgA from normal serum probably consists of molecules with Le-type
specificity. Exchange of IgA proteins between these groups showed that
they have found the same subclasses.

Another type of subclassification of IgA was established by Terry and
Robert (22) using monkey antiserum against a myeloma protein. Among
the 51 myeloma proteins studied, 7 proteins (Fu-type) contained an antigenic determinant which was lacking in the other 44 proteins (Ma-type).
Representative proteins in each class, Fu and Ma, belonged to the Le-type
established by Vaerman and Heremans, thus indicating that the subclassification of Terry and Robert is different from that described by other
groups.

Some possibility for the presence of IgM subclasses has been reported
for the M macroglobulin (23,24). No subclasses for IgD or IgE have
been described to date.

Immunoglobulins of Experimental Animals

Immunoglobulins of experimental animals and humans are similarly
classified. The discovery of transplantable plasma cell tumors and
leukemias in mice with serum myeloma proteins and urinary Bence-Jones
proteins made classification of mouse immunoglobulins possible (25,26).
Fahey et al. (27) reported four major classes of immunoglobulins: 7S
γ_2-, 7S γ_1-, IgA-, and IgM-globulins. Gamma$_2$ globulin probably corresponds
to γG in humans but 7S γ_1-globulin represents a unique immunoglobulin
class. All of the four major classes in the serum of mice immunized with
hemocyanin were shown to have antibody activity. In the course of
studies on γ_2 myeloma proteins, Fahey (28) has found that two γ_2
myeloma proteins differ from one another in antigenic composition, although both are identified as 7S γ_2-globulin class. Using the antiserum

specific for each myeloma protein, Fahey et al. (29) classified γ_2 myeloma proteins into two subclasses, i.e., γ_{2a}, γ_{2b}. Normal serum contained immunoglobulins of both subclasses, and antibody activity was detected among the γ_{2a}- and γ_{2b}-globulins of hyperimmune mouse serum. Along with the differences in antigenic determinants specific for each subclass, the genetically determined isoantigens Ig a-1 were present in γ_{2a} myeloma proteins but not in γ_{2b} myeloma proteins.

In guinea pigs, three immunoglobulin classes 7S γ_2-, 7S γ_1-, and IgM-globulins have been described (30). Rockey et al. (31) analyzed a specifically purified horse antibody preparation against p-azophenyl α-lactoside and identified six antigenically distinct immunoglobulins. They are γA-globulin, γM-globulin, a 10S γ_1-globulin, and three antigenically distinct 7S γ-globulins. The 7S γ-globulin group probably represents three IgG subclasses. They believe that their 7S γA-globulin probably corresponds to the T-globulin component of hyperimmunized equine serum. The 10S γ_1-globulin has not been reported in other animal species. Recently, Johnson and Vaughan (32) described six antigenically distinct immunoglobulins in canine serum.

PHYSICOCHEMICAL PROPERTIES OF IMMUNOGLOBULINS

IgG (γG-immunoglobulin)

The major fraction of immunoglobulins of human and other vertebrates is γG-globulin. In humans, this protein comprises about 85 percent of the total immunoglobulins. The major component of the protein has the slowest electrophoretic mobility of all serum proteins at pH 8.6. When the serum is fractionated by zone electrophoresis at the same pH and electrophoretically separated fractions are analyzed immunologically, γG-globulin is detected in the range of γ_2- to α_2-globulin region (33). The broad distribution of IgG was also demonstrated by immunoelectrophoresis (34). As shown in Fig. 3-1, the IgG precipitin band extends from the slow migrating γ_2 region into the α mobility range. These findings indicate that IgG is composed of a continuous range of molecules differing in their isoelectric points. Heterogeneity of IgG was also observed by diffuse spread on ion exchange chromatography (35). When human serum is applied to a diethylaminoethyl (DEAE) cellulose column equilibrated with either Tris-HCl or phosphate buffer of low ionic strength and proteins are eluted by a gradient of increasing ionic strength, IgG is detected in many of the fractions (36). If a fraction is eluted with a buffer of low ionic strength, however, the fraction contains a major part of IgG but none of the other serum proteins. Usually, pure human IgG is obtained

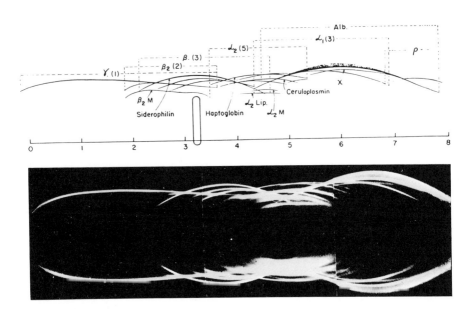

Fig. 3-1 Immunoelectrophoresis of normal human serum developed with a horse antiserum to whole normal serum. From Putnam (38) with permission.

using 0.005 M phosphate buffer or 0.05 M Tris buffer of pH 8.0. Rabbit IgG can be eluted with 0.02 M phosphate buffer.

The precise determination of the sedimentation coefficient of IgG indicates heterogeneity with an average sedimentation constant of 6.56 ± 0.32 Svedberg units (37). The molecular weight of IgG from different species ranges from 140,000 to 190,000 (38). However, recent measurements (39) suggest that the lower figure is probably correct. For example, Cammack (39) estimated the molecular weight of rabbit IgG as 137,000 from measurements of sedimentation constant and diffusion coefficient, and Marler et al. (40) gave the estimate of $145,000 \pm 5000$.

Normal IgG contains 2.6 percent carbohydrate by weight (41). As will be discussed, this value is significantly less than those of other immunoglobulins. Amino acid analysis of IgG from several species was also carried out (42). The characteristic features, distinguished from those of other proteins, are high values for the hydroxy and dicarboxylic amino acids. Particularly, the proline content of IgG is higher than that of any other globular protein.

IgM (γM-immunoglobulin)

This protein fraction has an average molecular weight of about 900,000 and constitutes 5 to 10 percent of the total γ-globulin. The study of

Waldenström-type macroglobulins, which are the pathological counterparts of normal IgM, has contributed greatly to the understanding of this class. IgM has also been found in many animal species such as mice, rabbits, horses, and chickens. The electrophoretic mobility of IgM at pH 8.6 is faster than that of the major components of IgG but slower than the β-globulin peak. Because of this electrophoretic mobility, the protein was originally called β_{2M}- or γ_{1M}-globulin.

Both normal and pathological IgM show a heterogeneity in the ultracentrifuge. The major component of this protein has a sedimentation constant of 19 Svedberg units. In addition to the major component, however, two heavier minor components exist. These components have sedimentation coefficients of approximately 29S and 38S and are thought to be polymeric forms (43). Recently, 7S protein with γM antigenic specificity was described (44). The total carbohydrate content of normal IgM and Waldenström-type macroglobulins is approximately 10 percent. The hexose content of the protein is 5.2 percent, and the hexosamine content is 2.9 percent by weight. The proteins contain small quantities of fucose, sialic acid, galactose, and mannose (45).

Antibody activity has been demonstrated in the IgM class in many antigen-antibody systems. It is believed that cold agglutinins (46) and antibodies to 0 antigens of *Salmonella* are confined to the IgM class (47). This conclusion, however, may be based on incomplete evidence. In general, IgM antibodies are demonstrated when animals are immunized with particulate antigens such as red cells and bacilli. The relative antibody activity in IgM and IgG fractions changes depending on the period after immunization when antibody is measured (see Chap. 8).

IgA (γA-immunoglobulin)

Most of the physicochemical and antigenic structures of this protein have been clarified through the study of A myeloma proteins. However, the protein comprises about 10 percent of the immunoglobulin in normal human sera and can be isolated by a combination of zinc sulfate, ammonium sulfate precipitation, and preparative electrophoresis (48). Electrophoretically, this protein has γ_1 mobility, but it is heterogeneous as is the case for other immunoglobulins.

Both normal IgA and A myeloma proteins show ultracentrifugal heterogeneity. The major component of normal serum IgA is 7S but usually contains polymeric forms such as 10.5S, 13S, and 17S components (49). In myeloma proteins, the relative concentration of the monomeric and polymeric forms is different depending on the samples. Although the monomeric form of IgA is quite similar to IgG with respect to ultra-centrifugal properties, these proteins can be separated by recycling gel filtration through a Sephadex G-200 column (50). Normal IgA is also chromatographically heterogeneous. When a serum sample was applied to a DEAE cellulose column which was equilibrated with a phosphate buffer of low ionic strength (pH 8.0) and eluted by either a stepwise or gradient increase of molarity, IgA was eluted in the 0.02 to 0.1 M range. However, the major component of IgA came off the column with 0.025 to 0.05 M buffer. The carbohydrate content of IgA is approximately 7 percent by weight. This value is higher than that of IgG but not as high as that of IgM. Proteins equivalent to human IgA have been described in the monkey (51), mouse (27), and rabbit (52). Horse IgA was also described by Rockey et al. (31).

Because of the difficulty in isolating this protein, antibody activity associated with it was not established for a long time. However, antibodies to *Brucella abortus suis*, diphtheria bacilli (53), probably antitoxin (54), and isoagglutinins (55–57) have been demonstrated in highly purified IgA preparations. IgA antibodies against insulin and ragweed antigen have been demonstrated by radioimmunoelectrophoresis (58).

Although IgG is the major immunoglobulin in serum, IgA is the predominant type of immunoglobulin in human parotid saliva, colostrum, and probably in nasal and bronchial fluids (59). The major immunoglobulin in the intestinal tract and urine is also IgA. The major component of IgA in these fluids is different from those in serum. The exocrine IgA isolated from human colostrum has a sedimentation coefficient of 11.4 to 11.6S (60,61). Furthermore, the 11S IgA in these fluids differs from the polymeric forms of IgA in serum. The polymeric protein in serum dissociates into monomeric form by reduction in aqueous solution, whereas the sedimentation coefficients of the exocrine IgA are not affected by the reduction. The protein also differs from serum IgA in carbohydrate content. It was also found by Hanson and Johansson (60) as well as by Tomasi et al. (61) that the exocrine IgA has antigenic determinants which are lacking in serum IgA. The extra antigenic determinants are due to an additional secretory piece that is attached to the IgA molecules.

The exocrine IgA was also detected in rabbits. Although IgA is a very minor component in rabbit serum (the concentration in serum was found to be 55 to 217 μg/ml), this immunoglobulin is the major component in colostrum (62). The protein, isolated by Cebra and Robbins (62), has a high sedimentation coefficient (10.8S) and a high carbohydrate content. Its molecular weight is approximately 370,000 (63).

IgD (γD-immunoglobulin)

The concentration of this protein in normal sera varies widely ranging from less than 3 μg to as high as 0.4 mg/ml. The median serum concentration is 0.03 mg/ml. IgD accounts for less than 1 percent of the normal serum immunoglobulins. Since IgD is a minor component and the physicochemical properties of the protein are similar to IgA, the protein has not been isolated from normal sera. Most of the physicochemical properties of the immunoglobulin were clarified using myeloma proteins. Electrophoretically, IgD migrates in the fast γ (γ_1) region and sediments at 7S in the ultracentrifuge. The protein comes off a Sephadex G200 column with IgA and slightly ahead of IgG. In chromatography of serum samples on diethylaminoethyl cellulose column, IgD can be separated from the major component of IgG, which is eluted by 0.015 M phosphate buffer (pH 8.0). The IgD protein remaining in the column is eluted in the region intermediate between transferrin and albumin and is close to IgA. Antibody activity associated with IgD has not been described.

IgE (γE-immunoglobulin)

This protein was first detected in atopic patients' sera in the course of studies on reaginic antibody (6). The physicochemical properties of the protein have been studied with the aid of radioimmunodiffusion techniques (7). The protein migrates in the γ_1-globulin region in preparative electrophoresis and is eluted from a Sephadex G200 column with IgA. The sedimentation coefficient of the protein is about 8.0S. By chromatography on DEAE cellulose column, IgE can be separated from the major component of IgG. The IgE and IgA are eluted close together; however, IgE appears in earlier eluate fractions and forms a narrower peak than IgA. An E myeloma protein was discovered recently (64). Physicochemical properties of this protein are similar to those of IgE in atopic patients' sera, i.e., 8.2S in ultracentrifuge and γ_1 in electrophoresis. The protein has a high carbohydrate content (11 percent by weight), which is definitely higher than that of IgA. Its concentration in normal human sera is 0.1 to 0.7 μg/ml, which is less than 0.01 percent of the total immunoglobulins (65). It was also found that monkeys (*Macaca mulatta* and *Macaca irus*) have a protein which is antigenically related to human IgE (66). So far, IgE antibodies against ragweed allergen [antigen E (67)], horse dander, and rye grass pollen have been detected in atopic patients' sera by radioimmunodiffusion and have been found to be responsible for reaginic activity of the sera (68).

Bence-Jones Proteins

Certain patients with multiple myeloma or Waldenström's macroglobuli-nemia excrete Bence-Jones proteins in their urine. This protein is char-acterized by precipitation with heating and redissolving upon boiling. The same protein (γL-globulin) was detected in urine and in the plasma of normal individuals (69,70). These proteins behave like Bence-Jones pro-tein upon heating. Bence-Jones proteins in urine are purified by precipi-tation with ammonium sulfate followed by chromatography on DEAE cellulose column. Electrophoretic mobility of this protein is in the β- to γ-globulin region. The sedimentation coefficient of highly purified Bence-Jones protein was reported to be 3.5 by van Eijk et al. (71). The molecu-lar weight of this protein is in the order of 43,000 (72). Gally and Edel-man (73), as well as Bernier and Putnam (74), found two populations in some Bence-Jones proteins of type K, a monomeric form of molecular weight of about 20,000, and dimers. Type L Bence-Jones protein is in the form of dimers.

Immunoglobulins in Experimental Animals

IgG, IgA, and IgM from animal species other than human are similar to human proteins in physicochemical properties. Therefore, only those im-munoglobulins which do not have a human counterpart will be described.

Guinea pig and mouse γ_1-globulin is different from human IgA. The carbohydrate content of γ_1-globulin is much less than that of IgA or IgE but comparable to that of IgG (75). The sedimentation coefficient of this protein is about 7S and its electrophoretic mobility is γ_1 (30). Biologi-cally, antibodies belonging to this protein sensitize homologous animals for anaphylactic reactions. Mouse 7S γ_1-globulin has physicochemical and biologic properties similar to guinea pig γ_1-globulin. Most of the protein can be separated from the bulk of γ_2-globulin by electrophoresis or DEAE cellulose column chromatography (27,30).

One of the major immunoglobulins in horse serum is the so-called T-globulin. In hyperimmune antitoxic serum, about 90 percent of the antibody activity is associated with this protein. On electrophoresis, the protein migrates in the β_2-globulin region. The protein can be isolated by combination of ammonium sulfate precipitation, DEAE cellulose column chromatography, and zone electrophoresis (76). After removal of the bulk of the γG-globulin by precipitation with 20 to 30 percent saturated ammonium sulfate, T-globulin can be precipitated at 45 percent saturation of the salt. The protein is eluted from a DEAE cellulose column with 0.02 to 0.05 M phosphate buffer at pH 7.4 but not with 0.005 M phosphate buffer. The sedimentation coefficient of the protein is 6.9, and its molecular weight is 160,000. The carbohydrate content of this protein is 4.9 percent, which is significantly higher than that of horse IgG (2.4 percent) but lower than that of human IgA.

BASIC STRUCTURE OF IMMUNOGLOBULINS

Major interest in the structure of immunoglobulins is derived from the fact that antibodies specifically combine with a number of antigens. Attempts to find chemical differences between antibodies against different antigens have been made for a long time by various ways such as analysis of amino acid composition, fingerprinting, or comparison of peptide patterns of enzymic digests. However, heterogeneity of antibody molecules against one antigen was too great to establish a difference due to combining sites. In order to overcome these difficulties, two methods have been used to split immunoglobulins into large fragments. These methods are enzymatic digestion and reduction of the interchain disulfide bonds with subsequent separation of the constituent polypeptide chains. Although the chemical structure of antibody combining sites was not clarified, fragmentation of immunoglobulins by the two methods provided much information on the basic structure of immunoglobulins. Since IgG has been studied extensively and the same principles applied to the other immunoglobulins, the structure of IgG will be described in detail followed by other immunoglobulin classes.

Structure of IgG

Enzymatic Splitting

The degradation of γ-globulin without loss of antibody activity was demonstrated many years ago. Pope (77) digested horse antitoxin with pepsin and obtained fragments of molecular weight of 100,000 without loss of precipitating activity. Porter (78) hydrolyzed rabbit IgG antibody by crystalline papain activated by cysteine and split the molecule into three fragments which together comprised 90 percent or more of the original molecule. The three fragments could be separated by chromatography on carboxymethyl cellulose and were designated as Fragments (Fr) I, II, and III (Fig. 3-2). Fragments I and II each had molecular weights of 45,000 and were similar in amino acid composition. These fragments did not precipitate with the homologous antigen but specifically inhibited the precipitation between antigen and original antibody, indicating that anti-

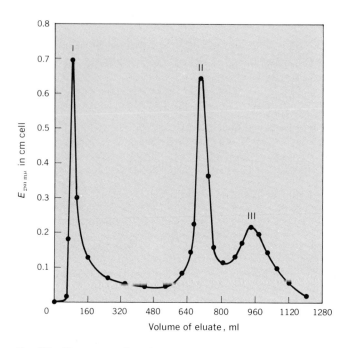

Fig. 3-2 Chromatography of papain digest of rabbit γ-globulin on carboxymethylcellulose. From Porter (78) with permission.

body combining sites exist in the fragments. Direct proof for the presence of a single antibody combining site in the fragments has been obtained by equilibrium dialysis (79) and by fluorescent quenching using antihapten antibodies (80). The third fragment, Fr III, with a molecular weight of about 50,000 (3.5S) was readily crystallized and contained most of the carbohydrate in the original molecule but no antibody activity. It was also found that the major antigenic determinants in the IgG molecule existed in Fr III but not in Fr I or II. On the other hand, the antigenic determinants responsible for cross-reactivity with different immunoglobulin classes (such as IgM) are present in Fr I and II but not in Fr III. However, the rabbit IgG (antibody) molecule was not composed of one of each piece. Palmer et al. (81) have shown that a single molecule is composed of two identical pieces I or II, together with III. When the electrophoretically fast-migrating (γ_1) portion of IgG was digested, I and III were obtained while the γ_2 portion of the same immunoglobulin gave II and III. The fragments having antibody combining sites (I and II) are now called *Fab* and the third piece is called *Fc*.

Papain digestion of IgG from various species gives pieces of molecular size similar to those obtained from rabbit IgG. Thus, the human IgG molecule is split into two Fab pieces of slow electrophoretic mobility (S) and an Fc piece of a more rapidly migrating fragment (F) (82). The ratio between Fab and Fc is 2:1.

Nelson (83) has described an intermediate product in the papain cleavage of rabbit IgG. He digested the protein with about 100 times less papain than that used in Porter's procedure in the presence of 0.01 M mercaptoethanol and then stopped the reaction by adding iodoacetamide. Under this condition a 5.2S fragment was obtained in addition to the 3.5S fragments and the whole molecule. After 2 to 3 hours of digestion the 5.2S fragment comprised 40 percent of the total protein. The fragment was found to be composed of one unit of Fab and one unit of Fc.

When IgG antibody is digested with pepsin at pH 5, one large piece of molecular weight approximately 100,000 is obtained together with several small peptides. The sedimentation constant of the large fragment is 5S. The fragments precipitate with homologous antigen and can be split into two equal pieces by reduction (84). These two halves possess one antibody combining site and are similar to the Fab obtained by papain digestion. In fact, Nisonoff et al. (85) showed that the two halves were connected by one disulfide bond. However, the univalent piece obtained by pepsin digestion and reduction was slightly different from Fab in amino acid composition and in molecular weight. The peptic fragment has a molecular weight of 92,000 (46,000 × 2), whereas the papain Fab fragment is 40,700. Therefore, the divalent 5S fragment obtained by pepsin digestion is called (Fab')$_2$. Formation of similar products by pepsin digestion and reduction and by papain digestion suggests that the cysteine used for the activation of papain might have split the disulfide bond to give Fab pieces by papain digestion. Cebra et al. (86) subsequently showed that activated insoluble papain which was free of cysteine split three to four peptide bonds in rabbit IgG but did not change the molecular weight. If cysteine was then added to treated IgG in the absence of papain, the globulin molecule split into three pieces identical to those prepared with soluble papain in the presence of cysteine.

Utsumi and Karush (85) have studied peptic fragments of rabbit IgG. In addition to (Fab')$_2$, they obtained three fragments. One had a molecular weight of 27,000, as compared with 50,000 for papain fragment Fc, and possessed some but not all of the antigenic determinants in Fc. The pepsin fragment did not contain carbohydrate and lacked interchain disulfide bonds. The second peptic fragment contained a carbohydrate moiety present in Fc but did not react with antiserum against Fc. The third fragment had a very small molecular weight, not exceeding 5000, but had antigenic determinants. In their experiments at least 50 percent of the antibody specific for heavy chain was capable of reacting with this fragment.

Multichain Structure

Another method of splitting IgG molecules was achieved by reduction of the molecules. In proteins having more than one peptide chain, the disulfide bonds of the cysteine residue are the common covalent linkage holding together the constituent chains. As the bond is split by reduction or oxidation, the consequent decrease in molecular weight gives a guide to the approximate number of peptide chains present. Edelman (87) demonstrated that the molecular weight of human IgG decreased to about 50,000 by reduction with mercaptoethanol in 6 M urea. IgG molecules of other animal species behaved similarly (88,89). This suggested that IgG of all mammalian species is composed of three to four polypeptide chains. Subsequently, Porter (90) separated two types of polypeptide chains from the reduced material by chromatography on carboxymethyl cellulose and by starch gel electrophoresis in buffer solution containing 6 M urea and designated them as heavy and light chains. These studies established that human IgG molecules are composed of multiple polypeptide chains. However, the chains separated from them were insoluble in aqueous solution and immunologically inactive. Fleischman et al. (91) attempted to split rabbit and human IgG by reduction under mild conditions to give products soluble in aqueous solution. They reduced the protein with mercaptoethanol in the absence of urea and then alkylated the products. Under these conditions a maximum of 5 of the 20 disulfide bonds in the molecule were split without changing the molecular weight. If the partially reduced alkylated protein was dialyzed against 1 N propionic or acetic acid at 3°C, and run through a Sephadex G 75 column under these conditions, two components were separated. The components, called A and B chains, corresponded to heavy and light chains obtained after more extensive reduction in the presence of urea. The heavy chains of IgG comprise three-fourths of the original molecule and have a molecular weight of 53,000. The light chains which make up one-fourth of the protein have a molecular weight of 20,000 (92). The relative yield of the heavy and light chains from a Sephadex G 75 column, the molecular weight of these chains, and the results of amino acid analysis (93) indicate that the IgG molecule is composed of two heavy and two light chains. In both human and rabbit IgG, the heavy and light chains have quite different amino acid compositions but the sum of the amino acids in the two heavy and two light chains is closely similar to that of the original molecule. It was also found by Fleischman et al. (91) that almost all of the carbohydrate in IgG is associated with the heavy chains.

The antigenic relationship between fragments obtained by papain digestion, i.e., Fab and Fc, and heavy and light polypeptide chains has been studied by Olins and Edelman (94) as well as by Fleischman et al. (91). Their results indicated that both heavy and light chains reacted with the antiserum against IgG but the precipitin lines of light and heavy chains mutually penetrate each other, thus representing a reaction of nonidentity. The antiserum specific for Fc precipitated heavy chains but not light chains. On the other hand, the light chains precipitated with anti-Fab and the precipitin band showed a reaction of partial identity with that of the Fab fragment. These findings indicate that (1) heavy and light chains have different antigenic determinants; (2) the antigenic determinants in Fc are present in heavy chains; (3) the light chains and Fab have common antigenic determinants, but the Fab fragments have the other antigenic determinants which are lacking in light chains. Olins and Edelman (94) could not show antigenic determinants shared by Fab and heavy chains. However, Fleischman et al. (91) observed the formation of a precipitin band between anti-Fab and the heavy chain preparation.

Finally, Fleischman et al. (95) reduced the Fab fragment of rabbit γG-globulin and obtained two components. One of them, called the B piece, was identified as a light (B) chain. Thus the B piece had the same N-terminal amino acid as the light chain and was indistinguishable from the light chain in antigenic structure and amino acid composition. The other component, called the A piece, had a molecular weight of 22,000 and a very low N-terminal amino acid content similar to that of whole heavy (A) chain. Furthermore, the A piece and A chain gave a single precipitin band of identical specificity against anti-Fab, which was previously absorbed with the light chain. Since the antiserum did not react with either light (B) chain or B piece, it became clear that the A piece came from heavy chain and therefore that Fab was composed of light chain and a portion of a heavy chain.

These findings have clarified the multichain structure of IgG molecules. The components, obtained by reduction followed by exposure to propionic acid, are the polypeptide chains because full reduction of the components in urea did not cause further splitting. The molecular weights of the components are in proportion to the yield. It is assumed that the IgG molecule is composed of two heavy (A) chains and two light (B) chains, which is in agreement with the molecular weight of the whole molecule. The amino acid and carbohydrate contents as well as the N-terminal amino acid of rabbit IgG are accounted for in terms of these two components. It is clear that papain and pepsin split heavy chains. Thus the Fc fragment is composed of a portion of each of the heavy chains and the Fab fragment is composed of a light chain and the rest of a heavy chain (95a). The portion of heavy chain, called the A piece, is now designated the *Fd* portion of the heavy chain (Fig. 3-3).

Bence-Jones protein was identified as light chain(s) by Edelman and Gally (96). The protein has light-chain antigenic determinants which are the same as the light-chain-type (K or L) of myeloma proteins from the same patients. The relative amino acid content of light chains and Bence-Jones proteins is almost identical. It was also found that light chains of γG-globulin have thermosolubility characteristics which are well known for Bence-Jones proteins.

Interchain Disulfide Linkages

Splitting of IgG molecules into polypeptide chains by reduction and alkylation indicates that the polypeptide chains are combined with each other by disulfide bonds to form the whole molecule. In order to visualize the configuration of the molecule, the number and allocation of interchain disulfide bonds have been studied. In the experiments by Fleischman et al. (95), five disulfide linkages per molecule were split by reduction with mercaptoethanol. Amino acid analysis of light chain showed one S-carboxymethyl cysteine present per light chain, thus indicating that a light chain was combined to an Fd piece through one disulfide linkage. As will be discussed, the presence of a single disulfide bond between light and heavy chains has been confirmed by Milstein (97,98). On the other hand, the Fd piece and heavy chain isolated by Fleischman contained 2 and 3.7 carboxymethyl cysteine groups per molecule. From these values they postulated that there were three interheavy chain disulfide linkages. However, subsequent work suggests that the number of interheavy chain disulfide linkages is probably one or two rather than three. Palmer et al. (99) reduced rabbit IgG in 0.03 M mercaptoethylamine and then alkylated the products. The reduced-alkylated molecule was then subjected to pH 2.4 to 2.5 with HCl, and the components were analyzed by ultracentrifugation and gel filtration. Under these conditions, 75 percent of the γG-globulin molecule split into two halves, each containing heavy and light chains. The molecular weight of the half molecule was 76,000 to 80,000. When the reduced-alkylated protein, which can be split to half molecules at pH 2.4, was dialyzed against 1 M propionic acid and applied to a Sephadex G 100 column, only 6 percent of the total protein was eluted as a light chain component. These results indicated that the disulfide bonds linking the half molecules are more labile to reduction by mercaptoethylamine than those holding light chains to heavy chains. By changing the conditions for reduction, Palmer and Nisonoff (100) demonstrated that one-half to two-thirds of rabbit IgG molecules can be dissociated into half molecules after reduction of one disulfide bond per molecule. There was only one S-carboxymethyl cysteine in the half molecule. Furthermore, Nisonoff and Dixon (101) showed that susceptibility of the disulfide bond linking half molecules to different concentrations of a reducing reagent is similar to that linking two Fab' fragments in (Fab')$_2$. On the other hand, Marler et al. (102), as well as Pain (92), showed that the molecular weight of the Fc fragment of a papain digest decreased to a value only half as great after reduction. The two sets of experiments suggest that the single disulfide bond linking the two heavy chains is in the region of Fc obtained by papain digestion and also in (Fab')$_2$. Therefore, papain and pepsin cleave on opposite sides of the disulfide bond. The idea is in agreement with the findings of Pain (92), Marler et al. (102), and Nisonoff et al. (84) that the molecular weight of Fab is somewhat lighter than that of Fab'. However, the scheme does not explain the findings of Cebra (103), who demonstrated that, by limited proteolysis with insoluble papain, rabbit IgG was dissociated into a soluble component with a molecular weight of 85,000 and an insoluble component. The soluble component retained the capacity to precipitate antigen dissociated into 3S by reduction, indicating that the component which is supposed to be (Fab')$_2$ contained at least one interheavy chain disulfide bond. Furthermore, the IgG digested with insoluble papain liberated a 5S component in sodium dodecyl sulfate. The slow reaction and the fact that the process was inhibited by sulfhydryl reagents suggest the occurrence of an intramolecular disulfide interchange. To account for the divergent evidence regarding the interheavy chain disulfide bonds, Utsumi and Karush (85) suggested the presence of two asymmetric interheavy chain disulfide bonds to be located in sufficient proximity so that interchange could occur between them.

Recently Steiner and Porter (104) have established the amino acid sequence in a portion of the heavy chain of a human IgG myeloma protein. They isolated a fragment containing sections of two heavy and two light chains and demonstrated that the immunoglobulin molecule contains four interchain disulfide bonds; one joins each heavy chain to a light chain and two bonds join the heavy chains to each other. Comparisons of amino acid sequence in the heavy chain portion of the myeloma protein and rabbit IgG indicate that rabbit IgG lacks a tripeptide containing a half cystine residue which forms an interheavy chain disulfide bond in the myeloma protein (105). This suggests that most rabbit IgG heavy chains are joined by a single disulfide bond, as proposed by Palmer and Nisonoff (100). Summarizing the information discussed above, the structure of IgG molecules can be visualized as shown in Figs. 3-3 and 3-4.

Although the polypeptide chains are combined with each other by disulfide bonds in the original IgG molecules, noncovalent bonds are present between light and heavy chains as well as between two heavy chains. In fact, the molecule does not dissociate after cleavage of interchain disulfide bonds unless it is subsequently exposed to denaturing solvents. Furthermore, if heavy and light chains are mixed in either propionic or acetic acid and the acid is gradually removed by dialysis, part of the chains reassociate to form 7S molecules, and if the chains are in the reduced state but not alkylated, the interchain disulfide bonds are reformed (106). The arrangement of the chains in the reconstituted molecules is similar to that of the native molecule because the digestion of the reconstructed molecule by papain resulted in the production of Fab and Fc fragments. Mixing of Fd fragment with light chain in propionic acid followed by dialysis also results in the formation of Fab fragment (107). It seems that a noncovalent bond is formed between a portion of the light chain and Fd. It was also found that half molecules formed by mild reduction and subsequent exposure to acid pH recombine at neutral pH without formation of a disulfide bond. By this procedure, Hong et al. (108) prepared hybrid molecules, half of which were derived from antibody and the other half from normal IgG; i.e., each half was derived from rabbit IgG molecules having a different genetic factor. As described previously, however, the 5S pepsin digest (Fab′)₂ dissociates into halves by reduction, and the Fab′ formed does not recombine naturally (84). These findings indicate that recombination of half molecules is due to interaction between the Fc portions of heavy chains.

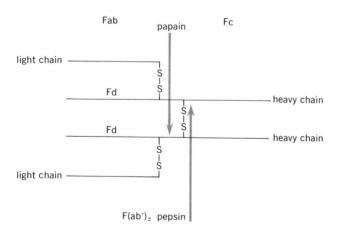

Fig. 3-3 Diagrammatic four-chain structure of the immunoglobulin molecule showing the probable sites of cleavage by papain and pepsin. From Cohen (95a) with permission.

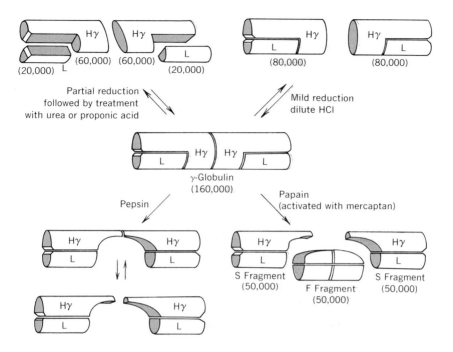

Fig. 3-4 Schematic diagram illustrating the ways in which the 7S antibody molecule may be degraded. Numbers in parentheses are approximate molecular weights. $H\gamma$ = heavy chain; L = light chain. Hatched areas indicate regions of noncovalent interchain bonding. Disulfide bonds or half-cystines are indicated in these regions. From Edelman and Gally (111) with permission.

Topographical Arrangement of Polypeptide Chains

The shape of IgG molecules has been estimated from hydrodynamic data, and evidence has been interpreted supporting an asymmetric molecule of a dimension of 250×42 Å (109). More detailed information from the angle x-ray scattering experiments of Kratkey et al. (110) suggests that the molecule is a cylinder of elliptical cross-section with dimensions of 240×19 Å. Based on these figures, Edelman and Gally (111) proposed the scheme shown in Fig. 3-4. In this model, the antibody combining sites were placed at the ends of the cylinder. However, Noelken et al. (112) pointed out that the data are equally compatible with a Y-shaped molecule. More direct evidence for the shape of the molecules was obtained from electron microscopy studies. For example, Almeida et al. (113) measured whole antibodies and Fab fragments attached to polyoma virus. The whole antibody was considered to be an elliptical cylinder $250 \times 41 \times 22.5$ Å, and the mean length of Fab was given as 67.5 ± 0.9 Å. Recently, Feinstein and Rowe (114) reported that the antibody showed little asymmetry with a maximum dimension of 105 Å when the molecule was not combined with antigen. However, the molecule opens about a control hinge portion and assumes a rod shape about 200 Å long after reacting with antigen. The flexible shape of the molecule was confirmed by Valentine and Green (115). Using rabbit IgG antibody against a dinitrophenyl group and divalent hapten, they observed the dimensions of the hapten-antibody complexes. The electron micrographs showed the antibody molecules joined together by the hapten and formed cyclic dimers, trimers, tetramers, and pentamers with a small projection at each corner of the various shapes. When the complex preparation was treated with pepsin, the conspicuous corner projections disappeared. The results indicated that the projection was an Fc fragment. If the pepsin-treated preparation was reduced with dithiothreitol, the rings fell apart. These findings demonstrate that the IgG antibody is Y-shaped and the hapten is bound very near the ends of the Fab fragments. The angle between the Fab fragments varied from 0 to 180°, and the mean length of Fab was 60 Å. A diagram of a hapten-linked trimer of the antibody molecules is shown in Fig. 3-5. If it is assumed that the fragments (both Fab and Fc) were cylinders, the calculated molecular weights were 50,000 for each fragment. All of the data are in agreement with the information on IgG structure and strongly suggest that IgG antibody molecules are flexible in shape and the three pieces are joined by a hinge.

Heterogeneity of Heavy and Light Chains

Both heavy and light chains from normal human IgG show a broad electrophoretic spread when analyzed in starch or acrylamide gels at alkaline pH. The relative mobility of heavy chains is related to that of the whole protein from which the chains were derived (116). The mobility of light chains is unrelated to that of their parent molecules. Cohen and Porter (116) have demonstrated that light chains from normal IgG resolve into 10 distinct components on starch gel electrophoresis in urea-glycine buffer, pH 7 to 8. When light-chain preparations of myeloma protein were analyzed, only one or two components were observed. These findings show that both heavy and light chains are electrophoretically heterogeneous.

As described in a previous section, myeloma and normal IgG can be classified into K and L types. The antigenic determinants responsible for the types are present in light chains but not in heavy chains. Light chains isolated from myeloma proteins are of a single antigenic type which is the same as that of Bence-Jones protein from the same patient. Amino acid composition and peptide maps after peptic digestion of light chains

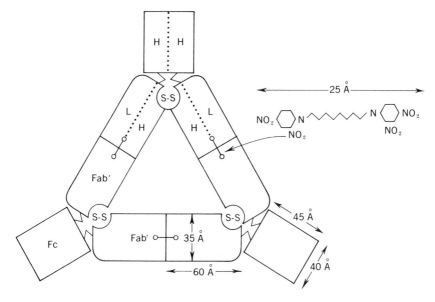

Fig. 3-5 Diagram of a hapten-linked trimer of IgG immunoglobulin molecules labeled according to current nomenclature. From Valentine and Green (115) with permission.

are different depending on the antigenic type. Antigenic structure of heavy chains is also heterogeneous.

Grey and Kunkel (16) and Terry and Fahey (17) found that the antigenic determinants responsible for the subclasses γG_1, γG_2, γG_3, and γG_4 are present in heavy chains. All of the γ chains possess major antigenic determinants for γG-globulin in the Fc portion of the chains. In addition to the determinants, γ chains from one subclass have determinants which are not shared by any other subclass. The determinants for γG_1, γG_2, and γG_4 are present in the Fc portion, whereas those for γG_3 are present in the Fd portion of the γ chains. Frangione et al. (117) and Grey and Kunkel (118) have digested the Fc piece of γG myeloma proteins with trypsin and observed that peptide maps of the Fc portion of γG_4-globulin differ markedly from the comparable fragment of γG_1, γG_2, and γG_3 proteins.

Both heavy and light chains are heterogeneous with respect to genetic factors. At the Gm locus, over 20 different genetically controlled antigens have been described. These are all localized in the heavy chain of human IgG (119). Each IgG subclass associates with its own independent group of genetic antigens (120). For example, Gm (1), Gm (4), Gm (22), and Gm (17) factors are present in γG_1 heavy chain but not in other subclasses. Genetic antigen Gm (n) was found in γG_2 but not in others (121). Factors Gm 5, 13, 14, and 21 were found only in the γG_3

heavy chain. So far no genetic factor has been found associated with γG_4 chain. All of the γG_1 molecules are positive for at least two Gm factors. Among Caucasians, either the pair of antigens Gm (1) and (17) or the pair (4) and (22) are present in the same molecule; i.e., each pair of genetic antigens characterizes one distinct variety of γG_1 heavy chain (122). When the γG_1 molecules are digested with papain, genetic antigens (1) and (22) are found in the Fc portion of the chain, whereas antigens (4) and (17) are present in Fab. The isolated light chain lacks Gm factor, and the heavy chain retains a little activity of Gm (17). In order to determine which chain contained the Gm (17) or Gm (4), Litwin and Kunkel (122) recombined isolated heavy and light chains from a different protein. The heavy chain from the Gm (17+) protein restored the Gm (17) antigen after recombination with any of the light chains from Gm (17+) and Gm (17−), whereas light chains from Gm (17+) protein did not get the antigen when it was recombined with a heavy chain from Gm (17−) protein. It was concluded that Gm (17) was specific for the Fd portion of heavy chain, but that the factor is not fully expressed unless the light and heavy chains are combined. Other than the four genetic antigens, factors Gm (2) and Gm (20) were variably associated with Gm (1). In a similar manner, some of the G3 myeloma proteins possess Gm (21), and the others contain Gm (5) in their heavy chains.

Light chains are also heterogeneous in genetic antigens. Two alleles at an independent locus Inv determine the factors Inv (1) and Inv (3) (119). These factors are limited to κ light chains, but approximately 40 percent of type K proteins were Inv (1–3). The rest of the proteins were either Inv (1+) or Inv (3+). It is also known that Inv factors were not detected in λ chain. Since the genetic antigens are present in κ-type light chains, they were detected not only in IgG but also in type K IgA and IgM molecules. As will be described later, evidence has been reported that the Inv (3) factor is correlated with the interchange of a single amino acid (valine-leucine) at a position in the carboxyl half of a κ chain.

Structure of IgM

One of the characteristic properties of IgM is its high molecular weight. However, this molecule dissociates into subunits by mild reduction. Deutsch and Morton (123) first observed that the Waldenström macroglobulin dissociated into 7S subunits by reduction in 0.1 M mercaptoethanol for 24 to 48 hours at pH 7.4, followed by alkylation with iodoacetamide. Removal of the reducing reagent by dialysis without alkylation resulted in reassociation of a part of the subunits, and the products were composed of a heterologous population of 7S-18S molecules. Their findings indicate that 18S IgM molecules are composed of 7S subunits which are combined with each other by disulfide linkages.

The dissociation of 19S IgM molecules to 7S subunits occurs under milder treatment. For example, Onoue et al. (124,125) have treated the protein in 0.1 M mercaptoethanol for 10 minutes at room temperature and obtained complete dissociation of the protein. Miller and Metzger (126) treated Waldenström macroglobulin with 0.05 M cysteine for 8 minutes at pH 8.6 and observed that 85 percent of the total protein split into 7S subunits. The 7S subunits (IgMs) separated from the pathological protein have a molecular weight of 185,000. Lamm and Small (127) reduced rabbit IgM and prepared subunits with molecular weights of 180,000. The percentage composition of each carbohydrate moiety, such as mannose, galactose, fucose, N-acetyl glucosamine, and sialic acid, was the same for IgM and its subunits. The molecular weight and absolute amount of carbohydrate in the 7S subunits indicated that the IgM molecule is composed of five subunits. The molecular weight of 185,000 for the subunits was only 4 percent higher than that expected for five equivalent subunits derived from an IgM of molecular weight 890,000.

IgM molecules are also composed of heavy (μ) and light chains. When IgM is reduced, alkylated, and subjected to gel filtration on Sephadex G100 columns equilibrated with 1 N propionic acid, two types of polypeptide chains are obtained. Light chains from IgM are comparable to those from IgG in electrophoretic mobility in starch gel electrophoresis and antigenic structure. Both κ-type and λ-type antigenic determinants were detected in IgM light chains, indicating the presence of κ- and λ-type light chains in the molecules. Heavy (μ) chains from IgM are different from γ chains from IgG in antigenic structure, amino acid composition, and electrophoretic mobility. The antigenic determinants for IgM are present in μ chains. Miller and Metzger (126) found that a μ chain is larger than a γ chain on the basis of Sephadex chromatography. Accurate measurements of molecular weights of μ and light chains from rabbit γM-globulin were carried out by Lamm and Small (127). They found that the μ chain has a molecular weight of 70,000, which is larger than the γ chain. The molecular weights of light chains from γM- and γG-globulins were comparable (22,000 to 23,000). The μ chain contained most of the carbohydrate in the IgM molecule. The molecular weights of μ chains and light chains from IgM indicate that the 7S subunits are composed of two heavy (μ) and two light chains and, therefore, that the IgM molecule is composed of ten heavy and ten light chains. Miller and Metzger (128) studied the interchain and intersubunit disulfide bonds in Waldenström macroglobulin by reducing the protein in aqueous solution followed by alkylation with C^{14}-iodoacetamide. They have found liberation of 49 to 50 new sulfhydryl groups per molecule, 40 of which were associated with the heavy chains and 10 with the light chains. Since the number of light chains in an IgM molecule would be 10, a light chain should be combined to a heavy chain by a single disulfide bond. The light chains therefore can be excluded as providing the linkage between subunits. From these results, they proposed six alternative symmetrical models for the IgM molecule (Fig. 3-6). Although the alternatives cannot be distinguished experimentally, the circular models illustrated in D, E, F in Fig. 3-6 were preferred because an IgM preparation is mostly pentamer and lacks dimers, trimers, and tetramers. Recently, Svehag et al. (129) have studied the shape of the IgM molecule by electron microscopy. Purified Waldenström macroglobulin and normal human and rabbit γM-globulins showed a spiderlike structure with five legs. These findings support a ring structure for the IgM molecule.

Partial hydrolysis of IgM by trypsin, papain, and pepsin was carried out by Deutsch et al. (130), Miller and Metzger (131), Onoue et al.

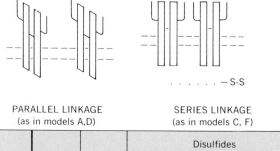

PARALLEL LINKAGE
(as in models A,D)

SERIES LINKAGE
(as in models C, F)

. . . . . . −S-S

Model	Array	Linkage	Disulfides			
			Interunit H—H	Intraunit		Total
				H—H	H—L	
A	linear	parallel	8	5	10	23
B	linear	series	4	10	10	24
C	linear	series	8	5	10	23
D	circular	parallel	10	5	10	25
E	circular	series	5	10	10	25
F	circular	series	10	5	10	25

Fig. 3-6 Upper, schematic models of IgM. Lower, tabulation of the most probable distribution of the interchain disulfides in IgM. From Miller and Metzger (128) with permission.

(124), and Harboe (132). When the molecules were digested by trypsin, 6.1S and 3.7S products were obtained (Fig. 3-7). Antigenic analysis of the products indicated that both fragments were composed of a light chain and part of a heavy (μ) chain. However, the 6.1S fragment contained additional antigenic determinants which were lacking in the 3.7S fragment, indicating that the 3.7S fragment was formed from the 6.1S fragment by removal of part of a μ chain. Reduction of the 6.1S fragment resulted in the formation of a 4.3S fragment which contained

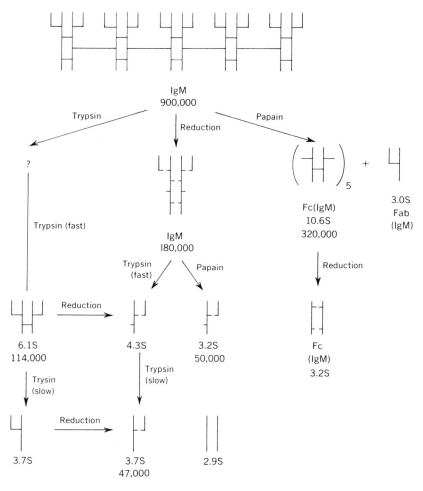

Fig. 3-7 Scheme for fragmentation of IgM by trypsin or papain digestion.

the antigenic determinant. The number of disulfide bonds in the fragments indicated that a portion of the μ chain contained an interheavy chain disulfide bond. When IgM subunits were digested by trypsin, both 4.3S and 3.7S components were obtained. The latter components (mol. wt 47,000) lacked heavy-light chain disulfide bonds and were very similar to the Fab fragment of IgG. The yield and molecular weight of the fragment suggested that one IgM molecule contained 10 of the 3.7S fragments.

Similar Fab-like fragments (3.2S) composed of a light chain and part of a μ chain were obtained by papain digestion of IgM subunits. The yield of the fragment was 10 per IgM molecule and 2 per subunit. In addition to the Fab-like fragment, Onoue et al. (124) obtained Fc-like fragments which did not contain light chains. The fragment carried the major antigenic determinants of μ chain and contained most of the hexose of the IgM subunits. The sedimentation coefficient of the fragment was 2.9S. Since this fragment is rapidly hydrolyzed by papain into small peptides, the fragment may not represent all of the remaining part of a μ chain other than that present in Fab. Onoue et al. (125) have digested whole molecules of a Waldenström macroglobulin by activated papain in the absence of reducing reagent and obtained 10.6S fragments which did not contain light chains. The fragment seems to be an Fc portion consisting of 10 heavy chains linked by intersubunit disulfide bonds (Fig. 3-7).

Structure of Other Immunoglobulins

The basic structure of the other three immunoglobulins, IgA, IgD, and IgE, is similar to that of IgG with respect to multichain structure. Because of the difficulties in the purification of the immunoglobulins in normal serum, myeloma proteins were employed in most of the structural studies.

All three immunoglobulins are composed of heavy chains, characteristic for each class, and light chains common to all classes. Both κ and λ light chains have been detected in the three immunoglobulins. After reduction and alkylation by the procedure of Fleischman et al. (91), heavy and light chains were isolated from A, D, and E myeloma proteins. Starch gel electrophoresis of the chain preparation in urea showed that electrophoretic mobility of heavy (α and ϵ) chains is different depending on the immunoglobulin class. Tryptic peptide maps of α chain were different from those of γ or μ chains (133). Carbohydrate in IgA and IgE is associated with heavy chains.

Antigenic determinants specific for each immunoglobulin class are present in heavy but not in light chains. Studies on E myeloma protein indicate that the γE antigenic determinants are present in the Fc portion of the heavy chains (64). In IgA, two types of subclasses have been described. Vaerman and Heremans (21) have classified myeloma IgA into two subclasses (Le and He types) using goat antisera against myeloma proteins. They found that α chains from Le proteins have antigenic determinants which are lacking in the chains from He type protein, indicating that their subclasses are related to structural difference in α chains. Another type of γA subclass, described by Terry and Robert (22), is not related to that reported by others. Using a monkey antiserum against normal IgA, they detected two subclasses (Fu and Ma types) in myeloma proteins. The antigenic determinants, present in Fu-type but not in Ma-type protein, were not detected in either α- or light (λ)-chain preparations of the original protein. The determinant was lost even by reduction and alkylation of the protein. It is interesting that all Fu-type myeloma proteins detected had λ-type light chains. Although localization of the antigenic determinants is not known, the results suggest that the determinants may include part of both the α and light polypeptide chains in the region of the molecule where the chains are in close proximity by interchain disulfide linkage.

As already described, human IgA has polymeric and monomeric forms. The polymeric form of IgA is dissociated into 7S subunits by reduction in 0.1 M mercaptoethanol. The 7S subunits do not associate at neutral pH when the reducing reagent is removed. However, they aggregate at pH 5 unless the reduced materials are alkylated. The findings indicate that disulfide linkages are involved in the formation of the polymeric forms (134). No antigenic difference has been detected between the polymeric and monomeric forms.

The Fc portion of IgA molecules is degraded into small peptides by papain digestion. The fragments obtained from human IgA by papain digestion are 3.5S and correspond to Fab fragments. Weir and Porter (76) have studied the structure of horse IgA (T-globulin) and IgG. A characteristic property of horse IgA is that the protein gives 5S fragments and small peptides following treatment with papain. The molecular weight of the 5S fragment was 97,000. When IgA diphtheria antitoxin was digested, the 5S fragments gave a precipitin reaction with toxoid. The 5S fragment splits into 3.5S fragments by reduction in 0.05 to 0.1 M mercaptoethanol. Amino acid analysis of whole heavy chain of IgA and of Fd fragment isolated from the protein indicated the presence of one disulfide linkage in the Fd portion of the molecule. It was also found that more than half of the carbohydrate in heavy chains is covalently bonded to the Fd fragment. This finding is different from the distribution of carbohydrate in the Fd and Fc portions of the γ chain. The difference in antigenic specificity between horse IgG and IgA is probably due to structural differences in the Fc portion of the two immunoglobulins.

The structure of human exocrine IgA has been studied by Tomasi and Zigelbaum (59), South et al. (135), and Hanson and Johansson (60,136) using the protein from colostrum. When the protein was reduced and alkylated and then exposed to 1 N acetic acid, the protein was dissociated into α and light chains. Hong et al. (137) found that a small fragment containing secretory piece specificity could be separated from colostral IgA by gel filtration after reduction and alkylation or in the presence of 5 M guanidine. They indicated that the secretory piece has antigenic determinants in common with light chains. However, Hanson and Johansson obtained secretory piece from secretions from individuals lacking IgA and showed that the preparations did not contain light-chain determinants.

Cebra and Small (63) have sudied the structure of exocrine IgA from rabbit colostrum. The protein was reduced with 0.1 M dithiothreitol in the presence of 7 M guanidine and was then alkylated. The polypeptide chains which were thus dissociated were then fractionated by gel filtration in the presence of guanidine into two major peaks. The first peak was composed of heavy (α) chains with a molecular weight of 64,000. This value was intermediate between γ (53,000) and μ chains (70,000), and a tryptic digest fingerprint for α chain was different from those for γ and μ chains obtained from rabbit IgG and IgM. The second peak was composed of light chains. However, comparisons of this material with light chains from IgG by disk electrophoresis showed that the light-chain-like material from exocrine IgA contained a fast migrating band which was lacking in light chains from IgG. This component could be obtained from exocrine IgA without reduction and alkylation. When the protein was dissolved in 5 M guanidine in the presence of 0.01 M iodoacetamide to eliminate disulfide interchange and passed through Sephadex G 200, a component having a molecular weight of 52,000 was separated from a major component which is composed of α and light chains. The molecular weight of this component decreased by reduction in 5 M guanidine. Disk electrophoresis of the reduced-alkylated material showed a high concentration of the fast-migrating component, and neither α nor light chain was detected in the preparation. It is apparent that the component, named T chain, represents a polypeptide chain present in exocrine IgA but not in serum IgA. Their studies indicate that secretory IgA is composed of three distinct kinds of polypeptide chains, an α chain, a light chain, and a T chain, and that it is composed of four pairs of the α and light chains and one or two of the T chains. Since the protein dissociates into 7.2S components, releasing a T piece in 5 M guanidine, it seems that the T piece (one or two T chains) causes or stabilizes dimerization of the monomeric form (7S) of IgA to yield the 10.8S exocrine IgA.

The molecular weight of heavy (ϵ) chain from E myeloma protein was calculated to be 75,500 from the data available for the whole molecule and its constitutent light chains (138). The value is considerably higher than those for γ chains. Chemical analysis of ϵ chain and Fc fragment has indicated the presence of six intrachain disulfide bonds and four methionine groups in the Fc part of the chain. As will be discussed later, the γ chain from rabbit γG-globulin probably has two intraheavy chain disulfide bonds in the Fc portion. The peculiar structure of the chain may be related to the function of the antibodies belonging to this immunoglobulin class.

AMINO ACID SEQUENCE OF IMMUNOGLOBULIN POLYPEPTIDE CHAINS

It is apparent from the basic structure of immunoglobulins that the five classes of immunoglobulins are made up of seven distinct polypeptide chains, as shown in Table 3-1. Furthermore, the individual chains exist in multiple distinct forms. In every individual, the IgG molecules have either κ or λ light chains. Similarly, the heavy chains exist in several forms in each individual. In addition, allelic variants are known for both

TABLE 3-1
Properties of Human Immunoglobulins

	IgG	IgA	IgM	IgD	IgE
Whole molecule					
Molecular weight	150,000	180,000 400,000 †	900,000	—	200,000
Carbohydrate	2.9	7.5	11.8	—	10.7
Heavy chain	γ	α	μ	δ	ϵ
Molecular weight	53,000	64,000	70,000	—	75,500
Light chain	κ λ	κ λ	κ λ	κ λ	κ λ
Molecular weight	22,000	22,000	22,000		22,000
Molecular formula	$\gamma_2\kappa_2$	$\alpha_2\kappa_2$	$(\mu_2\kappa_2)_5$	$\delta_2\kappa_2$	$\epsilon_2\kappa_2$
	$\gamma_2\kappa_2$	$\alpha_2\lambda_2$	$(\mu_2\lambda_2)_5$	$\delta_2\lambda_2$	$\epsilon_2\lambda_2$
		$\alpha_2\kappa_2$ T †			
		$\alpha_2\lambda_2$ T †			
Biologic function					
Antibody activity	+	+	+	?	+
Complement fixation	+	—	+	— ‡	— ‡
Skin sensitization					
Heterologous	+	—	—	—	—
Homologous	—	—	—	—	+

† Exocrine IgA.
‡ Aggregated immunoglobulin failed to fix C′.
SOURCE: From Cohen and Milstein (98a) with permission.

heavy and light chains. Antibody activity is usually found in IgG molecules of both κ and λ types, of all subclasses, and of the different allelic variants. Even purified antibody molecules against one antigen are quite heterogeneous with respect to light-chain, heavy-chain, and genetic factors. In contrast to the complexity of the IgG molecules in a normal individual, the myeloma proteins from one patient are usually homogeneous. Each protein belongs to one light-chain type, one subclass, and one allelic variant and is believed to be the product of a single clone of cells. Since the protein represents a single homogeneous sample of the many different kinds of IgG in normal serum, one can expect that the heavy and light chains of a myeloma protein have a single amino acid sequence. Thus, amino acid sequence of the polypeptide chains has been studied in myeloma proteins and Bence-Jones proteins.

Bence-Jones Proteins

In view of the findings that Bence-Jones proteins are identical to the light chains of myeloma protein in the same individual and analogous to the chains of normal immunoglobulins (111,133,139), amino acid analysis of Bence-Jones proteins was undertaken. By comparing peptide maps of the proteins, Putnam et al. (140) proposed the possibility that all Bence-Jones proteins of the same antigenic type share a common portion of their sequence. Further sequence studies have proven this hypothesis to be correct (133,141). When the tryptic peptides are placed in order in the sequence, the carboxyl half of the molecule is essentially constant, whereas the amino terminal half of the molecule differs from one protein to another. Titani et al. (142) worked out the complete amino acid sequence of a Bence-Jones protein. The type K Bence-Jones protein was composed of 214 amino acid residues. Subsequent studies in various laboratories on 20 other κ chains have shown that 43 variable positions have been found in residues 1 through 107 and only 1 in residues 108 through 214 (Fig. 3-8). This interchange is at position 191 and is correlated with the Inv genetic factor. Whenever residue 191 is valine, this genetic factor is Inv (b+), whereas it is Inv (a+) if the amino acid is leucine (143). Recent studies on Bence-Jones proteins of type L have also established that the sequence of the carboxyl half of the chains is constant (144,145). However, the amino acid sequence of the constant portions of the κ chains is very much different from that of the λ chains, indicating that the structure of the constant portion is related to antigenic differences of the light chains. Similar findings have been obtained in mouse Bence-Jones proteins which are also composed of 214 amino acids. As in human proteins, the variation in amino acid sequence occurs from position 1 through 107 in

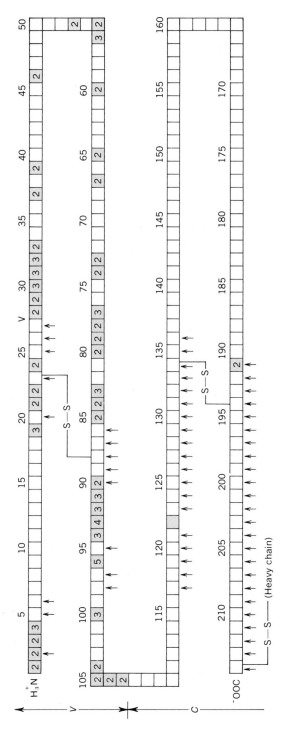

Fig. 3-8 Residue positions of human Bence-Jones protein type K. From Cohen and Milstein (98a) with permission.

mouse light chains, but there appears to be no sequence variation in the entire carboxyl terminal half. The carboxyl terminal halves of mouse and human κ chains show many differences, with a minimum of 45 changes out of 107. However, cysteine, histidine, proline, and tyrosine residues occupy identical positions in both proteins, indicating that the overall structures of the two proteins are very similar (146). The one exception is that positions 140 and 141 of mouse protein 41-A are tyrosine-proline, whereas the same positions of human protein are proline-tyrosine. The fixed structure of the carboxyl half of light chains is probably related to the affinity of the chains for heavy chains.

Milstein (97,98,98a) reported evidence that Bence-Jones proteins of type K have five cysteine residues, four of which are involved in the formation of two intrachain disulfide bonds and one in the interchain bridge to heavy chain. He found that the carboxyl terminal cysteine residue is involved in the interchain bridge. Determination of the sequence of this protein indicated that intrachain disulfide bonds are formed at positions 23-92 and 135-194 (143) (Fig. 3-8). This means that both the variable and constant portions of the light chain make a loop joined by one intra-chain disulfide bond and the length of the sequence in the loop is similar (66 residues for the amino terminal half and 61 residues for the carboxyl terminal half). The amino acid terminal part from the disulfide bond contained 22 amino acids, and the carboxyl terminal part from another bond contained 20 residues. Location of the half cystine and intrachain disulfide bond is exactly the same in κ-type Bence-Jones protein as well as in mouse-type protein (MOPC 41-A). These findings indicate that the overall structure of the light chain is very symmetrical (Fig. 3-8).

In the variable portion of light chains from 21 κ chains, 43 variable positions out of 107 residues have been found. This number may increase as more complete data become available. Milstein (147) observed that the interchanges frequently occur close to each of the two half cystine residues in the amino terminal half of the molecule (positions 19-33, 73-85, 90-96). Another major area of interchange is in residues 104 through 107, the so-called switch peptide which occurs just before the carboxyl half of the chain. Because of the presence of a disulfide bond, all of the regions are topographically the same region.

An interesting fact on the interchange is that the majority of interchanges involve homologous amino acid pairs such as valine and leucine, leucine and isoleucine, or aspartic acid and glutamic acid. In addition to these cases, many of the interchanges can be explained by a single nucleotide change in the codons for the corresponding pair of amino acids (one-step mutation). Putnam et al. (143) have pointed out that 20 out of 26 different amino acid pairings can be explained by a one-step mutation, and Milstein (148) claimed that 27 out of 32 positions are of the single-step mutation type. The ratio of one-step mutations in all interchanges could increase when sequences of new proteins are established. For example, the substitutions Asp/Asn and Asn/Thr are both possible by one-step mutation. This means that an ancestor protein containing Asn could give rise to Asp or Thr by a single-step mutation.

Heavy Chains

Determination of a full sequence of the heavy (γ) chain containing about 450 residues was quite difficult and depended on a technique to break the chain into relatively large pieces which could be aligned. For this purpose, the method of splitting of the chain with cyanogen bromide at the methionine residue was applied by Piggot and Press (149). This reagent breaks the peptide chain, giving a carboxyl terminal homoserine residue in place of methionine (150). The heavy chain of a G1 myeloma protein (Daw) was treated with cyanogen bromide and the product was fractionated on a Sephadex G 100 column in 6 M urea formate, pH 3.3. In this pathological IgG, there are four methionine residues in the heavy chain, and therefore reaction with cyanogen bromide would give four peptides terminating in homoserine and a fifth from the carboxyl end of the chain which terminates in the original carboxyl terminal amino acid. In fact, five fractions from a Sephadex G 100 column (Fig. 3-9) were obtained. Fraction 5 was composed of a small peptide containing 18 residues and terminating in glycine. All the other four fractions contained homoserine. However, the yield of Fr 1, with a molecular weight of about 29,000, was only 30 percent of that expected from its size and still contained a small amount of methionine. Further studies showed that Fr 1 was composed of fractions 2 and 4. Identification of four fragments (2, 3, 4, and 5) instead of five as expected from the number of methionines in a heavy chain suggested that a fifth fragment is held to one of the others by a disulfide bond. Complete reduction and refractionation of the fragments released a small component from fractions 1 and 2, leaving the major peptide 2a. The small peptide 2b contained 34 amino acids and had the amino terminal pentapeptide of the original heavy chain. Therefore, it is clear that 2b is derived from the amino terminal section of the chain. Fc and Fd fragments (papain digest fragments) were treated with cyanogen bromide. Fd gave fragments 2b, 4, and 2a', which had a similar size and composition with 2a but contained no homoserine. Fc fragment gave 5, 3, and a small peptide 2a'', which had a homoserine. Thus, Piggot and Press (149) proposed the alignment shown in Fig. 3-10. Fragment 3 contained carbohydrate. As already described, fragment 2b was combined

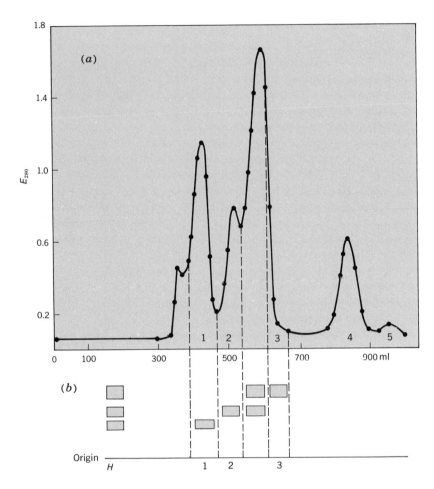

Fig. 3-9 (a) Gel filtration of the products of cyanogen bromide treatment of heavy chain of pathological IgG (Daw), on G 100 Sephadex column in 6 M urea formate buffer, pH 3.3 (135 × 3.3 cm). (b) Starch gel electrophoresis in 8 M urea formate buffer, pH 3.3, of the whole cyanogen bromide digest, H, and of the fractions (1, 2, 3) separated by gel filtration. From Piggot and Press (149) with permission.

with 2a through a disulfide linkage. Since 2b contained one S-carboxymethylcysteine residue, it is evident that the fragment is joined to 2a through one disulfide linkage. Fragment 4 also contained one S-carboxymethylcysteine residue and when the Fab fragment was treated with cyanogen bromide, no free fragment 4 was obtained. Estimation of the molecular weight of fragment 4 by amino acid analysis indicated that the fragment must be linked to fragment 2a′ by a disulfide bond rather than to a light chain. Analysis indicated that light chain is also linked to fragment 2a′ (see Fig. 3-10). The small fragment 2a″ also contained one S-carboxymethylcysteine residue. When the cyanogen bromide cleavage products of Fc were chromatographed without reduction, 2a″, 3, and 5 were obtained. Fragment 2a″ was recovered as a dimer, thus indicating that the S-carboxymethylcysteine residue in 2a″ is part of an interheavy chain disulfide bond in Fc. Fragment 3 was obtained as a monomer, and fragment 5 did not contain a cysteine residue. These findings indicate that the only interchain disulfide bond in the Fc portion of the myeloma protein is present in fragment 2a″. Amino acid sequences of carboxyl terminal peptides (fragment 5) of Daw IgG, normal human IgG (149,151), rabbit IgG (152), and horse IgG (153) have been clarified. The peptides from the two human γ chains have identical sequences. The only differences in the three species were at the fourth and sixth positions from the carboxyl terminal end. In connection with these findings variations were found in the 19 residues of human myeloma γ chains (154). The difference correlated with subclass and with one subclass the sequence was constant (Fig. 3-11).

The sequence of the Fc portion of rabbit IgG was studied by Hill et al. (155), who found that 27 of the soluble tryptic peptides, obtained in high yield from heavy chains or normal rabbit IgG, were derived from the Fc portion of the chain. Only three peptides were derived from the Fd portion. The total composition of these peptides almost accounts for the amino acid composition of the fragment. These findings indicate that the amino acid sequence of the Fc portion is fairly constant. Hydrolysis of the Fc fragment with chymotrypsin and cleavage of the fragment with cyanogen bromide were also employed to determine the sequence. Thus, 120 residues at the carboxyl terminal end, 27 residues at the amino terminal region of the Fc fragment, and 35 residues adjacent to the single aspartyl residue, to which the carbohydrate prosthetic group is linked, have been defined. Although about 65 residues contained in 5 different tryptic

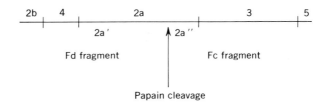

Fig. 3-10 Alignment in the heavy chain of the fragments derived from cyanogen bromide cleavage. From Piggot and Press (149) with permission.

Rabbit

   Met-His-Glu-Ala-Leu-His-Asn-His-Tyr-Thr-Gln-Lyo-Ser-*Lla*-Ser-*Ary*-Ser-Pro-Gly

Horse

   Met-His-Glu-Ala-Leu-His-Asn-His-Tyr-Thr-Gln-Lys-Ser-*Val*-Ser-*Lys*-Ser-Pro-Gly

Human γG_1 and γG_2

   Met-His-Glu-Ala-Leu-His-Asn-*His-Tyr*-Thr-Gln-Lys-Ser-*Leu*-Ser-*Leu*-Ser-Pro-Gly

γG_3

   Met-His-Glu-Ala-Leu-His-Asn-*Arg-Phe*-Thr-Gln-Lys-Ser-*Leu*-Ser-*Leu*-Ser-Pro-Gly

γG_1

   Met-His-Glu-Ala-Leu-His-Asn-His-Tyr-Thr-Gln-Lys-Ser-Leu-Ser-Leu-Ser-*Leu*-Gly

Fig. 3-11 Amino acid sequence of carboxyl terminal of γ chain.
From Press et al. (153) and Porter (154) with permission.

peptides have not been placed in order, a tentative sequence for 244 amino acids in the Fc region has been mapped. Four methionine residues at positions 19, 79, 96, and 211 from the carboxyl terminal end are present in Fc, and the half cystine residues are located at positions 22, 80, 126, 180, 220, and 244. Comparison of the sequence of κ and λ light chains has shown a certain homology between light chains and the Fc portion of rabbit IgG, suggesting an evolutionary relationship between heavy and light chains (155).

The second portion of heavy chains studied is the so-called hinge region which is exposed to enzyme attachment and, therefore, connects the Fd and Fc portion of a heavy chain. Structural studies have indicated that this region contains an interheavy chain disulfide bond. According to the provisional sequence proposed by Hill et al. (155), the amino terminal end of the Fc fragment was Cys-Pro-Pro-Glu. In view of the presence of a highly reactive disulfide bridge in the center of the hinge region, Smyth and Utsumi (156) reduced rabbit IgG or $(Fab')_2$ under mild conditions, blocked the released SH group with C^{14}-iodoacetate, and then digested the protein or $(Fab')_2$ with papain. By this procedure, they obtained the heptapeptide Cys-Pro-Pro-Pro-Glu-Leu and a mixture of peptides containing 9 to 13 amino acids. The sequence of the latter peptides was overlapping and concluded to be Ser-Lys-Pro-Thr-Cys-Pro-Pro-Pro-Glu-Leu. In all of these peptides, a single residue of galactosamine was attached to a threonine residue. Galactosamine is present on only 35 percent of the γ chain and appears to control the sites of papain cleavage, since the peptide bond between threonine and cysteine is attacked only when galactosamine is lacking.

The hinge region of human G myeloma (Daw) was studied by Steiner and Porter (104). Using C^{14}-iodoacetamide, the half cystine residues in the heavy chain were labeled. The chains were intensively reduced, alkylated, and then digested with trypsin. From the digest, a peptide containing three C^{14}-S-carboxymethylcysteines was isolated. The amino acid sequence of fragment 2a″, which was obtained by treating Fc fragment with cyanogen bromide (described above), overlapped that of the tryptic peptide. The amino terminal peptide from fragment 2a″ contained two out of the three S-carboxymethylcysteines present in the tryptic digest. Furthermore, a tetrameric peptide containing the equivalent section from both heavy and light chains still held together by disulfide bonds has been isolated. The tetramer was fragmented by digestion with trypsin into peptides containing the single disulfide bond between the heavy and light chains and into a symmetrical dimer containing two disulfide bonds joining the heavy chains to each other. It has been concluded that the four interchain disulfide bonds are the only interchain bonds in this protein. A summary of the sequence of the section of Daw IgG containing the interchain disulfide bonds is shown in Fig. 3-12. A comparison of the Daw protein with rabbit IgG shows an obvious homology in sequence. Of the 43 residues in this section of the Daw heavy chain, 29 residues are identical to rabbit IgG. An interesting observation is the deletion of a tripeptide Cys-Pro-Ala in rabbit IgG. The homology in position of the other two interchain half cystine residues in the Daw heavy chain with two half cystine residues in the rabbit chain suggests that rabbit IgG possesses a single interheavy chain disulfide bond.

The third portion of heavy chain studied is the amino terminal portion. The first problem was the N-terminal end of human and rabbit heavy chains, because the α amino group is unreactive in both proteins. Studies on Daw protein and rabbit IgG showed that the N-terminal amino acid is pyrrolid 2-1-5-carboxylic acid (PCA) in both molecules (151,157, 158). An amino acid sequence of the N terminal peptide (fragment 2b) obtained by cyanogen bromide treatment of Daw protein was shown by Piggot and Press (149). The sequence of the next cyanogen bromide fragment (4) was also completed by Press (159). Thus, 84 amino acids at the amino terminal end of the heavy chain have been mapped.

An important problem in amino acid sequencing of heavy chains is to find out whether the constant and variable portions are present in the chains. At present sufficient information on heavy chains of other myeloma proteins is not available. However, preliminary experiments on other myeloma γ chains suggested that variations would be found scattered over at least 100 positions in the Fd portion of heavy chains.

The sequence of the Fd portion of rabbit IgG was also studied (158). A mixed amino acid sequence of normal IgG follows PCA-Ser-Leu-Glu, 20 percent, and PCA-Glu (NH₂), 20 percent. This variation is unrelated

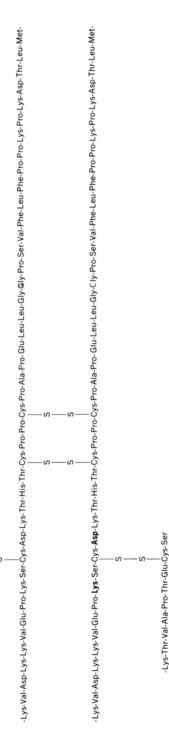

Fig. 3-12 Comparison of the amino acid sequences of Daw and rabbit IgG heavy chains in the region approximately 200 to 240 residues from the N-terminal end of these chains. Italics: Residues that correspond to codons differing in a single nucleotide base. Boldface: Residues that are not identical and do not correspond to "single base changes." From Steiner and Porter (104) with permission.

to either the allotypic specificity or the antibody specificity. The heavy chains of a purified antibody (antihuman serum albumin) and of IgG from a rabbit homozygous at the allotypic loci showed a similar mixed N-terminal sequence.

There are about five to six methionine residues in rabbit IgG heavy chain. The residues in the Fc portion are present in all molecules, although only one-third of the molecules have methionine at position 35. Much homology occurred between the N-terminal sequence of this section and the equivalent section of human IgG (Daw). There was variation in 5 positions out of 35 (154). When rabbit γ-chain is treated with cyanogen bromide, a large peptide C_1 is obtained from the remaining two-thirds of the molecule. This fragment covers the Fd portion of heavy chains and contains the N-terminal end of Fc. Six peptides were obtained from C_1 by tryptic digestion after blocking lysine residues. By this method, six arginine residues were hydrolyzed. These peptides accounted for 90 percent or more of fragment C_1. One of these peptides (T_2) corresponds to the C-terminal and another peptide (T_5) to the amino terminal section of C_1. Because of the yield and amino acid composition of these peptides, it is probable that the series of peptides will account for most of the sequence of fragment C_1 and therefore that the position of five of the six arginine residues is relatively constant in most molecules (160). Partial amino acid sequences of some of these peptides (T_2, T_3) are already known and suggest that they are from distinct sections of the Fd fragment. It is likely that a basic sequence can be established for 90 percent or more of the Fd portion of the heavy chain in the near future.

MOLECULAR BASES OF ANTIBODY ACTIVITY

Antibody Combining Site

One major purpose of the studies on immunoglobulin structure is to learn the basis of antibody specificity. As already described, much information has been obtained on the structure. However, immunochemical studies on antibodies have demonstrated a considerable heterogeneity in antibodies against one antigen. If an animal is immunized with a pure protein, antibodies against different antigenic determinants will be produced. Furthermore, evidence has been accumulated that antibodies against a single haptenic group are heterogeneous with respect to specificity. For example, antibodies of different specificity were found in anti-sym-azoisophthaloyl-glycine D, L-leucine (anti-GIL) rabbit serum (161). The antibodies were absorbed on an immunoadsorbent containing GIL and then eluted with various specific haptens. The binding properties of these separated anti-bodies with specific haptens showed some of the antibodies reacted with m-nitrobenzoyl leucine but not with m-benzoyl-glycine, whereas others reacted with m-nitrobenzoyl-glycine and not with m-nitrobenzoyl leucine, indicating that antibodies directed to different parts of the hapten exist in the antiserum. Similar findings have been obtained with antibodies against p-azobenzene arsonate (162). Eisen and Siskind (163) have reported that anti-DNP antibodies consisted of fractions which differed as much as ten thousandfold in the binding constant for a hapten. Thus the heterogeneity of the antibody combining site with respect to specificity and affinity with antigen has to be based on some structural differences in the antibody combining site.

The combining sites of antibody molecules are present in the Fab portion but not in the Fc portion. Nisonoff et al. (164) measured binding of hapten with Fab' fragment of purified antibody by equilibrium dialysis and found that affinity of the antibody combining site in the fragment with hapten is the same as that in the whole antibody. Since the Fab is composed of a light chain and the Fd portion of heavy chain, the combining site must be on one of these chains or be formed jointly by these chains. So far, conflicting results have been reported by many investigators. For example, Fleischman et al. (91) isolated heavy and light chains from horse diphtheria antitoxin and found that heavy chain but not light chain has antibody activity. In this experiment the heavy chain fraction appeared to be 100 percent as effective on a weight basis or 75 percent on a molar basis as the whole molecule. Similar results were reported by Utsumi and Karush (165) who reduced rabbit antibody specific for the p-azophenyl β-lactoside haptenic group and separated heavy and light chains on a Sephadex column in 0.03 M sodium dodecyl sulfate. Antigen binding activity of the isolated chains was evaluated by equilibrium dialysis. The unitary free energy for the binding of the hapten by the heavy chain was 87 percent of that of the reduced-alkylated antibody, whereas the light chain fraction did not combine with homologous hapten.

On the other hand, Edelman and Benacerraf (166) found that purified guinea pig antibodies gave a limited number of light-chain patterns in starch gel electrophoresis, as compared with the broad smudge shown by light chains of reduced normal IgG. A correlation was found between the electrophoretic pattern of light chain banding and specificity of the antibody. This correlation suggested that light chains contribute to the antibody combining site, although an alternate possibility remained that the band may be related to the cell types making the IgG molecules. If this is the case, the results suggest that different cell types are contributing unequally to the formation of the different kinds of antibody.

Another indirect evidence for the participation of light chain in forming antibody combining sites was obtained by Roholt et al. (167). They iodinated a rabbit antihapten antibody with I^{131} in the presence of the hapten and with I^{125} in the absence of hapten. The preparations were mixed, and heavy and light chains were separated. The chains were then digested with pepsin and the peptides separated by electrophoresis. Most of the peptides had the same relative labeling, but those fractions from the light chain showed preferential labeling with I^{125}, indicating that the tyrosyl residues in the peptides were partly protected from reaction with I^{131} by hapten. The results suggest that these parts of light chains are closely associated with the combining site. Metzger et al. (168) studied the problem using an affinity labeling technique which is based on two principles; i.e., a labeled reagent specifically binds to the combining site of certain antihapten antibodies and contains a functional group which can combine with one or more amino acid residues. Because of the complex formation between the reagent and the binding site, the local concentration of the reagent in the site becomes much higher than in free solution. Therefore, the reagent forms a covalent bond with residues in the site much faster than with the same residues elsewhere on the antibody molecule. Rabbit antihapten antibodies were treated with labeling reagent and light and heavy chains separated from the labeled antibodies. The label was present in both chains with about twice as much in heavy than in light chains, indicating that both heavy and light chains contribute one or more tyrosine residues to the active sites of both anti-p-azobenzene arsonate and anti-DNP antibodies.

Edelman et al. (169) found that separated heavy chains of guinea pig antiphage and antidinitrophenyl antibodies have much less activity than the reduced-alkylated antibody but the activity increased from 1.5- to 10-fold by recombination of homologous light chain to the heavy chain. Hybrids of the heavy chain with light chain derived from normal IgG showed less activity than homologous mixtures of chains from antibodies of the same specificity. Roholt et al. (170) showed similar results on rabbit antibenzoate antibody. With respect to recombination of heavy chain with light chain, Metzger and Mannik (171) added antibody heavy chain to the mixture of light chains from the antibody and normal γ globulin and found that anti-DNP antibody heavy chain preferentially interacts with the anti-DNP light chain in the presence of a specific hapten. Furthermore, antibody heavy chain–antibody light chain recombinants formed in the presence of hapten were more active than the corresponding recombinants formed in the absence of hapten. Subsequently, Roholt et al. (172) suggested that the recombination of heavy and light chains isolated from the same antibody are not random even when hapten is not present. They found that recovery of hapten binding activity by a mixture of heavy and light chains of the whole γG fraction from rabbit anti-*p*-azobenzene-arsonate serum is almost the same as that by a mixture of heavy and light chains from specifically purified antibody. On the other hand, recombination of heavy and light chains isolated from these antibodies with normal γG resulted in little recovery of hapten binding activity. Furthermore, mixtures of heavy or light chains from anti-*p*-azobenzoate antibody and the complementary chains from antibody-deleted γG-globulin showed little hapten binding activity. This suggests a preferential recombination of heavy and light chains from the same antibody. Extending these observations to recombination of Fd fragment and light chain, it was shown that the Fd fragment and light chain recombined to give an antibody binding site. Although the Fd fragment of antibody itself had little antigen binding activity, it was significantly enhanced by combination with antibody light chain derived from the same rabbit. The efficiency of forming combining sites also depends on the animal. When the Fd fragment and light chain for recombination were derived from different rabbits producing antibody against the same antigen, they still gave Fab fragments, but these did not have competent binding sites (107).

In any case, the findings described above indicate that light chains have some role in the formation of antibody binding sites. Direct evidence for the presence of antigen binding activity on light chain was recently obtained by Yoo et al. (173), who were able to combine hapten with light chain by fluorescence enhancement. Although heavy chain (Fd portion) plays a major role in the formation of binding sites, it is now apparent that light chain is also participating in the site. In summarizing all of these findings, it seems that both the Fd portion of heavy chain and the light chain participate in combining sites, although Fd may contribute more than light chains.

According to our present ideas on protein synthesis, the amino acid sequence of a protein determines its configuration and therefore its specific activity. Haber (174) as well as Whitney and Tanford (175) reduced the Fab fragment of antibody in 6 M guanidine to disrupt its steric structure and then recovered some specific antigen binding activity by reforming the disulfide bonds. The recovery of activity was only 10 to 15 percent of that of the original Fab fragment. However, these results suggest that the steric structure in Fab fragments is determined by amino acid sequence and, therefore, that specificity of the antibody combining sites is determined by sequence. If this is true, amino acid sequences in the Fd fragment as well as in the light chains would be characteristic of each antibody specificity. As already described, light chains are quite heterogeneous in starch gel electrophoresis and the sequence of the amino terminal half of Bence-Jones protein is variable. Studies of amino acid sequence in the Fd portion of myeloma heavy chain also suggest the presence of a variable section at the N-terminal portion (154). On the other hand, evidence has been accumulated that the antibody combining site against a single haptenic group is heterogeneous in both specificity and affinity to hapten. The problem is whether all heterogeneity of antibody molecules with respect to combining activity can be explained entirely on the basis of differences in amino acid sequence. Evidence suggests that the IgG of a normal animal is a mixture of many antibodies. Even when humans are immunized with antigen, the concentration of antibody against the antigen is less than 1 to 2 percent of the total IgG. If each antibody has a specific sequence in a part of Fd, one cannot expect to get a constant sequence for the section from such a complex mixture as normal IgG. In fact, Cebra (160) obtained seven peptides (T1 through T7) from the Fd portion of normal IgG, which will cover 90 percent of the Fd section. As complete alignment of the peptides has not been accomplished, it is still possible that about 20 amino acid residues, which are quite variable, may be missing. However, his data suggest that the variable section, in which sequence is varied from one antibody to another, cannot be large. Besides, some of the interchanges in sequence are known to be related to allelic variants. The present sequence data are not sufficient to establish whether amino acid sequence alone controls antibody specificity and affinity.

Structural Basis of Immunologic Properties

Valency of Antibodies for Precipitation and Agglutination

Both IgG and IgM antibodies give precipitin reactions with soluble antigens and agglutinate particulate antigens. If agglutinating activity of IgG and IgM antibodies is compared to the same particulate antigen, IgM antibodies have higher activity than IgG antibody (176). For example, human IgM anti-A isoagglutinins have about 20 times higher activity than IgG antibody on a weight basis (56). Since the polymeric form of IgA antibody (10S) has a significantly higher hemagglutinating activity than the monomeric form of IgA antibody, it is possible that the number of antibody combining sites may be related to the high agglutinating activity of IgM antibody. Onoue et al. (177) have shown that rabbit IgM antibody against a *p*-azobenzene arsonate group has five combining sites in a molecule. The 7S subunit of IgM antibody does not seem to agglutinate particulate antigen, although the subunit possesses an antigen binding site (178). Since the IgM molecule is composed of five subunits, one unit may have only one combining site if the combining sites are equally distributed to all subunits. Jacot-Guillarmod and Isliker (179) have reduced both anti-A and anti-B IgM isoagglutinins to dissociate them into subunits and oxidized a mixture of the reduced materials. Some of the reconstructed antibody had combining sites against both A and B cells.

The minimum number of antibody combining sites necessary to give precipitin and agglutinin reactions is probably two. (Fab')$_2$ fragments of antibody obtained by pepsin digestion give a precipitin reaction, whereas neither Fab nor Fab' does. Nisonoff and Palmer (180) have reported that the dissociation constant between hapten and Fab' of antihapten antibody is comparable to that of the combining site of the original antibody and the same hapten, indicating that the combining site did not change by the digestion. They also found that hybrid antibody, half of which is derived from normal γ-globulin and another half from anti-egg-albumin antibody, failed to give either a precipitin or agglutinin reaction. The same treatment of purified antibody does not impair the precipitating activity. When the purified antibody was dissociated into half molecules followed by recombination, the reconstructed antibody having two combining sites gave precipitin reactions.

However, it is not established whether all antibodies having two combining sites give precipitin reactions. Klinman et al. (181) purified IgA antibody from horse anti-p-azophenyl β-lactoside serum. The results of equilibrium dialysis showed that the antibody is divalent and has affinity comparable to IgG precipitating antibody. However, the IgA antibody did not give a precipitin reaction and inhibit the reaction when a sufficient amount of IgA antibody was mixed with the IgG antibody. It is possible that the physicochemical properties of an antibody may be important for giving precipitin reactions.

Biological Role of Fc Portion in IgG Antibody Molecule

The disappearance of complement (C') fixing activity of rabbit antibodies by pepsin digestion was found nearly 25 years ago. Taranta and Franklin (182) have shown that both (Fab')$_2$ and Fab failed to fix C' with antigen. These fragments from rabbit anti-sheep cell antibodies also lacked hemolytic activity (183). The presence of structures essential for C' fixation in the Fc portion of γG-globulin was reported by Ishizaka et al. (184). In view of the findings that nonspecific aggregates of γG-globulin fix C' and that mechanisms involved in inactivation of C' by aggregated γG-globulin are similar to those of C' fixation by antigen-antibody complexes (185), the activity of aggregated Fab and Fc was studied. Aggregated Fc fixed C' and aggregated Fab or (Fab')$_2$ did not do so (Table 3-2).

The Fc portion of γG-globulin is also essential for passive cutaneous anaphylaxis (PCA). The Fc fragment of rabbit γG-globulin induced

TABLE 3-2
Biologic Activity of Rabbit γG-globulin Fragments

Preparation	Aggre-gation	RPCA † (μg N)	C'F50 ‡ (μg N)	Direct skin reaction (μg N)
Whole molecule	—	0.01	624	32
	+		5.6	1.0
Fab	—	>10	>800	>35
	+		>800	>40
(Fab')₂	—	>8	≫200	>30
	+		≫200	>30
Fc	—	0.01	>800	>16
	+		7.8	2.0

† Minimum dose for a positive reversed PCA reaction.
‡ Dose required to fix 50 C'H50 out of 100.
SOURCE: From Ishizaka et al. (184) with permission.

reversed passive cutaneous anaphylaxis (RPCA) (186) and blocked passive sensitization of guinea pig skin with rabbit antibody when the mixture of the fragment and rabbit antibody was injected for passive sensitization (184). Whole γG-globulin has both sensitizing activity in RPCA reactions and blocking activity, but Fab fragments do not. These findings indicate that structures in IgG antibody essential for passive sensitization of guinea pig skin are present in the Fc portion of the molecule. It was also found that aggregated Fc increased permeability of guinea pig skin capillaries, whereas aggregated Fab did not (184). In view of the similarities between the skin reactions by antigen-antibody complexes and by aggregated γG-globulin and the fact that fixation of the aggregates is essential for the skin reactions, the results indicate that structures essential for PCA reactions in rabbit IgG antibodies are present in the Fc portion of the molecules. In connection with these findings, Goodman (187) found that the 5S fragment of rabbit antibody, obtained by papain digestion as an intermediate product, induced PCA reactions. Since the fragment is composed of one Fc and one Fab fragment and is univalent with respect to antibody combining site, positive reactions with the 5S fragment are due to the presence of the Fc portion of the molecule. These results, together with the fact that univalent hybrid antibody induces PCA reactions (188), indicate that a single antibody combining site in an antibody molecule is sufficient for the induction of the reactions. Paraskevas and Goodman (189) digested Fc fragment with crystalline pepsin and obtained fragments which were able to elicit reversed passive cutaneous anaphylaxis and block passive sensitization more effectively than did Fc. The sedimentation coefficient ($S_{20,w}$) of the active fragment was 3.3S, as compared to 3.6S for Fc in these experiments. Prahl (190) has isolated a peptide comprising the C-terminal 113 residues of rabbit IgG heavy chain by peptic digestion of Fc fragment. The purified fragment, as well as the mixture of fragments obtained by peptic digestion, failed to block the passive sensitization in their experiments. From these data they have suggested that the structures essential for the fixation of tissues may reside in the N-terminal 30 to 40 percent of the Fc portion.

Another role of the Fc portion of γG-globulin molecule is that of transmission across the fetal membrane. Brambell et al. (191) labeled papain fragments of rabbit γG-globulin and injected them into pregnant rabbits and found that Fc was transmitted at 70 percent of the rate of labeled IgG. The rate of Fab was one-sixth for piece II and one-eleventh for piece I. It is known that human IgM and IgA are barely transmitted (192,193) across the placental membrane. Failure of the two immunoglobulins to cross the placenta may be due to the absence of the necessary structure in their heavy chains. The Fc portion of the molecule may have the structures by which the catabolic rate of immunoglobulin is decided. Fahey and Robinson (194) found that the fractional breakdown rate of IgG can be increased in the mouse by injecting large amounts of either IgG or Fc fragments of the protein but not by IgA or IgM. It is known that the turnover rate differs depending on the immunoglobulin class (195,196). Little is known about the site and mechanisms of immunoglobulin catabolism; however, structures in the protein molecule probably play an essential role in the mechanism.

Immunochemical Properties of Antibodies Belonging to Different Immunoglobulin Classes

As the immunologic properties of IgG antibodies are based on certain structures in their heavy chains and the structures of heavy chains are different depending on the class of immunoglobulins, it can be expected that the immunologic properties of antibodies may be different depending on the immunoglobulin class. Several reports on this problem have revealed this to be the case in different animal species. In humans, anti-A isoagglutinins belonging to the three major immunoglobulins have been compared (56). On a weight basis, IgM and the polymeric form of IgA antibodies have the highest hemagglutinating activity and IgG antibody is the least active. All three antibodies gave precipitin reactions with A substance. Both IgM and IgG antibodies gave hemolysis of type A cells with either guinea pig or human complement, but IgA antibodies did not.

Hemolytic activity of IgM antibody was much higher than that of IgG antibody on a weight basis. Lack of hemolysis by IgA antibody suggests that the antibody does not fix C′. In fact, Heremans et al. (53) have reported that IgA antibody against *Bucella abortus* did not fix a detectable amount of C′ with the antigen, although the amount of antibody used in the experiment was unknown. Critical evidence for the lack of C′-fixing activity by IgA antibody was obtained by Ishizaka et al. (197) who demonstrated that human type A cells IgA-antibody complexes did not fix the first component of C′ (C′la). Among the 3 classes, only IgG antibody induced PCA reactions in guinea pigs. Failure of IgA and IgM antibodies for inducing PCA reactions is in agreement with the observations by Franklin and Ovary (198) that neither IgM- nor IgA-globulin gives reversed PCA reactions in guinea pigs. Biologic properties of human antibodies belonging to different classes are summarized in Table 3-1.

Differences in the immunochemical properties of antibodies depending on the immunoglobulin class were also found in rabbit antibodies (199). Similar to human antibodies, rabbit IgM antibodies have higher hemagglutinating and hemolytic activities than IgG antibodies, and IgM antibody does not give PCA reactions in guinea pigs. However, both IgG and IgM antibodies induce Arthus-type reactions (200). This finding is in agreement with the fact that complement is involved in Arthus reactions.

Biologic activities of guinea pig γ_1 and γ_2 antibodies have been studied (201–203). Both of these antibodies give precipitation with soluble antigen and agglutination of antigen-coated cells. Gamma$_2$ antibodies gave hemolysis, fixed C′, and induced Arthus reactions, along with hemorrhage, but gave no PCA reactions. On the other hand, γ_1 antibodies induced PCA reactions but neither C′ fixation nor Arthus reactions.

As already described, IgM antibodies against red cells have higher hemagglutinating and hemolytic activities than IgG antibodies. The high hemolytic activity of IgM antibody is probably related to high C′la fixing activity of the antibody on red cell surfaces. Borsos and Rapp (204,205), who established C′la fixation-transfer tests, studied the relationship between the concentration of antibodies added to particulate antigens, such as red cells or bacilli, and the number of C′la molecules fixed per antigen. When both the antibody concentration and the number of C′la molecules fixed were plotted in logarithmic scale, the slope of the dose response curve was 1.0 for IgM antibody and approximately 2.0 for IgG antibodies. This indicates that each IgM antibody molecule on the cell surface is capable of binding one molecule of C′la, whereas at least two IgG antibody molecules in the form of a doublet are required to generate one C′la fixation site. A direct proof was obtained using purified rabbit IgG and IgM anti-A antibody preparation. Assuming that a single molecule of IgM antibody on the cell surface fixes one C'1a molecule and that the molecular weight of IgM antibody is 900,000, the concentration of IgM antibody in the purified preparation was calculated. The concentration was in agreement with that of IgM antibody measured by a precipitin reaction, thus indicating that the assumption was correct (206). The requirement of only one IgM antibody molecule for generating one C'1a fixation site may explain why IgM antibody has a high hemolytic activity.

However, the high efficiency of IgM antibody for C'1a fixation is restricted to particulate antigen systems. With soluble antigen, IgM antibody was less effective than IgG antibody in C'1a fixation. It was also found that soluble antigen–IgM antibody complexes formed in excess antigen did not fix C'1a, indicating that a single IgM antibody complex with soluble antigen molecules does not have C'1a fixing activity. In the IgG system, C'1a fixing activity was not significantly different with either antigen. The results with cell antigens and insoluble A substance indicated that the difference of C'1a fixation of IgM antibody between a particulate and a soluble antigen system is ascribed to the number and distribution of antigenic determinants on the antigen involved. Since IgM antibody has five combining sites in a molecule, it seems that combination of IgM antibody molecule with antigen through multiple combining sites is essential for C'1a fixation. In the IgG antibody system, Ishizaka et al. (185) presented the hypothesis that IgG antibody molecules, combined with the same antigen, interact with each other, and distortion of the antibody molecules or consequent structural change in the Fc portion of the molecule is responsible for the initiation of C' fixation. The idea was supported by the facts that nonspecifically aggregated IgG-globulin and aggregated Fc fragments fixed C'. In fact, new antigenic determinants revealed in the Fc portion of IgG antibody molecules upon formation of antigen-antibody complexes or nonspecific aggregation (207) indicated that the structure of the Fc portion of IgG antibody actually changed by the formation of antigen-antibody complexes. If this idea is extended to the IgM antibody system, it seems that combination of the antibody through multiple combining sites may result in distortion of the molecule which is responsible for fixation of C'1a. Failure of C'1a fixation by soluble antigen–IgM antibody complexes formed in excess antigen may be explained by this idea because the combination of antibody combining sites with different antigenic molecules may not result in distortion of the antibody molecule. At any rate, characteristics of IgM antibody in C' fixation are probably related to the structure of the molecules.

Immunologic properties of human IgE antibodies are not completely resolved. It is known that the antibody sensitizes human and monkey skin for Prausnitz-Küstner reactions, whereas human antibodies belonging to other immunoglobulin classes do not (208,209). Nonantibody IgE-globulin blocks passive sensitization of human skin with reaginic antibody (8) and antibody specific for IgE induces reversed type allergic reactions (66). These findings indicate that IgE has structures essential for passive sensitization. The sensitizing activity of the IgE antibody was lost by heating at 56°C. The inactivation is due to degradation of the structure essential for the fixation to skin sites, rather than the antigen binding sites (210). The peculiar structure of heavy chains in this protein is probably responsible for its affinity to certain cells involved in human atopic hypersensitivity reactions.

Immunologic properties of antibodies are also related to subclasses. Terry (211), studying the ability of γG myeloma proteins to induce reversed PCA reactions in guinea pigs, found that γG$_1$, γG$_3$, and γG$_4$ globulins gave the reactions, whereas γG$_2$ did not. When these myeloma proteins were aggregated by coupling with bis-diazotized benzidine, γG$_1$, γG$_2$, and γG$_3$ globulins fixed C'1a, whereas aggregated γG$_4$ did not (212). The activities of these myeloma proteins did not have any correlation with light chain types of proteins. Apparently, the heavy chains of the γG$_2$ globulin have the structure essential for C'1a fixation, but do not have those involved in passive sensitization, while γG$_4$ globulin having the structure for sensitization does not have the structure for C'1a fixation. Although both of these structures are present in the Fc portion of γ chains, it is evident that structures for passive sensitization of guinea pig skin are different from those for initiation of C' fixation.

REFERENCES

1. Tiselius, A., and Kabat, E. A.: *J. Exp. Med.*, **69**:119, 1939.
2. Grabar, P., Fauvert, R., Burtin, P., and Hartmann, L.: *Rev. Franc. Etudes Clin. Biol.*, **1**:175, 1956.
3. Heidelberger, M., and Pedersen, K. O.: *J. Exp. Med.*, **65**:393, 1937.
4. Rowe, D. S., and Fahey, J. L.: *J. Exp. Med.*, **121**:171, 1965.
5. Rowe, D. S., and Fahey, J. L.: *J. Exp. Med.*, **121**:185, 1965.
6. Ishizaka, K., Ishizaka, T., and Hornbrook, M. M.: *J. Immunol.*, **97**:75, 1966.
7. Ishizaka, K., Ishizaka, T., and Hornbrook, M. M.: *J. Immunol.*, **97**:840, 1966.
8. Ishizaka, K., Ishizaka, T., and Terry, W. D.: *J. Immunol.*, **99**:849, 1967.
9. Johansson, S. G. O., Bennich, H., Ishizaka, K., and Ishizaka, T.: Unpublished data.
10. Korngold, L., and Lipari, R.: *Cancer*, **9**:183, 1956.

11. Heremans, J. F.: "Les Globulines Seriques du Systeme Gamma," Editions Ascia, S. A., Brussels, 1960.
12. Korngold, L., and Lipari, R.: *Cancer*, **9**:262, 1956.
13. Mannik, M., and Kunkel, H. G.: *J. Exp. Med.*, **116**:859, 1962.
14. Fahey, J. L., and Solomon, A.: *J. Clin. Invest.*, **42**:811, 1963.
15. Mannik, M., and Kunkel, H. G.: *J. Exp. Med.*, **117**:213, 1963.
16. Grey, H. M., and Kunkel, H. G.: *J. Exp. Med.*, **120**:253, 1964.
17. Terry, W. D., and Fahey, J. L.: *Science*, **146**:400, 1964.
18. Terry, W. D., Fahey, J. L., and Steinberg, A. G.: *J. Exp. Med.*, **122**:1087, 1965.
19. Mårtensson, L., and Kunkel, H. G.: *J. Exp. Med.*, **122**:799, 1965.
20. Kunkel, H. G., and Prendergast, R. A.: *Proc. Soc. Exp. Biol. Med.*, **122**:910, 1966.
21. Vaerman, J. P., and Heremans, J. F.: *Science*, **153**:647, 1966.
22. Terry, W. D., and Roberts, M. S.: *Science*, **153**:1007, 1966.
23. Harboe, M., Deverill, J., and Godal, H. C.: *Scand. J. Haematol.*, **2**.137, 1965.
24. Deutsch, H. F., and MacKenzie, M. R.: *Nature (London)*, **201**:87, 1964.
25. Potter, M., Fahey, J. L., and Pilgrim, H.: *Proc. Soc. Exp. Biol. Med.*, **94**:327, 1957.
26. Fahey, J. L., and Potter, M.: *Nature (London)*, **184**:654, 1959.
27. Fahey, J. L., Wunderlich, J., and Mishell, R.: *J. Exp. Med.*, **120**:223, 1964.
28. Fahey, J. L.: *J. Immunol.*, **90**:576, 1963.
29. Fahey, J. L., Wunderlich, J., and Mishell, R.: *J. Exp. Med.*, **120**:243, 1964.
30. Benacerraf, B., Ovary, Z., Bloch, K. J., and Franklin, E. C.: *J. Exp. Med.*, **117**:937, 1963.
31. Rockey, J. H., Klinman, N. R., and Karush, F.: *J. Exp. Med.*, **120**:589, 1964.
32. Johnson, J. S., and Vaughan, J. H.: *J. Immunol.*, **98**:923, 1967.
33. Slater, R. J.: *Arch. Biochem. Biophys.*, **59**:33, 1955.
34. Williams, C. A., and Grabar, P.: *J. Immunol.*, **74**:158, 1955.
35. Sober, H. A., Gutter, F. J., Wychoff, M. M., and Peterson, E. A.: *J. Amer. Chem. Soc.*, **78**:756, 1956.
36. Fahey, J. L., and Horbett, A. P.: *J. Biol. Chem.*, **234**:2645, 1959.
37. Cann, J. R.: *J. Amer. Chem. Soc.*, **75**:4213, 1953.
38. Porter, R. R.: in "The Plasma Proteins," F. W. Putnam (ed.), vol. 1, Academic Press, Inc., New York, 1960.
39. Cammack, K. A.: *Nature (London)*, **194**:745, 1962.
40. Marler, E., Nelson, C. A., and Tanford, C.: *Biochemistry*, **3**:279, 1964.
41. Müller-Eberhard, H. J., and Kunkel, H. G.: *J. Exp. Med.*, **104**:253, 1956.
42. Cohen, S., and Porter, R. A.: *Advan. Immunol.*, **4**:287, 1964.
43. Kunkel, H. G.: in "The Plasma Proteins," F. W. Putnam (ed.), vol. 1, Academic Press, Inc., New York, 1960.

44. Rothfield, N. F., Frangione, B., and Franklin, E. C.: *J. Clin. Invest.*, **44**:62, 1965.
45. Müller-Eberhard, H. J., and Kunkel, H. G.: *Clin. Chim. Acta*, **4**:252, 1959.
46. Fudenberg, H. H., and Kunkel, H. G.: *J. Exp. Med.*, **106**:689, 1957.
47. Robbins, J. B., Kenny, K., and Suter, E.: *J. Exp. Med.*, **122**:385, 1965.
48. Vaerman, J. P., Heremans, J. F., and Vaerman, C.: *J. Immunol.*, **91**:7, 1963.
49. Vaerman, J. P., Fudenberg, H. H., Vaerman, C., and Mandy, W. J.: *Immunochemistry*, **2**:263, 1965.
50. Killander, J.: in "Protides of the Biological Fluids," vol. 11, Elsevier, Amsterdam, 1963.
51. Picard, J., Heremans, J. F., and Vanderbroek, G.: *Vox Sanguinis*, **7**:100, 1962.
52. Onoue, K., Yagi, Y., and Pressman, D.: *J. Exp. Med.*, **123**:173, 1966.
53. Heremans, J. F., Vaerman, J. P., and Vaerman, C.: *J. Immunol.*, **91**:11, 1963.
54. Newcomb, R. W., and Ishizaka, K.: *J. Immunol.*, **99**:40, 1967.
55. Kunkel, H. G., and Rockey, J. H.: *Proc. Soc. Exp. Biol. Med.*, **113**:278, 1963.
56. Ishizaka, K., Ishizaka, T., Lee, E. H., and Fudenberg, H. H.: *J. Immunol.*, **95**:197, 1965.
57. Adinolfi, M., Mollison, P. L., Polley, M. J., and Rose, J. M.: *J. Exp. Med.*, **123**:951, 1966.
58. Yagi, Y., Maier, P., Pressman, D., Arbesman, C. E., and Reisman, R. E.: *J. Immunol.*, **91**:83, 1963.
59. Tomasi, T. B., and Zigelbaum, S.: *J. Clin. Invest.*, **42**:1552, 1963.
60. Hanson, L. A., and Johansson, B. G.: *Int. Arch. Allergy*, **20**:65, 1962.
61. Tomasi, T. B., Tan, E. M., Solomon, A., and Prendergast, R. A.: *J. Exp. Med.*, **121**:101, 1965.
62. Cebra, J. J., and Robbins, J. B.: *J. Immunol.*, **97**:12, 1966.
63. Cebra, J. J., and Small, P. A.: *Biochemistry*, **6**:503, 1967.
64. Johansson, S. G. O., and Bennich, H.: *Immunology*, **13**:381, 1967.
65. Johansson, S. G. O., Bennich, H., and Wide, L.: *Immunology*, **14**:265, 1968.
66. Ishizaka, K., and Ishizaka, T.: *J. Immunol.*, **100**:554, 1968.
67. King, T. P., Norman, P. S., and Connell, J. T.: *Biochemistry*, **3**:458, 1964.
68. Ishizaka, K., and Ishizaka, T.: *J. Allergy*, **42**:330, 1968.
69. Franklin, E. C., *J. Clin. Invest.*, **38**:2159, 1959.
70. Berggard, I., and Edelman, G. M.: *Proc. Nat. Acad. Sci. U.S.*, **49**:330, 1963.
71. van Eijk, H. G., Monfort, C. H., and Westenbrink, H. G.: *Koninkl. Ned Akad. Wetenschap., Proc. Ser. C*, **66**:363, 1963.
72. Holasek, A., Kratky, O., Mittelbach, P., and Wawra, H.: *J. Mol. Biol.*, **7**:321, 1963.

73. Gally, J. A., and Edelman, G. M.: *J. Exp. Med.*, **119**:817, 1964.
74. Bernier, G. M., and Putnam, F. W.: *Nature (London)*, **200**:223, 1963.
75. Oettgen, H. F., Binaghi, R. A., and Benacerraf, B.: *Proc. Soc. Exp. Biol. Med.*, **118**:336, 1965.
76. Weir, R. C., and Porter, R. R.: *Biochem. J.*, **100**:63, 1966.
77. Pope, C. G.: *Brit. J. Exp. Pathol.*, **19**:245, 1938.
78. Porter, R. R.: *Biochem. J.*, **73**:119, 1959.
79. Nisonoff, A., Wissler, F. C., and Woernley, D. L.: *Arch. Biochem. Biophys.*, **88**:241, 1960.
80. Velick, S. F., Parker, C. W., and Eisen, H. N.: *Proc. Nat. Acad. Sci. U.S.*, **46**:1470, 1960.
81. Palmer, J. L., Mandy, W. J., and Nisonoff, A.: *Proc. Nat. Acad. Sci. U.S.*, **48**:49, 1962.
82. Edelman, G. M., Heremans, J. F., Heremans, M. T., and Kunkel, H. G.: *J. Exp. Med.*, **112**:203, 1960.
83. Nelson, C. A.: *J. Biol. Chem.*, **239**.3727, 1964.
84. Nisonoff, A., Markus, G., and Wissler, F. C.: *Nature (London)*, **189**:293, 1961.
85. Utsumi, S., and Karush, F.: *Biochemistry*, **4**:1766, 1965.
86. Cebra, J. J., Givol, D., Silman, H. I., and Katchalski, E.: *J. Biol. Chem.*, **236**:1720, 1961.
87. Edelman, G. M.: *J. Amer. Chem. Soc.*, **81**:3155, 1959.
88. Edelman, G. M., and Poulik, M. D.: *J. Exp. Med.*, **113**:861, 1961.
89. Franek, F.: *Biochem. Biophys. Res. Commun.*, **4**:28, 1961.
90. Porter, R. R.: in "Basic Problems of Neoplastic Disease," A. Gellhorn and E. Hirschberg (eds.), Columbia University Press, New York, 1962.
91. Fleischman, J. B., Pain, R. H., and Porter, R. R.: *Arch. Biochem. Biophys.*, Suppl. **1**:174, 1962.
92. Pain, R. H.: *Biochem. J.*, **88**:234, 1963.
93. Crumpton, M. J., and Wilkinson, J. M.: *Biochem. J.*, **88**:228, 1963.
94. Olins, D. E., and Edelman, G. M.: *J. Exp. Med.*, **116**:635, 1962.
95. Fleischman, J. B., Porter, R. R., and Press, E. M.: *Biochem. J.*, **88**:220, 1963.
95a. Cohen, S.: *Proc. Roy. Soc. (Biol.)*, **166**:115, 1967.
96. Edelman, G. M., and Gally, J. A.: *J. Exp. Med.*, **116**:207, 1962.
97. Milstein, C.: *Biochem. J.*, **101**:338, 1966.
98. Pink, J. R. L., and Milstein, C.: *Nature (London)*, **214**:92, 1967.
98a. Cohen, S., and Milstein, C.: *Nature (London)*, **214**:449, 1967.
99. Palmer, J. L., Nisonoff, A., and Van Holde, K. E.: *Proc. Nat. Acad. Sci. U.S.*, **50**:314, 1963.
100. Palmer, J. L., and Nisonoff, A.: *Biochemistry*, **3**:863, 1964.
101. Nisonoff, A., and Dixon, D. J.: *Biochemistry*, **3**:1338, 1964.
102. Marler, E., Nelson, C. A., and Tanford, C.: *Biochemistry*, **3**:279, 1964.
103. Cebra, J. J.: *J. Immunol.*, **92**:977, 1964.
104. Steiner, L. A., and Porter, R. R.: *Biochemistry*, **6**:3957, 1967.
105. Cebra, J. J., Steiner, L. A., and Porter, R. R.: Unpublished data.

106. Olins, D. E., and Edelman, G. M.: *J. Exp. Med.*, **119**:789, 1964.
107. Roholt, O. A., Radzimski, G., and Pressman, D.: *J. Exp. Med.*, **123**:921, 1966.
108. Hong, R., Palmer, J. L., and Nisonoff, A., *J. Immunol.*, **94**:603, 1965.
109. Neurath, H.: *J. Amer. Chem. Soc.*, **61**:1841, 1939.
110. Kratky, O., Porod, G., Sekora, A., and Paletta, B.: *J. Polymer Sci.* A1, **16**:163, 1955.
111. Edelman, G. M., and Gally, J. A.: *Proc. Nat. Acad. Sci. U.S.*, **51**:846, 1964.
112. Noelken, M. E., Nelson, C. A., Buckley, C. E., and Tanford, C.: *J. Biol. Chem.*, **240**:218, 1965.
113. Almeida, J. D., Cinader, B., and Naylor, D.: *Immunochemistry*, **2**:169, 1965.
114. Feinstein, A., and Rowe, A. J.: *Nature (London)*, **205**:147, 1965.
115. Valentine, R. C., and Green, N. M.: *J. Mol. Biol.*, **27**:615, 1967.
116. Cohen, S., and Porter, R. R.: *Biochem. J.*, **90**:278, 1964.
117. Frangione, B., Franklin, E. C., Fudenberg, H., and Koshland, M.: *J. Exp. Med.*, **124**:715, 1966.
118. Grey, H. M., and Kunkel, H. G.: *Biochemistry*, **6**:2326, 1967.
119. Steinberg, A. G.: in "Advances in Immunogenetics," T. J. Greenwalt (ed.), J. B. Lippincott Company, Philadelphia, 1967.
120. Kunkel, H. G., Allen, J. C., and Grey, H. M.: *Cold Spring Harbor Symp. Quant. Biol.*, **29**:443, 1964.
121. Kunkel, H. G., Yount, W. J., and Litwin, S. D.: *Science*, **154**:1041, 1966.
122. Litwin, S. D., and Kunkel, H. G.: *J. Exp. Med.*, **125**:847, 1967.
123. Deutsch, H. F., and Morton, J. I.: *Science*, **125**:600, 1957.
124. Onoue, K., Kishimoto, T., and Yamamura, Y.: *J. Immunol.*, **98**:303, 1967.
125. Onoue, K., Kishimoto, T., and Yamamura, Y.: *J. Immunol.*, **100**:238, 1968.
126. Miller, F., and Metzger, H.: *J. Biol. Chem.*, **240**:3325, 1965.
127. Lamm, M. E., and Small, P. A.: *Biochemistry*, **5**:267, 1966.
128. Miller, F., and Metzger, H.: *J. Biol. Chem.*, **240**:4740, 1965.
129. Svehag, S. E., Chesebro, B., and Bloth, B.: *Science*, **158**:933, 1967.
130. Deutsch, H. F., Stiehm, E. R., and Morton, J. I.: *J. Biol. Chem.*, **236**:2216, 1961.
131. Miller, F., and Metzger, H.: *J. Biol. Chem.*, **241**:1732, 1966.
132. Harboe, M.: *Scand. J. Clin. Lab. Invest.*, **17**(Suppl. 84):233, 1965.
133. Bernier, G. M., Tominaga, K., Easley, C. W., and Putnam, F. W.: *Biochemistry*, **4**:2072, 1965.
134. Deutsch, H. F.: *J. Mol. Biol.*, **7**:662, 1963.
135. South, M. A., Cooper, M. D., Wollheim, F. A., Hong, R., and Good, R. A.: *J. Exp. Med.*, **123**:615, 1966.
136. Hanson, L. A., and Johansson, S. G. O.: in "Gamma Globulins: Struc-

ture and Control of Biosynthesis," J. Killander (ed.), Interscience-Wiley, New York, 1967.

137. Hong, R., Pollara, B., and Good, R. A.: *Proc. Nat. Acad. Sci. U.S.*, **56**:602, 1966.

138. Bennich, H., and Johansson, S. G. O.: in "Gamma Globulins: Structure and Control of Biosynthesis," J. Killander (ed.), Interscience-Wiley, New York, 1967.

139. Cohen, S.: *Biochem. J.*, **89**:334, 1963.

140. Putnam, F. W., Easley, C. W., and Helling, J. W.: *Biochem. Biophys. Acta*, **78**:231, 1963.

141. Putnam, F. W., Kozuru, M., and Easley, C. W.: *Acta Med. Scand. Suppl.*, **445**:109, 1966.

142. Titani, K., Whitley, E., Jr., and Putnam, F. W.: *Science*, **152**:1513, 1966.

143. Putnam, F. W., Titani, K., and Whitley, E., Jr.: *Proc. Roy. Soc. (Biol.)*, **166**·174, 1966.

144. Titani, K., Wikler, M., and Putnam, F. W.: *Science*, **155**:828, 1967.

145. Milstein, C., Clegg, J. B., and Jarvis, J. M.: *Nature (London)*, **214**:270, 1967.

146. Gray, W. R., Dreyer, W. J., and Hood, L.: *Science*, **155**:465, 1967.

147. Milstein, C.: *Nature (London)*, **209**:370, 1966.

148. Milstein, C.: *Proc. Roy. Soc. (Biol.)*, **166**:138, 1966.

149. Piggot, P. J., and Press, E. M.; *Biochem. J.*, **104**:616, 1967.

150. Gross, E., and Whitkop, B.: *J. Amer. Chem. Soc.*, **83**:1510, 1961.

151. Press, E. M., Piggot, P. J., and Porter, R. R.: *Biochem. J.*, **99**:356, 1966.

152. Givol, D., and Porter, R. R.: *Biochem. J.*, **97**:32C, 1965.

153. Press, E. M., Givol, D., Piggot, P. J., Porter, R. R., and Wilkinson, J. M.: *Proc. Roy. Soc. (Biol.)*, **166**:150, 1966.

154. Porter, R. R.: *Biochem. J.*, **105**:417, 1967.

155. Hill, R. L., Delaney, R., Lebovitz, H. E., and Fellows, R. E.: *Proc. Roy. Soc. (Biol.)*, **166**:159, 1966.

156. Smyth, D. S., and Utsumi, S.: *Nature (London)*, **216**:332, 1967.

157. Porter, R. R., and Press, E. M.: *Biochem. J.*, **97**:32P, 1965.

158. Wilkinson, J. M., Press, E. M., and Porter, R. R.: *Biochem. J.*, **100**:303, 1966.

159. Press, E. M.: *Biochem. J.*, **104**:30C, 1967.

160. Cebra, J. J.: *Cold Spring Harbor Symp. Quant. Biol.*, **32**:65, 1967.

161. Kreiter, V. P., and Pressman, D.: *Immunochemistry*, **1**:151, 1964.

162. Kitagawa, M., Yagi, Y., and Pressman, D.: *J. Immunol.*, **95**:455, 1965.

163. Eisen, H. N., and Siskind, G. W.: *Biochemistry*, **3**:996, 1964.

164. Nisonoff, A., Wissler, F. C., Lipman, L. N., and Woernley, D. L.: *Arch. Biochem. Biophys.*, **89**:230, 1960.

165. Utsumi, S., and Karush, F.: *Biochemistry*, **3**:1329, 1964.

166. Edelman, G. M., and Benacerraf, B.: *Proc. Nat. Acad. Sci. U.S.*, **48**:1035, 1962.

167. Roholt, O. A., Radzimski, G., and Pressman, D.: *Science*, **141**:726, 1963.
168. Metzger, H., Wofsy, L., and Singer, S. J.: *Proc. Nat. Acad. Sci. U.S.*, **51**:612, 1964.
169. Edelman, G. M., Olins, D. E., Gally, J. A., and Zinder, N. D.: *Proc. Nat. Acad. Sci. U.S.*, **50**:753, 1963.
170. Roholt, O., Onoue, K., and Pressman, D.: *Proc. Nat. Acad. Sci. U.S.*, **51**:173, 1964.
171. Metzger, H., and Mannik, M.: *J. Exp. Med.*, **120**:765, 1964.
172. Roholt, O. A., Radzimski, G., and Pressman, D.: *J. Exp. Med.*, **122**:785, 1965.
173. Yoo, T. J., Roholt, O. A., and Pressman, D.: *Science*, **157**:707, 1967.
174. Haber, E.: *Proc. Nat. Acad. Sci. U.S.*, **52**:1099, 1964.
175. Whitney, P. L., and Tanford, C.: *Proc. Nat. Acad. Sci. U.S.*, **53**:524, 1965.
176. Franklin, E. C.: *Progr. Allergy*, **8**:58, 1964.
177. Onoue, K., Yagi, Y., Grossberg, A. L., and Pressman, D.: *Immunochemistry*, **2**:401, 1965.
178. Onoue, K., Yagi, Y., Stelos, P., and Pressman, D.: *Science*, **146**:404, 1964.
179. Jacot-Guillarmod, H., and Isliker, H.: *Vox Sanguinis*, **7**:675, 1962.
180. Nisonoff, A., and Palmer, J. L.: *Science*, **143**:376, 1964.
181. Klinman, N. R., Rockey, J. H., and Karush, F.: *Science*, **146**:401, 1964.
182. Taranta, A., and Franklin, E. C.: *Science*, **134**:1981, 1961.
183. Amiraian, K., and Leikhim, E. J.: *Proc. Soc. Exp. Biol. Med.*, **108**:454, 1961.
184. Ishizaka, K., Ishizaka, T., and Sugahara, T.: *J. Immunol.*, **88**:690, 1962.
185. Ishizaka, T., Ishizaka, K., and Borsos, T.: *J. Immunol.*, **87**:433, 1961.
186. Ovary, Z., and Karush, F.: *J. Immunol.*, **86**:146, 1961.
187. Goodman, J. W.: *Biochemistry*, **4**:2350, 1965.
188. Ovary, Z.: *Federation Proc.*, **24**:94, 1965.
189. Paraskevas, F., and Goodman, J. W.: *Immunochemistry*, **2**:391, 1965.
190. Prahl, J. W.: *Biochem. J.*, **104**:647, 1967.
191. Brambell, F. W. R., Hemmings, W. A., Oakley, C. L., and Porter, R. R.: *Proc. Roy. Soc. (Biol.)*, **151**:478, 1960.
192. Franklin, E. C., and Kunkel, H. G.: *J. Lab. Clin. Med.*, **52**:724, 1958.
193. Gitlin, D., Rosen, F. S., and Michael, J. G.: *Pediatrics*, **31**:197, 1963.
194. Fahey, J. L., and Robinson, A. G.: *J. Exp. Med.*, **118**:845, 1963.
195. Cohen, S., and Freeman, T.: *Biochem. J.*, **76**:475, 1960.
196. Wochner, R. D., Barth, W. F., Waldmann, T. A., and Fahey, J. L.: *Clin. Res.*, **11**:231, 1963.
197. Ishizaka, T., Ishizaka, K., Borsos, T., and Rapp, H. J.: *J. Immunol.*, **97**:716, 1966.
198. Franklin, E. C., and Ovary, Z.: *Immunology*, **6**:434, 1963.
199. Onoue, K., Tanigaki, N., Yagi, Y., and Pressman, D.: *Proc. Soc. Exp. Biol. Med.*, **120**:340, 1965.

200. Tada, T., and Ishizaka, K.: *J. Immunol.*, **96**:112, 1965.
201. Ovary, Z., Benacerraf, B., and Bloch, K. J.: *J. Exp. Med.*, **117**:951, 1963.
202. Bloch, K. J., Kourilsky, F. M., Ovary, Z., and Benacerraf, B.: *J. Exp. Med.*, **117**:965, 1963.
203. Bloch, K. J., Ovary, Z., Kourilsky, F. M., and Benacerraf, B.: *Proc. Soc. Exp. Biol. Med.*, **114**:79, 1963.
204. Borsos, T., and Rapp, H. J.: *J. Immunol.*, **95**:559, 1965.
205. Borsos, T., and Rapp, H. J.: *Science*, **150**:505, 1965.
206. Ishizaka, T., Tada, T., and Ishizaka, K.: *J. Immunol.*, **100**:1145, 1968.
207. Henney, C. S., and Ishizaka, K.: *J. Immunol.*, **100**:718, 1968.
208. Ishizaka, K., and Ishizaka, T.: *J. Immunol.*, **99**:1187, 1967.
209. Ishizaka, K., Ishizaka, T., and Arbesman, C. E.: *J. Allergy*, **39**:254, 1967.
210. Ishizaka, K., Ishizaka, T., and Menzel, A. E. O.: *J. Immunol.*, **99**:610, 1967.
211. Terry, W. D.: *J. Immunol.*, **95**:1041, 1965.
212. Ishizaka, T., Ishizaka, K., Salmon, S., and Fudenberg, H.: *J. Immunol.*, **99**:82, 1967.

4
Development of the Immune Response

The phylogeny, or the evolution of development, of the adaptive immune response has been investigated for many years. A number of studies of vertebrate species have demonstrated that birds, reptiles, amphibians, and higher fishes are capable of exhibiting adaptive immune responses. However, only recently have these studies been extended to the lower marine vertebrates. Interest in the defense mechanisms of invertebrates has been rejuvenated, and earlier reports which suggested that immune responses could be demonstrated in some invertebrate species are currently being reinvestigated.

Adaptive immunity can be represented as a series of responses to foreign materials (antigens) in which specific combining substances (antibodies) are produced. To be considered immunocompetent, an organism must demonstrate the ability to exhibit certain characteristic responses. These responses include the production of circulating antibody (immunoglobulin) after antigenic stimulation, the ability to reject foreign tissue from an unrelated donor of the same species (homograft rejection), the capacity to develop delayed hypersensitivity, the proliferation of immuno-competent cells following antigenic stimulation, and finally, immunologic memory as measured by either the second-set homograft rejection or anamnestic response to secondary exposure to an antigen.

The steps involved in measuring the level of immunocompetence of an organism include the following: the response characteristics enumerated above can be tested and evaluated. In addition, the presence or absence of the structural components (lymphoid tissues and immuno-globulins) of the immune system can be determined. Careful histologic studies demonstrate the presence or absence of lymphoid organs, tissues, or cells as well as their state of complexity or degree of development. These studies also demonstrate the types of lymphoid cells present. Study of the body fluids by electrophoresis and immunoelectrophoresis shows the presence or absence of immunoglobulins. If immunoglobulins are present, their physical properties can be determined by density gradient ultracentrifugation and other techniques.

As will be demonstrated later, the degree of lymphoid tissue development correlates well with the level of immune responses. As the degree of lymphoid development increases, the level of immune responses also increases as evidenced by an ability to react to a wider range of antigens, to produce a more rapid response following antigenic stimulation, and to produce larger amounts of antibody following antigenic stimulation.

IMMUNITY IN INVERTEBRATES

Adaptive immunity does not appear to exist in invertebrates. Definitive lymphoid tissues or cells have not been observed in any invertebrate species studied to date, nor, with one possible exception, have gamma globulins been detected in these organisms. Pollara et al. (1), in 1965, discovered that the body fluids of the keyhole limpet, a mollusk, contained a fraction that electrophoretically resembles gamma globulin. However, the functional properties of this protein remain unknown. Early reports (2) that invertebrates could produce substances capable of reacting specifically with the immunizing agent have not been confirmed (3).

Homotransplantation immunity generally has been lacking in most invertebrate species tested to date. However, the recent work of Cooper (4–6) reports that integumental allografts exchanged between individuals of two different populations of the same species of earthworm show chronic rejection 18 to 20 days after grafting in 50 percent of the cases. When grafts are exchanged between earthworms of the same population, rejection occurs much less frequently. In addition, second-set integumental allo-grafts between the same first-set donor and host are rejected at an acceler-ated rate, while grafts between different first-set donors and hosts are rejected at the same rate as first-set grafts.

There are no reports suggesting that delayed hypersensitivity can develop in invertebrates, but two early studies indicate that anaphylactic-type reactions may occur in both earthworms and crayfish (7,8). How-ever, according to Good and Papermaster (9) these results have not been substantiated.

While adaptive immunity in the classical sense has not been described in invertebrates, recent evidence suggests that, at least in certain species, a specific protective response does occur following bacterial vaccination. The larva of the wax moth, *Galleria mellonella*, can be protected for a short time against infection with the homologous organism following vaccination (10). Protection starts very soon after vaccination and remains for only a few days. The protective substance is not similar to mammalian anti-body. The protection apparently takes the form of bacteriostatic action until the invading organisms can be dispensed with by phagocytosis and intracellular digestion. However, the protection is only afforded against the species of bacteria used in the vaccine.

Recently an immunologic response of male cockroaches to *Tetrahymena pyriformis* has been reported (11). Within 24 hours after injection of antigen, hemolymph from immunized cockroaches has been found to immobilize living *Tetrahymena*. The immobilizing factor ap-pears to be a protein which is sensitive to heat and acid treatment. The material is protective, and protection can be conferred passively to non-immune cockroaches.

Nevertheless, invertebrate defense mechanisms generally appear to be nonspecific and consist primarily of phagocytosis, encapsulation, and intra-cellular digestion. In some species nonspecific humoral substances exist which will combine with a variety of antigens. For example, in the sea anemone there is a substance which binds with various protein antigens and can be measured by the degree to which it interferes with antigen-antibody reactions (12,13). Nonspecific agglutinating, bactericidal, and lytic substances have been found in various insect and marine invertebrates (3,14–18). The exact chemistry of most of these substances remains unknown. Insect lysins have been reported to be proteins (19) which are heat stable (20), dialyzable, unaffected by trypsin, and weakly acidic (21).

In summary, invertebrate species studied to date generally lack immunocompetence as judged by current criteria. The rejection of allo-grafts by earthworms and the induction of specific immunity in the wax moth and cockroach are notable exceptions. Whether or not these examples of invertebrate immunity are curious artifacts or whether they can be tied together and taken as evidence for a different but specific parallel protective system remains unknown.

EVOLUTION OF THE ADAPTIVE IMMUNE RESPONSE IN VERTEBRATES

Immunologic competence appears to have developed in the lower marine vertebrates. The most primitive of these, the Ostracodermi, seem to have evolved during the Ordovician period (Fig. 4-1). Living forms are represented today by the order Cyclostomata, of which the hagfishes and lampreys are members. More advanced, but still quite primitive, are the Chondrichthyes (sharks and rays), often called the elasmobranchs, and chondrostean fish (paddlefish). These fish represent independent lines of development from the Placodermi during the Paleozoic period. The most advanced of the fishes are the holostean and teleostean fishes. By this stage of evolution the adaptive immune responses are well developed. A few important evolutionary changes involving the immune system occur in amphibians, reptiles, birds, and mammals.

Adaptive Immunity in Cyclostomes

The cyclostomes, an order of vertebrates in the superclass Agnatha, are the most primitive vertebrates presently inhabiting the earth. These animals are characterized by a lack of true jaws or paired appendages, by thin cylindrical bodies possessing only median fins, smooth and scaleless skins, a two-chambered heart, single nasal opening, and a suctorial mouth possessing horny teeth. The two suborders making up the order Cyclostomata are the Myxinoidia (hagfishes) and the Petromyzontia (lampreys). Hagfishes are entirely marine, but lampreys may be found in both fresh and salt water (22).

Hagfish Lymphoid Tissues

Until very recently hagfish were thought to be immunoincompetent (9,23). However, the recent studies of Hildemann and Thoenes (24) demonstrated that hagfish maintained in an ideal environment are quite immunocompetent. However, there is no thymus or other obvious lymphoid organ known in the hagfish. A primitive spleen consisting of islands of erythropoietic cells is present. Nevertheless, there is a cell present in the circulation of these animals which morphologically appears

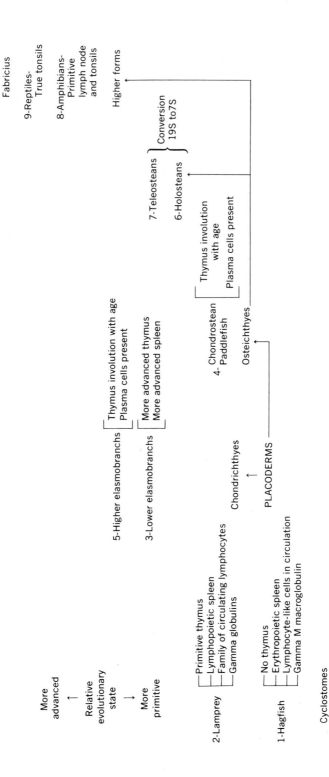

Fig. 4-1 Schematic diagram illustrating the major evolutionary steps in the development of vertebrate immune systems.

to be a lymphocyte (25) (Fig. 4-2). In addition, Hildemann reports an abundance of mononuclear cells at the site of homograft rejection.

Hagfish Immune Responses

Good et al. (25,26) have reported the failure of hagfish to respond immunologically to a variety of particulate (T2 bacteriophage, killed *Brucella abortus*) and soluble antigens (BSA, keyhole limpet hemocyanin). Furthermore, they could not detect clearance of either type of antigen from the circulation or the presence of globulins in hagfish sera by electrophoresis or immunoelectrophoresis (27). In addition, they could find no experimental difference in the acceptance rate between autografts and homografts and thus concluded that hagfish were unable to initiate the homograft reaction (27).

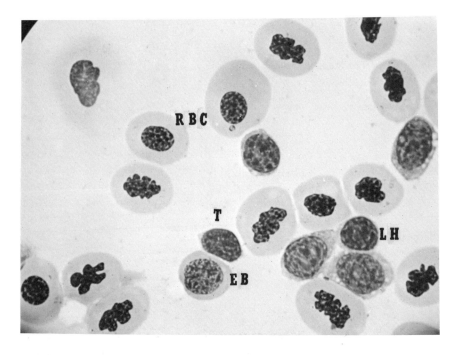

Fig. 4-2 Cell types found in the peripheral blood of the California hagfish (*Eptatratus stouti*). Red blood cells, thrombocytes, and protogranulocytes can be seen in various stages of development. Of special interest is the hagfish hemoblast, which closely resembles a mammalian small lymphocyte. LH = lymphoid hemoblast; T = thrombocyte; EB = erythroblast; RBC = red blood cell (Wright-Giemsa; × 1000). Photograph courtesy R. A. Good.

However, Hildemann and Thoenes (24) have reported a series of experiments the results of which contradict those reported by Good et al. The essential point of difference in procedure between the two groups of experiments was that Hildemann and Thoenes attempted to provide an ideal environment in which to maintain these animals for the duration of the experiments. To achieve these conditions, they utilized the facilities of the Marineland of the Pacific in California. They found that hagfish immunized with sheep erythrocytes under these conditions produced a hemagglutinin which was associated with a macroglobulin fraction similar to mouse IgM on immunoelectrophoresis. Although neutralizing antibody to coliphages has not been detected, hagfish do manage to clear these particles from their circulation. Hagfish have a well-developed capacity to recognize and reject skin homografts; first-set grafts have a mean survival time of 72 days, while second-set grafts remain viable for an average of 28 days. The first-set rejection is chronic in nature and resembles that which occurs when grafts are exchanged across weak histocompatibility loci in higher forms.

Therefore, it now appears that hagfish are immunologically competent by current standards and that perhaps further studies should be undertaken in an attempt to uncover in this species an organ or tissue equivalent to the thymus of higher vertebrates.

Lamprey Lymphoid Tissue

The lamprey possesses a primitive nonencapsulated thymus primarily made up of epithelial cells and a few lymphoid cells (25) (Fig. 4-3). Foci of lymphocytes are found in the adult spleen and primitive bone marrow (protovertebral arch) (Fig. 4-4) and the peripheral blood contains lymphoid cells (Fig. 4-5). Although the complete morphological spectrum of lymphocytes is present (small, medium, and large), members of the plasma cell series have not been demonstrated in the lamprey (25).

Lamprey Immune Responses

Of the various particulate (e.g., *Brucella abortus*, F2 bacteriophage, and SRBC) and soluble (e.g., BSA and BGG) antigens injected into the lamprey, antibody activity (an agglutinin) developed only against killed *Brucella abortus* (28) and bacteriophage (29). Lampreys do reject homografts, but very feebly. The first-set rejection time ranges between 20 and 40 days. The second-set rejection process occurs much more rapidly, rejection generally being complete within 5 days of grafting (28).

Complete Freund's adjuvant induces a necrotizing lesion at the site of injection, and the injection of old tuberculin 29 days later will elicit a

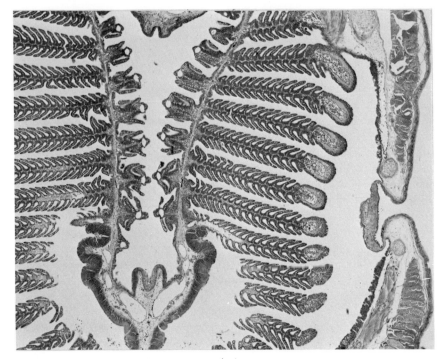

(a)

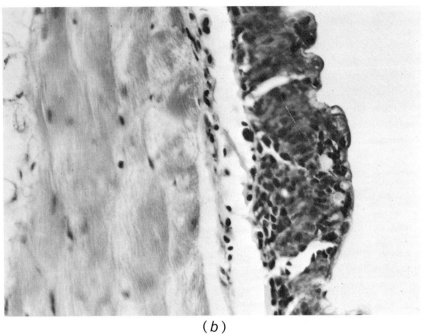

(b)

delayed hypersensitivity reaction in lampreys (28). Evidence for immuno-logic memory in the lamprey has also been described (28). Following the first injection of killed *Brucella abortus* a very weak agglutinating activity is demonstrated in lamprey serum. However, following a second injection of antigen, there is a rapid rise of agglutinating activity in the serum. In addition to this type of memory (anamnestic response) the accelerated second-set homograft reaction mentioned above (28) also occurs.

Immunoelectrophoresis of whole lamprey serum demonstrates two distinct proteins with the electrophoretic mobility of gamma globulin as well as seven other serum components with alpha and beta globulin mobili-ties (30). By use of sucrose density gradient centrifugation procedures, the antibody against *Brucella* was found to have a sedimentation constant of 9S; it was also shown to be 2-mercaptoethanol sensitive. The gamma globulin sedimenting at 7S appears to be immunologically inactive, since no anti-*Brucella* antibody activity could be demonstrated in this fraction (30). The implications of these results are not clear, since 7S gamma globulins are very important immunologically in higher forms. Lamprey serum also contains a natural agglutinin to SRBC which has been defined as a 16S macroglobulin. The titer of this agglutinin remains constant in any given animal, and repeated injections of SRBC have failed to increase the agglutinating activity (30).

Marchalonis and Edelman (29) found antibodies to F2 bacteriophage which sedimented in the 6.6S and 14S fractions of lamprey serum. They obtained evidence which suggests that the 6.6 immunoglobulins consist of light components (mol. wt 25,000) and heavy components (mol. wt 70,000). These polypeptide chains are linked by weak interactions but not by interchain disulfide bonds. In this respect, the lamprey antibody differs from the immunoglobulins of other vertebrates which require cleavage of disulfide bonds prior to dissociation. The heavy chain mobility corresponded to that of μ chains and resembled that of heavy chains of shark and sting ray immunoglobulins. This finding is consistent with the hypothesis that μ chains were the earliest of the heavy chain classes to emerge. It further supports the view that the multichain structure of

Fig. 4-3 (a) Gill region of the sea lamprey (*Petromyzon marinus*) showing pharyngeal gutter region. Primitive lymphoepithelial thymus is scattered throughout this tissue from the second to the fifth gill arch (Hematoxylin-eosin; × 25).
(b) Scattered lymphoepithelial thymus cells in the epithelial lining of the pharyngeal gutter of the gill region of the sea lamprey (Hematoxylin-eosin; × 400). Photographs courtesy R. A. Good.

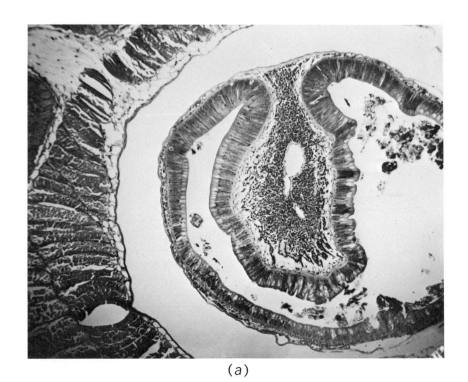

(a)

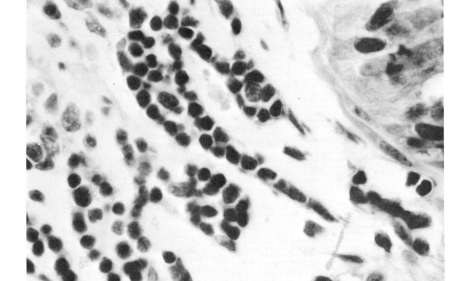

(b)

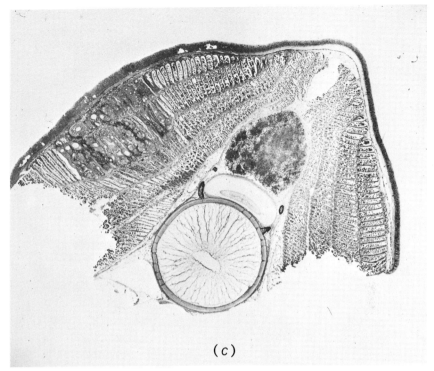

(c)

Fig. 4-4 (a) Spleen of the sea lamprey located in an invagination of the anterior gut. Lymphoid cell accumulations are located along the periphery of this tissue (Hematoxylin-eosin; × 25).
(b) Lymphoid cells located along the periphery of the sea lamprey spleen. The medullary portion of the spleen is comprised of reticulum cells (Hematoxylin-eosin; × 800).
(c) Bone marrow of the sea lamprey located in the protovertebral arch. This tissue is primarily hematopoietic, but some lymphoid cells are present. Cells proliferate in this region following intense antigenic stimulation (Hematoxylin-eosin; × 8). Photographs courtesy R. A. Good.

immunoglobulins is a fundamental feature of antibody molecules (see Chaps. 3 and 10).

Mononuclear cell proliferation has been reported in the lamprey following antigenic stimulation. Following an injection of bovine serum albumin in Freund's adjuvant, Finstad and Fichtelius (26) observed that there was an increase in uptake of the tritiated thymidine, a DNA precursor, in the protovertebral arch. Unfortunately, no detectable circulating antibody to this antigen has been described in the lamprey.

While the immune responses of cyclostomes may be considered weak by mammalian standards, they nevertheless are present. Table 4-1 summarizes the present knowledge of immune responses of Cyclostomes.

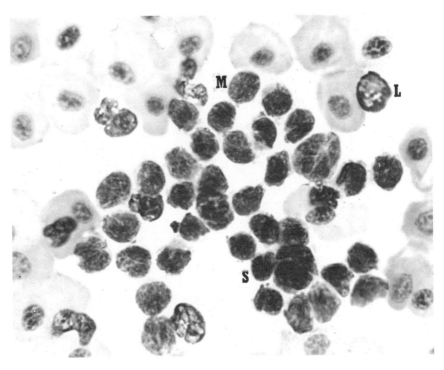

Fig. 4-5 Peripheral blood of the lamprey illustrating mononuclear cell types. L = large lymphocyte; M = medium lymphocyte; S = small lymphocyte (Wright-Giemsa, × 1000). From Good et al. (25) with permission.

Adaptive Immunity in Lower Elasmobranchs

The elasmobranchs (Chondrichthyes) represent one of the two independent lines of development from the Placodermi (Fig. 4-1). This class is made up of the cartilaginous fishes (sharks and rays), almost all of which are marine species. Sharks first appeared during the Carboniferous period (about 250 million years ago), and the rays first appeared during the Triassic period (about 175 million years ago). Sharks and rays are perhaps the most primitive of the jawed vertebrates living today and are characterized by a cartilaginous skeleton, presence of both upper and lower jaws with enamel-capped teeth, persistent notochord, tough skin, and a two-chambered heart (22).

Elasmobranch Lymphoid Tissues

Both sharks and rays have a fairly well-developed thymus which is encapsulated and organized into a cortex and medulla (Fig. 4-6). A few primitive Hassall's corpuscles have also been observed. The thymus of

104

TABLE 4-1

Adaptive Immunity in Cyclostomes

Species	Lymphoid tissues	Immune responses	Serum globulins
Hagfish	1. No thymus	1. Agglutinins against SRBC	1. IgM macroglobulin
	2. Erythropoietic spleen	2. Coliphages cleared	
	3. Lymphoid cells in circulation	3. Homograft rejection	
		4. Memory	
Lamprey	1. Epithelial thymus	1. Agglutinins against *Brucella abortus*	1. Two gamma types
	2. Lymphocytic foci (spleen and bone marrow)	2. Neutralizing antibodies against F2 bacteriophage	2. Seven alpha and beta types
	3. Family of lymphocytes	3. Homograft rejection	
	4. No plasma cells	4. Delayed allergy	
		5. Memory	
		6. Cell proliferation	

primitive elasmobranchs does not involute with age, but the thymus of more advanced sharks and rays does involute during adult life. The spleen is a discrete encapsulated organ at birth, and foci of lymphocytes appear in the spleen a few weeks after birth (Fig. 4-7). Foci of lymphocytes are also found in the gut, gonads, and renal parenchyma. Primitive rays (guitarfish) and sharks (horned sharks) do not possess plasma cells. However, more advanced rays (sting rays) and sharks (leopard and nurse sharks) possess cells in the spleen and gonads which by morphological criteria are similar to the plasma cells seen in mammals and birds (25) (Fig. 4-8).

Elasmobranch Immune Responses

The response of primitive elasmobranchs to injected antigens has been variable. No response was elicited against either BGG or BSA, although BSA was cleared from the circulation. Antibody titers have been obtained following injection of bacteriophage, hemocyanin, and *Brucella* antigens. When the animals respond to antigens, there is a very weak primary response but a more vigorous secondary response (28). The higher elasmobranchs are capable of a more vigorous response to a wider variety of antigens than more primitive species (25).

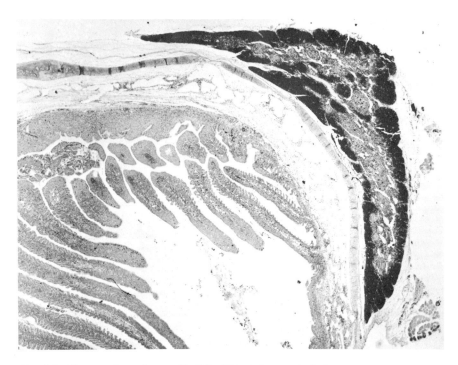

Fig. 4-6 Thymus of newborn guitarfish (*Rhinobatus productus*) which is located over the gills. The organ is well developed and encapsulated. Both cortex and medulla are present. Note the large numbers of well-developed lymphocytes in the cortex (Hematoxylin-eosin; × 10). Photograph courtesy R. A. Good.

These animals develop severe delayed hypersensitivity reactions following injections of BGG in complete Freund's adjuvant. Death usually results from the ultimate breakdown of epithelial integrity caused by the severe inflammatory reaction. The causes behind this uncontrolled progression of events have not been defined (28).

Sharks and rays have no difficulty in rejecting homografts. While autografts heal and remain in place indefinitely, homografts initially heal but are rejected 3 to 6 weeks later. The rejection is accompanied by a vigorous inflammatory reaction (28).

Immunoelectrophoresis of shark and ray sera reveals several gamma globulin fractions (30). Again no antibody activity has been demonstrated in the 7S gamma globulin. The antibody produced against *Brucella abortus* antigens is a 2-mercaptoethanol-sensitive 19S macroglobulin as demonstrated by sucrose density gradient centrifugation procedures (30).

The immune responses of elasmobranchs are summarized in Table 4-2.

Adaptive Immunity in Chondrostean Fish

The chondrostean fish (primitive bony fish of the order Chondrostei) first evolved during the lower Jurassic period about 160 million years ago. Living members of this class of vertebrates are the sturgeon and paddlefish, or spoonbill. These species, like the more primitive fish, have a persistent notochord. The skeleton of these animals, while partially bony, is largely cartilaginous. Chondrostean fish have neither scales nor teeth (22). The species studied most extensively is the paddlefish, *Polyodon spathula.*

Chondrostean Lymphoid Tissues

The thymus of the paddlefish is organized into definitive lobes and lobules, and Hassall's corpuscles are present throughout the tissue (Fig. 4-9). Whereas the thymus in the more primitive species discussed above persists throughout the life of the animal, the thymus in the paddlefish involutes

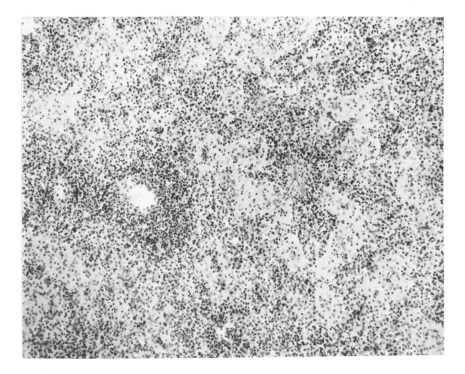

Fig. 4-7 Spleen of one-month-old guitarfish. Lymphoid foci are developing around small vessels, and a division between red and white pulp can be seen (Hematoxylin-eosin; × 250). From Good et al. (25) with permission.

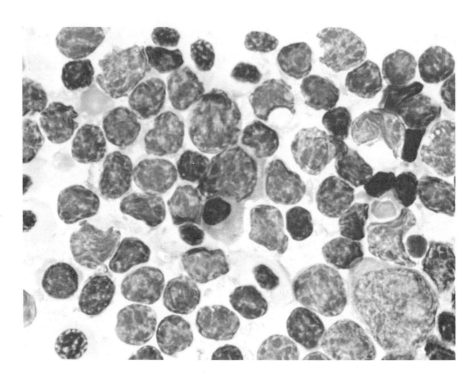

Fig. 4-8 Imprint of spleen of leopard shark (*Triakis semifasciata*) showing mature plasma cells (Wright-Giemsa; × 1000). Photograph courtesy R. A. Good.

TABLE 4-2
Adaptive Immunity in Elasmobranchs

Species	Lymphoid tissues	Immune responses	Serum globulins
Guitarfish and horned shark	1. Well-developed thymus	1. Variable to injected antigens Poor primary Good secondary	1. Several gamma types
	2. Involution of thymus in higher forms	2. Homograft rejection	2. Several alpha and beta types
	3. Spleen	3. Delayed allergy (severe)	
	4. Lymphocytic foci	4. Memory	
	5. Family of lymphocytes		
	6. No plasma cells in lower forms		
	7. Plasma cells in higher forms		

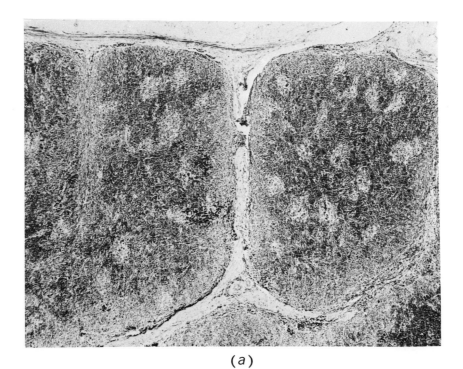

(*a*)

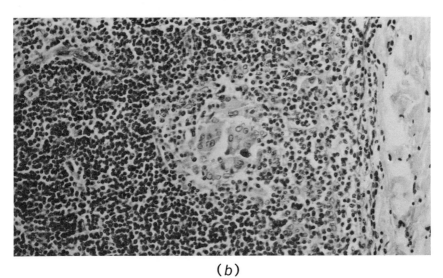

(*b*)

Fig. 4-9 (*a*) Paddlefish (*Polyodon spathula*) thymus showing division into lobes and lobules and primitive Hassall's corpuscles (Hematoxylin-eosin; × 25).
(*b*) Primitive Hassall's corpuscle from paddlefish thymus. Note the solidly packed thymocytes in the thymic cortex (Hematoxylin-eosin; × 400).

during adult life. The spleen is well developed, having both red and white pulp (Fig. 4-10). The white pulp is made up of dense collections of lymphocytes, and the red pulp contains numerous cells which appear to be morphologically similar to plasma cells. Hematopoietic tissue, both erythropoietic and lymphopoietic, is present over the base of the heart and extends down over both the atrium and the ventricle. This tissue has an organization which appears to be similar to that of mammalian bone marrow (Fig. 4-11). Cells of both the lymphocyte and plasma cell series can be found in all stages of development. While many lymphocytic foci are also found throughout the gut, plasma cells have only been observed in the spleen and pericardial hematopoietic tissue (26).

Chondrostean Immune Responses

Compared to the more primitive species, the paddlefish responds to a wide range of antigens (BSA, BGG, hemocyanin, T2 bacteriophage, and *Brucella abortus*) with a more vigorous response following both primary and secondary antigen exposures. Unlike the elasmobranch fishes, paddlefish do not develop a complete breakdown of skin following intramuscular injections of BGG in complete Freund's adjuvant but instead exhibit a much less severe reaction consisting of inflammation without integumental breakdown. During the secondary response to antigens a marked proliferation of plasma cells has been observed. Plasma cells may also be found in the infiltrate around the homograft site during the rejection process (28).

Chondrostean Serum Proteins

Immunoelectrophoresis of paddlefish serum has revealed several gamma globulins. However, the 7S fraction is still inactive immunologically. Antibody to *Brucella* has been demonstrated in the 19S fraction, but it is not sensitive to treatment with 2-mercaptoethanol (31). The cause of its resistance is not definitely known but probably is related to the tertiary and quaternary structure of the molecules. Our present knowledge of the immune responses among the chondrostean fishes is summarized in Table 4-3.

Adaptive Immunity in More Advanced Species

Immunity in Holostean and Teleostean Fish

The living forms of the holostean (e.g., gar, bowfin) and teleostean (e.g., trout, goldfish, bass) fish are the most advanced of the fishes. In both of these groups of fish there is a definitive thymus which involutes with

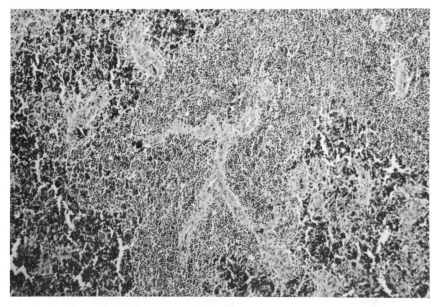

(a)

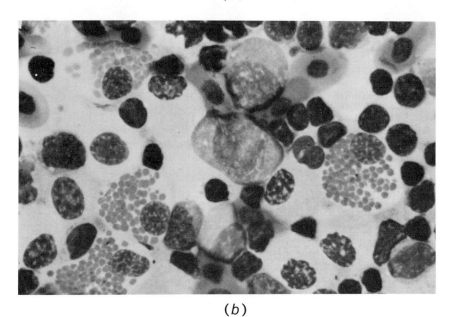

(b)

Fig. 4-10 (a) Spleen of paddlefish showing well-developed lymphoid tissues with division into red and white pulp (Hematoxylin-
eosin; × 100).
(b) Plasma cells, plasmablasts, and eosinophils in the paddlefish
spleen. (Wright-Giemsa; × 1000). Photographs courtesy R. A.
Good.

111

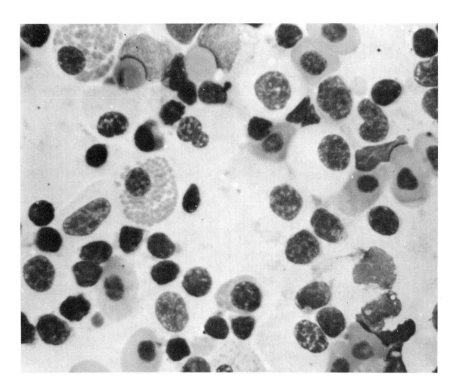

Fig. 4-11 Hematopoietic tissues resembling bone marrow found in the pericardial tissue of the paddlefish. Note the plasma cells and large eosinophils with coarse granules (Wright-Giemsa; × 1000). Photograph courtesy R. A. Good.

age. It was believed that some teleosts did not possess circulating gamma globulin. However, the use of sensitive immunoelectrophoretic techniques has revealed that these fish contain small amounts of circulating gamma globulins (23,32). These species also lack large numbers of plasma cells which can be correlated with the low levels of circulating gamma globulin. The deficiency in the Teleostei of both plasma cells and circulating gamma globulin may be due to low levels of antigenic stimulation. However, following injection with such antigens as rabbit red blood cells, freshwater teleosts produce detectable levels of immunoglobulin directed against this immunogen (33). An antibody activity attributable to the 7S fraction of gamma globulins occurs in these groups. For example, following antigenic stimulation, goldfish will initially produce 19S antibody, but if the water temperature is raised, a conversion to 7S antibody production occurs (34).

TABLE 4-3
Adaptive Immunity in Chondrostean Fishes

Species	Lymphoid tissues	Immune responses	Serum globulins
Paddlefish	1. Highly organized	1. Good to wide range of antigens	1. Several gamma types
	2. Well-developed spleen	2. Homograft rejection	2. Several alpha and beta types
	3. Family of lymphocytes	3. Delayed allergy	
	4. Many lymphocytic foci	4. Memory	
	5. Plasma cells in spleen and bone marrow	5. Plasma cell proliferation	

Immunity in Reptiles and Amphibians

Reptiles and amphibians have inhabited the earth since upper Devonian and lower Permian times. However, present living forms have evolved from the Cretaceous period of the Mesozoic era, through the Cenozoic era, to comparatively recent times. In both groups the thymus involutes with age. Primitive lymph nodes, made up of encapsulated lymphoid follicles, are present in a few amphibian species such as the marine toad. The center of these follicles contains relatively dense collections of lymphoid cells which become less dense toward the periphery (35). Some amphibians (e.g., mud puppy) have primitive tonsillar tissue consisting of lymphoid nodules in the sublingual region which are characterized by accumulations of small- and medium-sized lymphocytes. However, these nodules do not contain any lymphoepithelial organization as seen in true tonsils (25). The first true lymphoepithelial tonsils are found in the pharyngeal region of the alligator. Reptiles and amphibians are the lowest forms containing plasma cells in the lamina propria of the gut (25) (Fig. 4-12). The conversion of 19S to 7S antibody synthesis has been described in many species of amphibians and reptiles (34).

Immunity in Birds and Mammals

In addition to the thymus, birds apparently have a second central or primary lymphoid organ called the *bursa of Fabricius*. Anatomically the bursa is situated near the cloaca and apparently functions as a central lymphoid organ directing maturation of humoral antibody productivity,

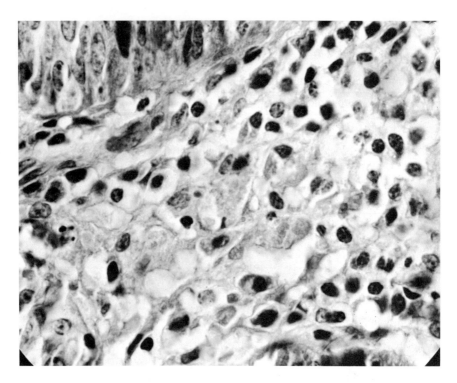

Fig. 4-12 Lamina propria of amphibian mud puppy (*Necturus maculosa*) gut with plasma cells (Hematoxylin-eosin; × 800). Photograph courtesy R. A. Good.

while the thymus of birds is responsible for maturation of cellular immunity. The thymus and bursa of the birds will be discussed in detail later. The phylogenetic origin of the bursa is not known. Both the rectal gland of the elasmobranchs and the anal sac of turtles have been suggested as evolutionary precursors of the bursa (25). The bursa present in very primitive birds persists throughout life, as does the thymus of the more primitive marine vertebrates. The bursa does involute with age in the more advanced avian species (25).

True lymph nodes first appear in mammals and are possibly dependent on tonsillar tissue for their development (25).

Summary

The major transitional points of the phylogenetic development of the immune system can be summarized as follows: First is the development in the hagfish of a lymphocyte-like cell capable of participation in chronic inflammatory responses, homograft rejection, and antibody formation. Next, beginning in the lamprey, the evolution of a primitive thymus and spleen coincides with the appearance of a family of lymphoid cells along with rather weak immunologic responses. These responses become stronger as the thymus becomes more highly developed. With the advent of the plasma cell system in the higher elasmobranchs and paddlefish comes much stronger immune responses along with the involution of the thymus with age. In reptiles the development of tonsils and tonsillar-dependent lymphoid tissue begins, while in birds is observed the development of the bursa of Fabricius and bursa-dependent lymphoid tissue. The first true lymph nodes appear in the mammals.

The chondrostean paddlefish may represent the end of the first line of evolution of the immune system. By this stage of development most of the immune responses seen in mammals have evolved to more or less efficient states. Perhaps the only response missing is the conversion of 19S to 7S antibody production. The adaptive immune response therefore is in a rather sophisticated stage of development in species which have been present on the earth for at least 170 million years. This is comparatively recent by geologic standards, as life has been present on the earth for at least 1 billion years. The innovation of tonsils, the bursa, and lymph nodes in the higher forms represents a second line of evolution and perhaps serves to make the immune system function more efficiently and diversely. Important in the evolution of the immune response is the ability of lymphoid cells to recognize and interpret structural differences among antigens and to respond to these discrete differences by the production of specific antibody.

ONTOGENESIS OF THE ADAPTIVE IMMUNE RESPONSE

The differentiation and maturation of the immune response during fetal and neonatal life take place gradually and pass through several phases. However, no immunologic responses can be elicited until a minimal maturation of lymphoid organs occurs. Indeed, the entire adaptive immune response, both phylogenetically and ontogenetically, appears to keep pace with the differentiation and maturation of the lymphoid organs.

Morphology of the Thymus and Bursa

The mammalian thymus is a paired organ which originates embryologically from the ventral portions of the third and fourth pharyngeal pouches and generally consists of two or more lobes on each side of the midline (36). The organ is encapsulated, and each lobe is made up of many lobules separated by septa of connective tissue (see Fig. 4-13). Each lobule is

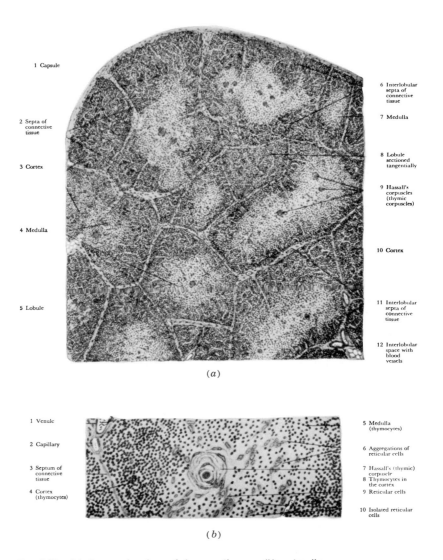

1 Capsule

2 Septa of connective tissue

3 Cortex

4 Medulla

5 Lobule

6 Interlobular septa of connective tissue

7 Medulla

8 Lobule sectioned tangentially

9 Hassall's corpuscles (thymic corpuscles)

10 Cortex

11 Interlobular septa of connective tissue

12 Interlobular space with blood vessels

(a)

1 Venule

2 Capillary

3 Septum of connective tissue

4 Cortex (thymocytes)

5 Medulla (thymocytes)

6 Aggregations of reticular cells

7 Hassall's (thymic) corpuscle
8 Thymocytes in the cortex
9 Reticular cells

10 Isolated reticular cells

(b)

Fig. 4-13 (a) Panoramic view of human thymus (Hematoxylin-eosin; × 40).
(b) Higher power illustrating finer structure. Note the architecture of the Hassall's corpuscle (Hematoxylin-eosin; × 250). From *An Atlas of Human Histology* (3d ed.) by M. S. H. Di Fiore. Lea and Febiger, Philadelphia, 1967, with permission.

divided into a cortex with dense collections of lymphoid cells and a medulla which contains more diffuse lymphoid tissue. Hassall's corpuscles, found in the medulla, are made up of laminated layers of epithelial cells. Reticular cells are scattered throughout the medulla (37,38). See Chap. 6.

Neither light nor electron microscopy has revealed the functional significances of either the thymus cortex or medulla. In addition, no function has been definitely attributed to the Hassall's corpuscles.

The bursa of Fabricius, a lymphoepithelial organ like the thymus, probably arises by differentiation of hindgut epithelium. The bursa is a saclike organ attached by a stalk to the proctodaeal region of the cloaca. The mucous membrane of the bursa is lined with pseudostratified epithelium. The inside wall contains several folds which, on microscopic observation, contain numerous lymphoid follicles. Each lymphoid follicle contains a central medullary portion and an outer cortical portion (Fig. 4-14). The cortex is separated from the medulla by a row of basal undifferentiated epithelial cells. The medulla primarily contains small lymphocytes, while the cortex contains compact masses of larger, more immature lymphocytes. Lymphopoiesis occurs in the bursa until late in its phase of involution following sexual maturity (39).

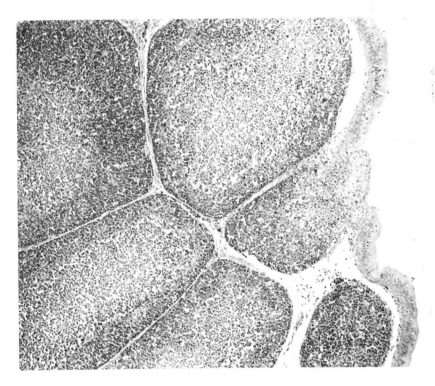

Fig. 4-14 Bursa of Fabricius of sixty-day-old chicken (Hematoxylin-eosin; × 100). Photograph courtesy R. A. Good.

Development and Role of the Thymus and Bursa of Fabricius

In most vertebrate species studied the thymus is the first lymphoid organ to develop. The fetal human thymus is well developed and lymphoid by the third gestational month (37). However, the fetal human spleen is not lymphopoietic until the fifth gestational month (40). Lymph nodes begin to develop during the first year of postnatal life, and this development continues until puberty. The mouse thymus is epithelial on day 12 of gestation, lymphopoietic on day 14 of gestation, and becomes primarily lymphoid by day 16 (41). Lymph nodes and spleen do not become lymphoid until after birth. The chicken thymus is epithelial on the ninth day of incubation and is lymphoid by the twelfth day. (Fig. 4-15). The bursa of Fabricius begins to form on day 12 and becomes lymphoid from days 15 through 18 (Figs. 4-16, 4-17) At the same time the spleen is entirely erythropoietic and myelopoietic; there is no follicular lymphoid tissue in the intestine nor are cutaneous lymphoid follicles present. These tissues become lymphoid during the last days of incubation and the first few days after hatching (42). A similar sequence of development is observed in the rabbit (43), dog (44), and opossum (45); that is, appearance of a lymphoid spleen, central lymph nodes, and finally peripheral lymph nodes. However, in the cat, lymphocytes appear in the lymph nodes before they appear in the thymus (46).

Ball and Auerbach (41) have suggested that the lymphoid cells of the thymus arise from the epithelium. Experimental evidence supporting this viewpoint has been obtained. Rudimentary epithelial thymuses taken from 12-day mouse embryos, when cultured in the presence of mesenchyme in vitro, will differentiate into a lymphoid organ. Differentiation will even occur when the epithelial tissue is separated from mesenchyme by a filter designed to prevent any exchange of cells between the two types of tissue (41). More recent experiments demonstrate the effect of the thymus on other potentially lymphoid tissues (47,48). So far mouse embryonic spleen has failed to become lymphoid when cultured alone in vitro. However, when embryonic spleen and embryonic thymus are cultured together, marked synergism occurs, with the development of a complex lymphoid organ system. The degree of lymphoid development in embryonic thymus alone is much less than when two organs are cultured together. A combination of embryonic marrow, thymus, and spleen has demonstrated additional interaction (48). Neither embryonic spleen nor bone marrow cultured separately or together will produce lymphocyte development. Some differentiation of granulopoietic elements occurs in the bone marrow, but growth soon ceases and the explant degenerates. On the other hand, when thymus is added to one or both of these organs, a

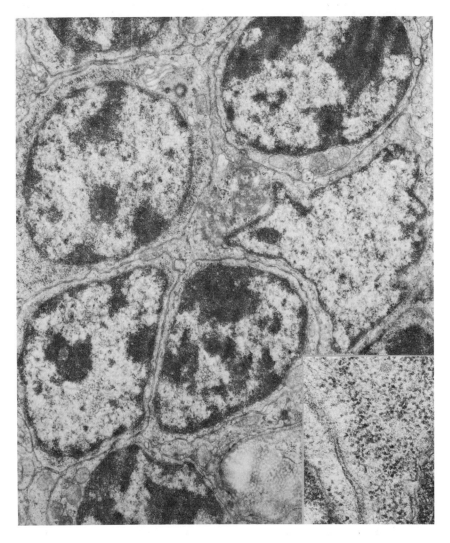

Fig. 4-15 Electron micrograph of lymphocytes from the thymus of a normal antigen-stimulated chicken (× 16,000). Insert shows the cytoplasm of a thymus lymphocyte (× 55,000). The ribosomal population and lack of polysome organization in these cells may be contrasted with the bursal lymphocyte shown in Fig. 4-16. Photograph courtesy R. A. Good.

marked lymphoid development occurs and the cultures continue to thrive for long periods. The ability of these differentiating organ systems to produce antibody following antigenic stimulation has not been reported. However, the pairing of neonatal mouse thymus and spleen in culture resulted in small amounts of antibody formation following stimulation with

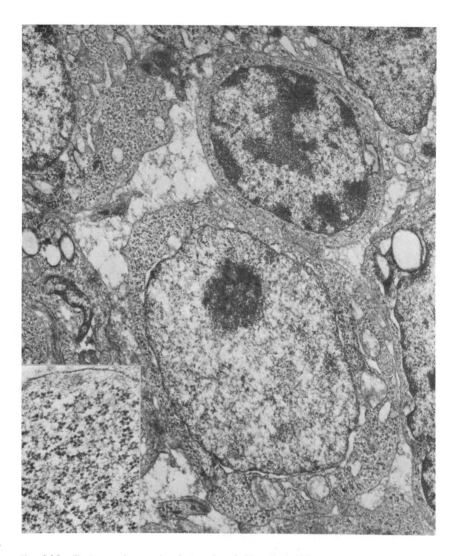

Fig. 4-16 Electron micrograph of two lymphoid cells within a follicle of the bursa of Fabricius (× 16,000). Insert shows the cytoplasm of a bursal lymphocyte. These cells contain a large population of ribosomal particles which are usually arranged in clusters or polysomes from four to six particles (× 55,000). This appearance may be contrasted with the ribosomal configuration of the thymic lymphocyte in Fig. 4-15. Photograph courtesy R. A. Good.

R17 bacteriophage, while neither organ cultured separately with the antigen produced detectable antibody (49).

Another view, experimentally supported, states that the first lymphocytes develop outside of the thymus and are later transported to it. Maximow (50) observed that primitive basophilic lymphoblasts have migrated into the endodermal epithelium of the third and fourth branchial pouches, from which the epithelial rudiment of the thymus is derived, before the rudiment actually begins to differentiate. Just where these precursor cells arise is unknown. Ackerman (46) has shown that in the embryonic cat, the lymph nodes become lymphoid a few days before any lymphoid cells can be found in the thymus. However, no wandering lymphoblasts were seen.

Recently Hoshino et al. (50a) have published electron microscope observations which depict lymphoblasts in the mesenchyme surrounding the third pharnygeal pouch (from which the thymus differentiates) of 11-day-old mouse embryos. If these observations are valid, some doubt is cast on the conclusions drawn by Ball and Auerbach (41) from their experimental results since these workers used thymus rudiments from 12-day-old mice during their investigation.

Only recently has the relationship of the thymus to immunocompetence been realized. Earlier experiments involving removal of the thymus and evaluation of its effects on immune competence have been unsuccessful for two reasons. First, the animals used were not young enough and secondly, the experiments were too short. Miller (51), who studied mouse leukemia, pioneered the studies of thymus function by observing that mice thymectomized at birth failed to become fully immunocompetent; in fact they were relatively incompetent. These mice were unable to reject skin homografts and responded at low levels to many injected antigens. However, some antigens such as hemocyanin, tetanus toxoid, and *Salmonella* flagella antigen elicited almost normal immune responses. These experiments have been extensively repeated and have been expanded to other species as well. Decreased immunologic responsiveness has been observed following neonatal thymectomy in the rabbit, rat, guinea pig, and chicken. The effects of thymectomy vary with the animal's age at the time of surgery. Further development of thymus-dependent tissues usually ceases and for a time remains at the level reached when the thymus is removed. However, such tissues degenerate with time.

Neonatal thymectomy in the mouse results in the depletion of small lymphocytes in the circulatory pool, lymphocytic fields of lymph nodes, and periarteriolar lymphocyte sheaths of the spleen (52). The deficiency of lymphocytes in the circulatory pool reaches over 90 percent of normal by four months of age. Thus these areas can be considered as being thymus-dependent. Lymphoid follicles and germinal centers have been found in young neonatally thymectomized mice but become less active with age and are often absent in older mice. In addition, plasma cells are not deficient and tend to accumulate in thymus-dependent areas in thymectomized mice older than six weeks (52). It is therefore conceivable that follicle cell production, germinal center formation, and plasma

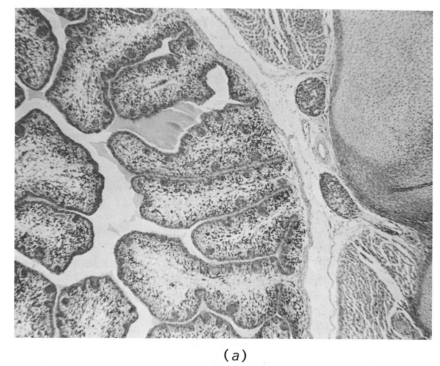

(a)

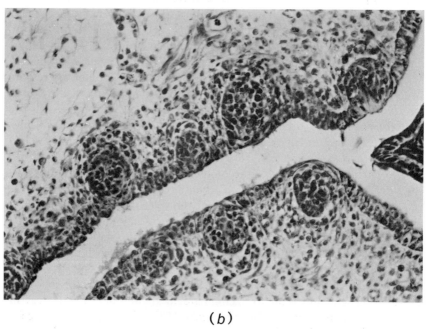

(b)

cell differentiation are not thymus-dependent processes. However, it is also possible that the thymus exerted some influence in these areas during the last few days of gestation. As will be discussed later, these areas of maturation in the chicken are bursa-dependent.

Results of thymectomy in adult mice, while not so profound as those in neonatal mice, are nevertheless functionally important (52). Again, there is a depletion of lymphocytes from thymus-dependent areas. Circulatory levels of small lymphocytes usually decline to 60 to 70 percent of normal levels, while spleen and lymph nodes decrease in mass in concurrence with decreased mitotic activity. Thymectomy followed by irradiation results in the partial failure of regeneration of the lymphoid system while regeneration will occur when the thymus is intact. Following both irradiation and thymectomy, these animals will not respond to a new antigen but will produce responses to antigens encountered before treatment.

Adult thymectomized mice appear to respond normally to injected antigens and reject allografts vigorously when these procedures are performed a few weeks after surgery. Some degree of impairment of the secondary response has been reported in some cases. However, antigenic stimulation following a period of rest after thymectomy elicits impaired responses, at least to BSA and SRBC (52). Such results indicate that the thymus exerts an influence on the development of the population of immunocompetent cells and that when this pool is depleted by senescence and death of its cells, defects in immune capacity of thymectomized animals manifest themselves.

Whether the activity of the thymus is due primarily to cellular or humoral factors has not been resolved. Neonatally thymectomized mice become competent following either injections of syngeneic thymus cell or tissue implants. However, these mice will also become competent following injections of syngeneic spleen, bone marrow, thoracic duct, and lymph node cells (52–55). In fact, spleen, lymph node, and thoracic duct cells are more efficient than thymus or bone marrow cells in reversing effects of neonatal thymectomy. On the other hand, thymus tissue placed in cell-tight diffusion chambers and implanted into the peritoneum will

Fig. 4-17 (a) Bursa of Fabricius of twelve-day-old chick embryo. Note the budding follicles which arise from the epithelium (Hematoxylin-eosin; × 25).
(b) Bursa of Fabricius of fourteen-day-old chick embryo showing intimate association of the follicles with the epithelium and beginning lymphoid development (Hematoxylin-eosin; × 400). Photographs courtesy R. A. Good.

restore competence to thymectomized mice, presumably by some humoral mechanism, e.g., a thymus hormone (56,57).

Thymus extracts have been prepared which will induce lymphopoieses when injected into normal recipients (58). In addition, some efforts to prepare a thymus extract capable of restoring immunological competence have been successful. A purified fraction derived from calf thymus (thymosin) has been shown to restore the graft-versus-host reaction in neonatally thymectomized mice (58a,58b).

More recently the interaction of thymus cells with bone marrow cells has been intensely investigated. Studies by Claman et al. (59) demonstrated that injections of both marrow and thymus cells into heavily irradiated mice followed by injection of antigen (SRBC) resulted in the production of more hemolysin-producing cells than either cell type injected alone. This was not just an additive effect; the increase was absolute. Using a cell transfer system with chromosome and isoantigenic markers in irradiated animals Davies et al. (60,61) reported that while the cells derived from a thymus graft divided rapidly following antigenic stimulation, the marrow cells were actually the immediate precursors of antibody-producing cells. Recent work by Mitchell and Miller (62) supports this conclusion and implies that thymus cells must react with antigen before their interaction with bone marrow cells can induce significant maturation of immunocompetent marrow cells. Furthermore, irradiation of the thymus cells or use of a thymus cell-free extract prevented this interaction suggesting that dividing cells are necessary. However, Osoba (62a) claims to have rapidly restored competence to lethally irradiated mice using a combination of injected syngeneic bone marrow cells and thymus cells placed in peritoneal cell-tight diffusion chambers, which again suggests a humoral thymus influence. Mitchell and Miller also found that thoracic duct lymphocytes could be substituted for thymus cells and concluded that thoracic duct lymphocytes and thymus lymphocytes may be derived from the same cell lineage. Experiments of this type indicate the probable presence of precursor cells in bone marrow which attain the capacity to differentiate into antibody-producing cells only after exposure to either thymus cells or thoracic duct lymphocytes. Mitchell and Miller (62) suggest that thoracic duct and thymus lymphocytes may be derived from the same cell lineage.

The above findings that thymectomy leads to a reduction of the population of small lymphocytes and to a deficiency of immunologic responsiveness, especially cell-mediated responses, although plasma cells, lymphoid follicles, germinal centers, and circulating immunoglobulin levels are less affected give support to the idea that two control systems may be operating. Cooper et al. (63) have proposed that the thymic system is primarily responsible for the development of the circulating small lymphocytes and for cellular immunity, while another central system is responsible for plasma cell and follicular cell development as well as for immunoglobulin synthesis and humoral antibodies.

The best evidence for a thymus-dependent system is found in the chicken through bursectomy and/or thymectomy experiments (63–66). Complete removal of the thymus in newborn chickens is a difficult procedure since small amounts of thymic tissue are often left behind. However, complete thymectomy causes a deficiency of small lymphocytes both in the blood and the spleen. Thymectomized birds do not normally reject allografts, nor do they exhibit normal delayed hypersensitivity responses. Some deficiency in thymectomized birds to produce humoral antibody exists but is incomplete. These birds possess the normal complement of germinal centers and plasma cells, as well as normal levels of immunoglobulins.

Bursectomized birds lack germinal center development and plasma cells and are markedly deficient in IgG and IgM immunoglobulins. Detectable antibody following antigenic stimulation in such animals is lacking, but these animals can reject homografts and participate in other delayed hypersensitivity reactions. Both bursectomy and thymectomy in a chicken result in a totally deficient immunologic system.

Thus, in the chicken there is a rather distinct separation of the functional components of the immune system. This model has led to the search for a comparable organ to the bursa in mammals. The tonsils and gut-associated lymphoid tissue have been suggested as possibilities (67). Appendectomy and thymectomy in the rabbit lead to more striking defects in antibody response than thymectomy alone (68,69). However, both plasma cell development and the ability to synthesize immunoglobulins remain. Rabbits which have had tonsils, sacculus rotundus, and Peyer's patches removed, in addition to the thymus and appendix, exhibit increased deficiencies, but these deficiencies are by no means complete (70).

In a recent study Perey et al. (71) have demonstrated that complete removal of the gut-associated lymphoepithelial tissues (Peyer's patches, sacculus rotundus, and appendix), when coupled with lethal x-radiation followed by reconstitution with rabbit fetal liver cells, will prevent the immunologic recovery of rabbits. These animals are unable to produce humoral antibody against killed *Brucella abortus* antigen. However, lethally irradiated, reconstituted animals in which the gut-associated lymphoepithelial tissue was left intact but the thymus or spleen was removed recovered the ability to produce humoral antibody to this antigen. These experiments suggest that rabbit intestinal lymphoepithelial tissues are responsible for the differentiation of those cells involved in producing specific antibody.

ONTOGENESIS OF GAMMA GLOBULIN FORMATION

Until recently it was believed that fetal and most neonatal animals were incapable of synthesizing gamma globulins and that any of these proteins present were of maternal origin. However, by using sensitive labeling methods, recent experiments have shown that immunoglobulin synthesis occurs in several mammalian species during fetal and neonatal life (72). In these experiments fetal lymphoid tissues, usually the spleen, were exposed to C^{14}-labeled amino acids in vitro and the incorporation of these amino acids into gamma globulins was measured. It must be emphasized that the animals used were not stimulated antigenically before the incubation period. Intrauterine immunization can induce a wider range of responses (73). For example, sheep immunized in utero as early as the ninetieth day of gestation will produce a spectrum of immunoglobulins, including IgM, gamma 1 and gamma 2 (IgG), and IgA. However, in the labeling experiments described above the unstimulated spleen tissue produced only IgM immunoglobulin.

In all species studied to date, the onset of immunoglobulin formation closely follows morphological differentiation of lymphoid organs. It is of interest that the onset of IgM synthesis precedes the onset of IgG synthesis. Such a sequence has been seen phylogenetically, as discussed previously, and is also true of adult animals. The development of the capacity to produce immunoglobulins does not render an organism fully immunocompetent. There appears to be a definite progression in time from noncompetence through partial competence to full immunocompetence. The fetal opossum, for example, will attain the capacity to form antibodies against the flagellar antigens of *Salmonella typhi* by the twentieth day after conception (eighth day of life in the pouch), at which time it has developed a lymphoid thymus and at least one lymph node. It is comparable to an 8-week human fetus or an 11-day rat fetus (74,75). Immunization with BGG, however, fails to elicit an immune response in these animals (76). Moreover, the antibody against *S. typhi* is primarily of the 19S type. The fetal lamb can produce antibody to bacteriophage ϕX174 following immunization as early as 38 to 40 days of gestation (73,77). At the same stage of development responses to other immunogens could not be elicited. At 66 days of gestation an antibody response can be obtained against ferritin. Homograft rejection can occur only after the eightieth day of gestation. Antibodies against crystalline egg albumin could not be obtained until the one hundred twenty-first day of gestation. Responses to some antigens, e.g., *Salmonella typhosa*, could not be obtained until after birth. Similar studies (73) with the rhesus monkey fetus have yielded similar results, implying that this progression of competence may occur in other mammalian species. That is, for any given species at any given time in its development the individual may respond to one immunogen but not to others. However, once immune competence is developed to such antigens as SRBC and bacteriophage ϕX174, the response to the immunogen is comparable to the response to the same immunogen in a fully immunocompetent animal (73,78,79). The sequential development of antigen recognition has been suggested to be due to the differentiation and maturation of the clones of antigen target cells (73). Clones responsive to different immunogens may arise at different times. The possibility also exists that the ability to process different immunogens before their exposure to target cells may develop at other times. However, no difference was seen in the rate of catabolism of ovalbumin in the fetal lamb during early gestation compared to late gestation (73). While these explanations are in keeping with current concepts of the genetic regulation of immunocompetence, the data obtained in the opossum suggest that some species differences may be present which require further investigation.

As has been described, immunoglobulin synthesis can occur in fetal and neonatal animals, but the level of synthesis usually remains quite low until some time following birth. This low level of synthesis can be ascribed to several causes, the most important of which are probably a combination of lack of full antigenic stimulation and repression of synthesis due to the presence of circulating maternal antibodies. The cause of spontaneous immunoglobulin synthesis in fetal animals is not clear, since at least two possibilities exist. First, the synthesis may represent normal functional differentiation of the lymphoid system and does not depend on antigenic stimulation. Secondly, the synthesis of these proteins may be a direct result of intrauterine antigenic stimulation.

A system of passive transfer of maternal antibody to the fetus has been evolved to protect the fetus before immunocompetence is attained (9). Antibody protein transfer occurs in various ways, depending on the species. In the chicken, β-globulins are transferred from the hen to the ovum before ovulation and via the yolk sac to the developing chick. In equine, porcine, caprine, and bovine genera, in which there is a highly developed placenta, the passive antibody transfer occurs via lactoglobulins present in the dam's colostrum. For a few days after birth the newborn animal is able to absorb these proteins via the intestinal tract. In rabbits and guinea pigs, the transfer is via the fetal yolk sac. Mice and rats utilize the fetal yolk sac as well as colostrum. In primates, transfer occurs solely by the placenta and begins early in gestation. The importance of colostrum in those animals which have highly developed placentas cannot be overemphasized; these animals, due to lack of antigenic stimulation in utero, are essentially agammaglobulinemic at the time of birth and as such are highly susceptible to the multitude of organisms in their surroundings.

While passive antibody provides protection to the fetal and infant animal there is some evidence that this antibody inhibits the initiation of native immune responses (80–83). Other experiments have shown that administration of serum containing antibody may also stop the production of antibody once the active immune process has been initiated (78). Part of this effect may be due to the inactivation of antigen, but these studies suggest the possibility of a feedback mechanism.

In the newborn human the gamma globulin level is usually equal to that of the mother. For a period from 3 to 10 weeks the level declines, then levels off and rises until adult levels are reached, between 1 and 4 years. The decline after birth can be ascribed to failure of synthesis, natural decay of the maternal protein, and an increase in blood volume due to growth of the infant (9).

The preceding section may be summarized by repeating the observations that maturation of the immune system occurs sequentially. However, in all cases there first must be a minimum morphological differentiation of the lymphoid cell systems. Regardless of the state of the lymphoid system at birth, maturation continues for some time after birth; in man this maturation lasts until puberty. Plasma cells are not usually present at birth but develop as a consequence of antigenic stimulation after birth. Indeed, the studies cited in this section indicate that part of the development of competence depends on the presence of adequate external stimuli. As a matter of fact, animals reared and maintained in a germ-free environment have very low levels of circulating immunoglobulins as well as very poor morphological development of secondary lymphoid organs (83–85). Prior to birth, sufficiently intense stimulation with certain immunogens will induce both plasma cell proliferation and antibody production in various mammalian species. However, the characteristic immune responses to antigenic stimulation are largely postnatal events due primarily to lack of exposure to antigens and the inhibiting influence of maternal antibody.

IMMUNOLOGIC DEFICIENCY STATES

In some instances human beings are born who do not possess or develop normal competence, or who may have normal competence but lose partial or total immunocompetence later in life. In lower animals these deficiency states probably also exist, but are usually not detected because of the inability of these animals to survive past the first few days or weeks of life. The cause of early postnatal death in lower animals is not usually studied as well as in the case of humans. Immunologic deficiency states in humans take three forms: (1) lack of the ability to synthesize circulating gamma globulin; (2) lack of the ability to produce cellular antibody; and (3) lack of the ability to produce both circulating and cell-bound antibody. These deficiency states can be either congenital or acquired.

Bruton-type Agammaglobulinemia

Bruton-type agammaglobulinemia is a sex-linked recessive disease affecting males (86). The disease is usually suspected only after the child has experienced several bouts of recurrent chronic septic illnesses, which usually begin to occur when the child is three to six months old. At this time maternal antibody reaches critically low levels (87). The disease is characterized by very low levels of circulating antibody (less than 25 mg per 100 ml), a severe deficiency of germinal centers in lymph nodes and spleen, and the virtual absence of plasma cells (88,89). Circulating small lymphocytes are not deficient and appear morphologically normal (88,90). The thymus is present and appears to be morphologically normal (87,88); however, pharyngeal lymphoid tissue is absent (91). The lymph nodes undergo hypertrophy following antigenic stimulation, and the proliferation of reticular cells and of some lymphocytes occurs, but no plasma cells are found (92). Patients with this disease show a remarkable ability to resist most viral infections (93). Since resistance to viral infections is associated with the small lymphocyte and cell-bound antibody, it would be expected that these individuals would exhibit normal delayed hypersensitivity reactions (88,91). However, homograft survival time is greatly prolonged, but rejection eventually occurs (94).

Thymus-dependent lymphoid tissue is relatively normal, and the delayed hypersensitivity functions attributed to thymus-dependent tissues are present. In this disease the defect is apparently a failure of development of the central lymphoid tissue responsible for plasma cell differentiation and humoral antibody synthesis. Treatment of the infections occurring as a result of this deficiency has been somewhat successful using a combination of antibiotic and gamma globulin therapy (95).

Mauer-Sorenson Agammaglobulinemia

The components of this disease include a normal gamma globulin concentration in the blood and apparently normal antibody production following antigenic stimulation. The characteristics of this disease have recently been reported in detail (88). The prime deficiency is a decrease in the absolute count of small lymphocytes, while the overall lymphocyte count is almost normal; that is, only 6 percent of the total lymphocytes are small lymphocytes compared to their normal preponderance. The plasma cell system is not visibly affected. These patients do not exhibit delayed hypersensitivity reactions, nor can they reject homografts. Diagnosis of this disease is often made following smallpox vaccination when the vaccinia lesion fails to heal and progression of the lesion occurs locally, with new lesions developing throughout the body. Resistance to viral disease rests largely with the delayed hypersensitivity system. The thymus of individuals afflicted with this disease is quite underdeveloped and depleted of both lymphoid elements and Hassall's corpuscles, and the lymph nodes consist largely of stromal elements. The disease occurs in both sexes and is attributable to a defect in thymus differentiation and lack of subsequent development of thymus dependent lymphoid tissues (88).

The characteristics of the two foregoing deficiency states give support to the theory that the delayed hypersensitivity and the immunoglobulin production systems can be separated in man as well as in the chicken. That is, the thymus is apparently responsible for the development of delayed hypersensitivity capacities while some other tissue, perhaps the gut-associated lymphoid nodules, is responsible for the maturation of immunoglobulin synthesizing abilities.

Swiss-type Agammaglobulinemia

Both humoral and cellular mediated antibody reactions are deficient in this disease. The disease is transmitted as an autosomal recessive and as such affects either sex; however, in some families only males are affected (90,91,96,97). Both the plasma cell series and lymphocyte series of cells are depleted (91,97). Circulating gamma globulin levels are less than 25 mg/100 ml (91). Since both cell series are deficient, persons with this disease are highly susceptible to both viral and septic infections. Smallpox vaccination is invariably fatal (98,99). Pathological findings include aplastic thymus, spleen, and lymph nodes and absence of tonsils (91,97). The thymus is not organized into cortical and medullary areas, nor are Hassall's corpuscles present. The most common thymus cell type found is a large primitive epithelial cell. In some cases the thymus rudiment is found totally undeveloped in its embryonic position in the neck (87,88, 96). Unlike the Bruton-type agammaglobulinemia, this form is generally fatal. Once recurrent illness sets in during the first year of life, the course of the disease is quite malignant, usually resulting in death by the end of the second year of life. All forms of treatment tried to date have been unsuccessful. Gamma globulin and antibiotic therapy have proven fruitless (96). Thymus grafts from healthy donors have also been tried without success (97). The graft is not rejected but except for a slight rise in lymphocyte levels no other significant effects have been observed. The total lack of development of lymphoid elements is obviously responsible for the complete immunoincompetence of these patients.

Acquired Agammaglobulinemia

Primary Acquired Agammaglobulinemia

Primary acquired agammaglobulinemias are usually due to either a late expression of genetic deficiency or to defects occurring in the thymus, such as thymoma (90,100,101). The onset of the disease, generally occurring between thirty to fifty years of age, is defined by persistent recurring respiratory tract infections. Blood levels of gamma globulin are usually at low levels but most often are not so low as those in congenital forms of the disease. A deficiency of plasma cells is seen in the bone marrow and lymph nodes; lymph nodes often lack germinal centers (91). Gamma globulin therapy along with antibiotics can usually control the condition.

Secondary Acquired Agammaglobulinemia

In addition to genetic and thymus defects, agammaglobulinemia can be acquired as a result of other diseases such as malignancies of the reticulo-endothelial system and protein-depleting diseases such as the nephrotic syndrome (90,91,102,103). Where the primary disease can be successfully treated, gamma globulin levels will eventually return to normal. However, where malignancy is present and not controlled, supplementary gamma globulin therapy must be given. Drugs used in treating malignant diseases will also severely depress normal immunologic functions as well as control the malignancy, and again gamma globulin therapy is often useful.

Dysgammaglobulinemias

Dysgammaglobulinemia represents a deficiency in one or two types of gamma globulins while other types are present in normal or elevated quantities. These deficiencies can be either congenital or acquired and are usually characterized by the patient's increased susceptibility to infection (89,104). In congenital cases thymus organization is often abnormal (87). Treatment with whole gamma globulin often helps to control this disease.

REFERENCES

1. Pollara, B., Hakin, C. M., and Condie, R. M.: *Federation Proc.*, **24**:504, 1965.
2. Huff, C. G.: *Physiol. Rev.*, **20**:68, 1940.

3. Bang, F. B.: *Federation Proc.*, **26**:1680, 1967.
4. Cooper, E. L.: *Amer. Zool.*, **5**:254, 1965.
5. Cooper, E. L.: *Sobretiro de Acta Medica*, **2**:1, 1966.
6. Cooper, E. L.: *Abstr. Premier Congr. Int. Soc. Transplant.* Paris, June, 1967.
7. Krafka, J.: *Amer. J. Hyg.*, **10**:261, 1929.
8. Ramsdell, S. G.: *J. Immunol.*, **13**:385, 1927.
9. Good, R. A., and Papermaster, B. W.: *Advan. Immunol.*, **4**:1, 1964.
10. Stephens, J. M.: *Canad. J. Microbiol.*, **5**:203, 1959.
11. Seaman, G. R., and Robert, N. L.: *Science*, **161**:1359, 1968.
12. Phillips, J. H., *Ann. N.Y. Acad. Sci.*, **90**:760, 1960.
13. Phillips, J. H., and Yardley, B. J.: *Nature (London)*, **188**:728, 1960.
14. Tripp, M. R.: *J. Invertebr. Pathol.*, **8**:478, 1966.
15. Stephens, J. M.: *Canad. J. Microbiol.*, **8**:491, 1962.
16. Jakowska, S., and Nigrelli, R. F.: *Ann. N.Y. Acad. Sci.*, **90**:913, 1960.
17. Cushing, J. E.: *Federation Proc.*, **26**:1666, 1967.
18. Feng, S. Y.: *Federation Proc.*, **26**:1685, 1967.
19. Briggs, J. D.: *J. Exp. Zool.*, **138**:155, 1958.
20. Zernoff, V.: *Ann. Inst. Pasteur (Paris)*, **46**:565, 1931.
21. Stephens, J. M., and Marshall, J. H.: *Canad. J. Microbiol.*, **8**:719, 1962.
22. Romer, A. S.: "The Vertebrate Body," 3d ed., W. B. Saunders Company, Philadelphia, 1962.
23. Papermaster, B. W., Condie, R. M., Finstad, J., and Good, R. A.: *J. Exp. Med.*, **119**:105, 1964.
24. Hildemann, W. H., and Thoenes, G. H.: *Transplantation*, **7**:506, 1969.
25. Good, R. A., Finstad, J., Pollara, B., and Gabrielsen, A. E.: in "Phylogeny of Immunity," R. T. Smith, P. A. Miescher, and R. A. Good (eds.), University of Florida Press, Gainesville, 1966.
26. Finstad, J., and Fichtelius, K. E.: *Federation Proc.*, **24**:491, 1965.
27. Papermaster, B. W., Condie, R. M., and Good, R. A.: *Nature (London)*, **196**:355, 1962.
28. Finstad, J., and Good, R. A.: in "Phylogeny of Immunity," R. T. Smith, P. A. Miescher, and R. A. Good (eds.), University of Florida Press, Gainesville, 1966.
29. Marchalonis, J. J., and Edelman, G. M.: *J. Exp. Med.*, **127**:891, 1968.
30. Pollara, B., Finstad, J., and Good, R. A.: in "Phylogeny of Immunity," R. T. Smith, P. A. Miescher, and R. A. Good (eds.), University of Florida, Gainesville, 1966.
31. Fish, L. A., Pollara, B., and Good, R. A.: in "Phylogeny of Immunity," R. T. Smith, P. A. Miescher, and R. A. Good (eds.), University of Florida Press, Gainesville, 1966.
32. Sorvachev, K. F., Zadvorochnov, S. F., and Isayev, F. A.: *Biokhimiya*, **27**:202, 1961.
33. Hodgins, H. O., Ridgway, G. J., and Utter, F. M.: *Nature (London)*, **208**:1106, 1965.
34. Uhr, J. W., Finkelstein, M. S., and Franklin, E. C.: *Proc. Soc. Exp. Biol. Med.*, **111**:13, 1962.

35. Kent, S. P., Evans, E. E., and Attleberger, M. H.: *Federation Proc.*, **23**:189, 1964.
36. Patten, B. M.: "Embryology of the Pig", 3d ed., McGraw-Hill, New York, 1948.
37. Hammar, J. A.: *Endocrinology*, **5**:731, 1921.
38. Smith, C.: in "The Thymus in Immunobiology," R. A. Good and A. E. Gabrielsen (eds.), Harper & Row, New York, 1964.
39. Ackerman, G. A., and Knouff, R. A.: in "The Thymus in Immunobiology," R. A. Good and A. E. Gabrielsen (eds.), Harper & Row, New York, 1964.
40. Knoll, W.: Z. *Mikrosk. Anat. Forsch.*, **18**:199, 1929.
41. Ball, W. D., and Auerbach, R.: *Exp. Cell Res.*, **20**:245, 1960.
42. Papermaster, B. W., and Good, R. A.: *Nature (London)*, **196**:838, 1962.
43. Archer, O. K., Papermaster, B. W., and Good, R. A.: in "The Thymus in Immunobiology," R. A. Good and A. E. Gabrielsen (eds.), Harper & Row, New York, 1964.
44. Kelly, W. D.: *Federation Proc.*, **22**:600, 1963.
45. Block, M.: *Ergeb. Anat. Entwicklungsgesch.*, **37**:237, 1964.
46. Ackerman, G. A.: *Anat. Rec.*, **158**:387, 1967.
47. Auerbach, R.: in "Symposium on Organ Culture," Nat. Cancer Inst. Monograph 11, 1963.
48. Auerbach, R.: in "The Thymus: Its Experimental and Clinical Studies," Ciba Foundation Symposium, Little, Brown and Company, Boston, 1966.
49. Saunders, G. C., and King, D. W.: *Science*, **151**:1390, 1966.
50. Maximow, A.: *Arch. Mikroskop. Anat.*, **74**:525, 1909.
50a. Hoshino, T., Takada, M., Abe, K., and Ito, T.: *Anat. Rec.*, **164**:47, 1969.
51. Miller, J. F. A. P.: *Proc. Roy. Soc. (London), Ser.* **B 156**:415, 1962.
52. Miller, J. F. A. P., and Osoba, D.: *Physiol. Rev.*, **47**:437, 1967.
53. Miller, J. F. A. P.: *Lancet*, **I**:43, 1963.
54. Parrott, D. M. V., and East, J.: in "The Thymus in Immunobiology," R. A. Good and A. E. Gabrielsen (eds.), Harper & Row, New York, 1964.
55. Dalmasso, A. P., Martinez, C., Sjodin, K., and Good, R. A.: *J. Exp. Med.*, **118**:1089, 1963.
56. Osoba, D., and Miller, J. F. A. P.: *J. Exp. Med.*, **119**:177, 1964.
57. Levey, R. H., Trainin, N., and Law, L. W.: *J. Nat. Cancer Inst.*, **31**:199, 1963.
58. Metcalf, D.: *Brit. J. Cancer*, **10**:31, 1956.
58a. Goldstein, A. L., Slater, F. D., and White, A.: *Proc. Nat. Acad. Sci. U.S.*, **56**:1010, 1966.
58b. Law, L. W., Goldstein, A. L., and White, A.: *Nature (London)*, **219**:1391, 1968.
59. Claman, H. N., Chaperon, E. A., and Triplett, R. F.: *J. Immunol.*, **97**:828, 1966.

60. Davies, A. J. S., Leuchars, E., Wallis, V., and Koller, P. C.: *Transplantation*, **4**:438, 1966.
61. Davies, A. J. S., Leuchars, E., Wallis, V., Marchant, R., and Elliott, E. V.: *Transplantation*, **5**:222, 1967.
62. Mitchell, G. F., and Miller, J. F. A. P.: *Proc. Nat. Acad. Sci. U.S.*, **59**:296, 1968.
62a. Osoba, D.: *Proc. Soc. Exp. Biol. Med.*, **127**:418, 1968.
63. Cooper, M. D., Gabrielsen, A. E., and Good, R. A.: in "Ontogeny of Immunity," R. T. Smith, R. A. Good, and P. A. Miescher (eds.), University of Florida Press, Gainesville, 1967.
64. Glick, B., Chang, T. S., and Jaap, R. G.: *Poult. Sci.*, **35**:224, 1956.
65. Cooper, M. D., Peterson, R. D. A., and Good, R. A.: *Nature (London)*, **205**:143, 1965.
66. Cooper, M. D., Peterson, R. D. A., South, M. A., and Good, R. A.: *J. Exp. Med.*, **123**:75, 1966.
67. Cooper, M. D., Peterson, R. D. A., and Good, R. A.: in "Phylogeny of Immunity," R. T. Smith, P. A. Miescher, and R. A. Good (eds.), University of Florida Press, Gainesville, 1966.
68. Archer, O. K., Sutherland, D. E. R., and Good, R. A.: *Nature (London)*, **200**:337, 1963.
69. Archer, O. K., Sutherland, D. E. R., and Good, R. A.: *Lab. Invest.*, **13**:259, 1964.
70. Cooper, M. D., Perey, D. Y., McKneally, M. F., Gabrielsen, A. E., Sutherland, D. E. R., and Good, R. A.: *Lancet*, **I**:1388, 1966.
71. Perey, D. Y. E., Cooper, M. D., and Good, R. A.: *Science*, **161**:265, 1968.
72. Thorbecke, G. J., and van Furth, R.: in "Ontogeny of Immunity," R. T. Smith, R. A. Good, and P. A. Miescher (eds.), University of Florida Press, Gainesville, 1967.
73. Silverstein, A. M., Parshall, C. J., and Prendergast, R. A.: in "Ontogeny of Immunity," R. T. Smith, R. A. Good, and P. A. Miescher (eds.), University of Florida Press, Gainesville, 1967.
74. La Via, M. F., Rowlands, D. T., Jr., and Block, M.: *Science*, **140**:1219, 1963.
75. Rowlands, D. T., Jr., La Via, M. F., and Block, M. H.: *J. Immunol.*, **93**:157, 1963.
76. La Via, M. F.: Unpublished observations.
77. Silverstein A. M., Uhr, J. W., Kramer, K. L., and Lukes, R. J.: *J. Exp. Med.*, **117**:799, 1963.
78. Silverstein, A. M., Parshall, C. J., and Uhr, J. W.: *Science*, **154**:1675, 1966.
79. Saunders, G. C.: In preparation.
80. Uhr, J. W., and Baumann, J. B.: *J. Exp. Med.*, **113**:935, 1961.
81. Osborn, J. J., Dancis, J., and Julia, J. F.: *Pediatrics*, **10**:328, 1952.
82. Perkins, F. T., Yetts, R., and Gaisford W.: *Brit. Med. J.*, **I**:1083, 1959.

83. Thorbecke, G. J., Gordon, H. A., Wostman, B., Wagner, M., and Reyniers, J. A.: *J. Infect. Dis.*, **101**:237, 1957.
84. Wostman, B. S.: *Ann. N.Y. Acad. Sci.*, **78**:254, 1959.
85. Gustafsson, B. E., and Laurell, C. B.: *J. Exp. Med.*, **110**:675, 1959.
86. Bruton, O. C.: *Pediatrics*, **9**:722, 1952.
87. Peterson, R. D. A., Good, R. A., and Gabrielsen, A. E.: *Postgrad. Med.*, **36**:505, 1964.
88. Fulginiti, V. A., Pearlman, D. S., Reiquam, C. W., Claman, H. N., Hathaway, W. E., Blackburn, W. R., Githens, J. H., and Kempe, C. H.: *Lancet*, **II**:5, 1966.
89. Thomas, O. C., and McGovern, J. P.: *Southern Med. J.*, **57**:498, 1964.
90. Rosen, F. S., and Janeway, C. A.: *New Engl. J. Med.*, **275**:769, 1966.
91. Peterson, R. D. A., Cooper, M. D., and Good, R. A.: *Amer. J. Med.*, **38**:579, 1965.
92. Good, R. A.: *J. Lab. Clin. Med.*, **46**:167, 1955.
93. White, C. M.: *Lancet*, **I**:969, 1963.
94. Schubert, W. K., Jowler, R., and Martin, L. W.: *Transplant. Bull.*, **26**:125, 1960.
95. Wallenborn, P. A.: *Laryngoscope*, **70**:1, 1960.
96. Gitlin, D., and Craig, J. M.: *Pediatrics*, **32**:517, 1963.
97. Hitzig, W. H., Kay, H. E. M., and Cottier, H.: *Lancet*, **II**:151, 1965.
98. Flewett, T. H., and Ker, F. L.: *J. Clin. Pathol.*, **16**:271, 1963.
99. Jarkowski, T. L., Mohagheghi, H. A., and Nolting, W. S., *Clin. Pediat.*, **2**:332, 1963.
100. Wollheim, F.: *Lancet*, **I**:316, 1961.
101. Fudenberg, H. H., and Hirschhorn, K.: *Med. Clinics N. Amer.*, **49**:1533, 1965.
102. Martin, N. H., and Squire, J. R.: *Proc. Roy. Soc. Med.*, **57**:749, 1964.
103. Gitlin, D., Gross, P. A. M., and Janeway, C. A.: *New Engl. J. Med.*, **260**:72, 1959.
104. Huntley, C. C., Lafferty, J. W., and Lyerly, A.: *Pediatrics*, **32**:407, 1963.

5
Antibody Induction and Production

The chapter on the nature of antigenicity has presented some of the current knowledge concerning antigens and their structure. It is apparent that antigens are usually fairly large, complex molecules and that in such large structures more than one antigenic determinant is present. The antigenic determinant usually consists of only a small portion of the molecule. Small molecules, called *haptens*, are also capable of exercising an antigenic effect. It is apparent that any discussion of antigen without a concomitant discussion of its biologic effects would be meaningless, since the main effect of antigens is to induce antibody production. Therefore this chapter will examine some of the ways in which antigen might induce an immune response.

In what way do antigenic determinants on an antigen molecule interact with the immunologically competent cell (antigen target cell) to stimulate the production of a specific antibody? This is the basic question to be answered. It is apparent that several possibilities exist. The simplest way would be that the antigen enters the cell, interacts with its protein-

136

synthesizing mechanism (DNA, mRNA, polyribosomes), and stimulates it to produce a specific antibody. Another possibility is that antigen may interact with the outer surface of the immunocompetent cell and through some membrane phenomenon, the nature of which is not well known, induce this cell to start antibody production. Another way may be that antigen is taken up by a cell which processes it and then releases a product capable of inducing the antigen target cell to produce antibody; this product may be part of the antigen, a preexisting inducer which is now liberated, a newly synthesized inducer, or a combination of two or more of these. The final possibility is that antigen interacts with preexisting antibody present in extremely minute amounts, thus removing a repressor of further synthesis of antibody. In this chapter the present status of the knowledge of antigen uptake and processing mechanisms will be discussed to determine which one of these possibilities is most likely to occur.

ANTIGEN METABOLISM

Metabolic Fate of Antigen

Antibody does not appear immediately in the circulation following exposure of the animal to antigen, nor does the animal become at once immune. Instead, a latent period occurs in which most of the antigenic material is rapidly catabolized before the ensuing antibody response. The disappearance of antigen from the circulating system during this latent period is readily followed by using I^{131}-labeled antigens, as was done by Dixon (1,2) and Weigle (3). They followed the disappearance rates of iodinated rabbit gamma globulin, bovine gamma globulin, and bovine serum albumin in rabbits following intravenous injections of these antigens. The homologous rabbit γ-globulin equilibrated between the intravascular and extravascular compartments of the plasma protein pool in 2 days (equilibrium phase) and then was catabolized at a logarithmic rate characteristic of the antigen and the species (Fig. 5-1). The antigenic proteins BGG and BSA undergo similar equilibrations, indicating that they have free access to the same tissues and fluid compartments as do homologous proteins. After equilibration the antigens are catabolized at a logarithmic rate prior to the production of significant amounts of antibody (nonimmune catabolism). With the onset of antibody production, the fourth day after injection of BGG and the eighth day after BSA, the antigens are rapidly catabolized and disappear from the circulation (immune catabolism), after which free antibody appears in the circulation. The rate of elimination during this phase varies from species to species with a given antigen and from antigen

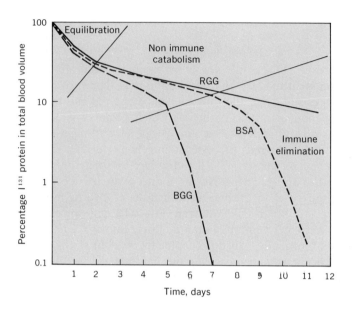

Fig. 5-1 Rates of disappearance of I[131] proteins from the blood of rabbits. From Dixon (2) with permission.

to antigen within any given species (Table 5-1). For example, the half-life of the rate of elimination of BSA is 4.1 days in the rabbit, 2.3 days in the guinea pig, and 1.5 days in the mouse. Also, in the guinea pig, the half-life of the rate of elimination of rabbit γ-globulin is 5.1 days whereas it is 1.8 days for bovine γ-globulin.

It has been shown that antigens combine with antibody as it is formed and the resulting soluble complexes are then taken out of circulation and rapidly catabolized. Using ammonium sulfate precipitation techniques, Dixon (1) was able to show that the amount of antigen bound to antibody increases sharply, and in the final stages of elimination, virtually all of the circulating antigen is bound (Fig. 5-2). Active cellular sensitization does not appear to play an essential role in the immune elimination of antigen from the circulation, since actively and passively sensitized rabbits with comparable levels of circulating antibody eliminated and degraded antigen at comparable rates. The availability of antibody capable of forming suitable complexes with the circulating antigen seems to be the essential element in immune elimination of antigen. Circulating antigen or antigen-antibody complexes have not been observed in the circulating system following the appearance of free antibody.

Immune elimination of labeled antigens can be used to detect the presence of trace amounts of antibody in passively immunized animals, animals injected with labeled antigen-antibody complexes, and presumably,

TABLE 5-1
Half-lives of Homologous and Heterologous Serum
Proteins

Species	Protein †	Average half-life, in days
Guinea pig	GPGG(P)	5.4 ± 0.3
	GPGG	5.4 ± 0.9
	GPSA(P)	2.8 ± 0.2
	GPSA	2.6 ± 0.2
	RGG(P)	5.1 ± 0.2
	RGG(A)	4.8 ± 0.4
	RGG	4.5 − 4.7
	BGG(A)	1.8 ± 0.1
	HGG(L)	1.9 ± 0.2
	RSA(P)	2.3 ± 0.1
	RSA(A)	2.2 ± 0.1
	BSA(P)	2.3 ± 0.1
Rat	Rat SA	1.9 − 2.2
	Rat GG	5.5 ± 0.6
	RGG(P)	6.7 ± 0.7
	BGG	3.0
	RSA(P)	1.1 ± 0.1
	BSA(P)	1.3 ± 0.1
Rabbit	RGG(A)	4.6 ± 0.8
	RGG	5.7 ± 1.2
	RSA(A)	5.7 ± 0.3
	BGG(A)	2.2 ± 0.3
	HGG(L)	3.0 ± 0.4
	GPG(P)	1.6 ± 0.3
	HSA(A)	4.1 ± 0.4
	BSA(A)	4.3 ± 0.6
Mouse	Mouse GG	1.9
	Mouse SA	1.2
	RGG	5.3 ± 0.2
	RGG	5.1
	BGG(A)	1.5
	HSA(L)	1.5 ± 0.1

† BSA = bovine serum albumin, BGG = bovine gamma globulin, HSA = human serum albumin, HGG = human gamma globulin, RSA = rabbit serum albumin, RGG = rabbit gamma globulin, GPSA = guinea pig serum albumin, GPGG = guinea pig gamma globulin, GPG = guinea pig globulin; (A) = Armour and Co., (P) = Pentex, Inc., (L) = Lederle Laboratories.
SOURCE: Adapted from Weigle (3) with permission.

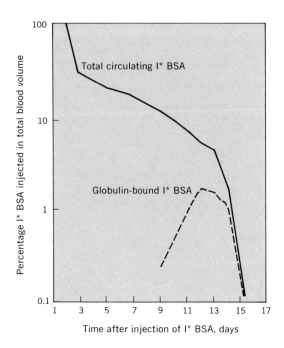

Fig. 5-2 Immune elimination of antigen during a primary immune response. From Dixon (2) with permission.

actively sensitized animals. The level of antibody which can be detected by the immune elimination technique is limited by the smallest amount of labeled antigen that can be traced in vivo, which is determined by the specific activity of the antigen. This is limited by the amount of label which can be conjugated to protein without denaturation. Using this technique Patterson et al. (4) have detected immune elimination in passively sensitized rabbits in which the antibody levels were as low as 0.0033 μg antibody N per ml of plasma.

Antigen Distribution at the Organ Level

It is apparent from early in vivo work on antigen distribution that particulate antigens (in this case *Salmonella typhi*), when given intravenously, are phagocytosed and distributed throughout the organism (5). During the first few hours following injection, the spleen contained the highest concentration of antigen. By 24 hours, however, the amount of antigen present in this organ, as well as in the liver, was very small. Excretion of antigen by-products in the urine increased rapidly so that by 48 hours about 80 percent of the antigen was excreted. Ada et al. (6) subsequently

140

examined the pattern of localization of S. *typhi* flagella in the rat after injection in the footpad. Although their data did not include findings during the early hours after injection, it was apparent that the pattern of localization of this antigen was similar to that observed in rats injected intravenously. With the administration of soluble antigens, these authors found that 48 hours after injection only a small amount of the injected dose was still retained. However, a notable difference occurred between the localization of particulate and soluble antigens, the latter being dependent upon the route of injection of antigen. While intravenous injection led to a high concentration of antigen in the spleen with little antigen present in lymph nodes, footpad administration was followed by heavy deposition in the draining lymph node with little antigen in the spleen.

Antigen clearance from the bloodstream, in the case of intravenous administration, appears to be similar for both particulate and soluble antigens (5,7). Intravenously injected antigens appear to localize quickly in organs where lymphoreticular cells are abundant and are phagocytosed by these cells and deposited in these organs (5). Therefore, the distribution is usually heavy in the liver, spleen, bone marrow, kidney, and lungs, with small amounts in lymph nodes, since by the time antigen reaches the nodes much has been removed from the bloodstream (Fig. 5-3). Depositions of antigen in the lung and kidney occur because of mechanical trapping. The subcutaneous administration of antigen on the contrary will send most of the antigen to be deposited in the regional lymph nodes, and only a small amount will escape and move beyond this first station (6). A brief review of the structure of lymphoid organs will help in understanding antigen localization. These organs are described more fully in Chap. 6. The lymphoid organs can be divided generally into a cortical and a medullary area (8). There is some difference between the spleen and the other lymphoid organs, since the spleen is made up of typical lymphoid areas, the white pulp, surrounded by atypical lymphoid parts, the red pulp (Fig. 5-4). The typical lymphoid portion is arranged in follicles much as the ones seen in lymph node cortex. The follicle is surrounded by a mantle of medium and large lymphocytes and then by areas bounded by the splenic trabeculae which contain lymphoid and myeloid series elements. Very important in antigen metabolism is the perifollicular sinus which surrounds the white pulp follicles.

The lymph nodes are usually subdivided into several compartments by the trabeculae which delve into the organ from the capsule (Fig. 5-5). Each portion contains a cortical area which is made up of small tightly packed lymphocytes and a medullary area surrounded by the cortical area consisting of less loosely packed lymphocytes with many medium and large

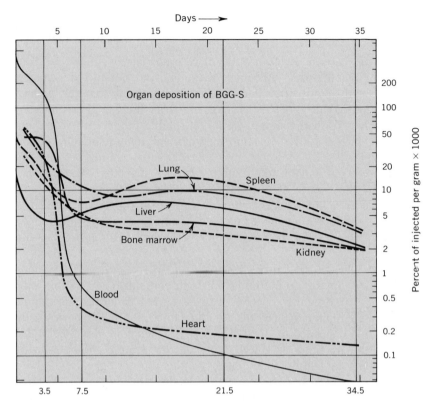

Fig. 5-3 Organ distribution of BGG labeled by traces of diazotized S[35]-sulfanilic acid in rabbits following intravenous injection. From Haurowitz (43) with permission.

lymphocytes. The medullary area is crisscrossed by sinusoids; a perifollicular sinus is also found in the lymph node (8).

Antigen Distribution at the Cell Level

It has been established that a portion of the injected antigen is transported to lymphoid organs and taken up by phagocytosis or pinocytosis (5,6). Whether the antigenic association with phagocytic cells is essential or whether this merely represents a phenomenon which has nothing to do with the production of antibodies is still a debated question.

Much has been learned about antigen distribution in vivo, by using soluble and particulate, naturally occurring, and chemically synthesized antigens. The pattern which has emerged is that the immunogenic portion of antigens, when injected for the first time, will localize in two principal modes (9,10). The macrophages in the medullary cords of lymph nodes

142

and in the red pulp of the spleen pick up much of the injected antigen (Fig. 5-6). This antigen enters macrophages by pinocytosis or by direct penetration of the plasmalemma without vacuole formation (11). Lysosomes form around this antigen, which is then slowly digested. Lymphocytes are shown to make contact with macrophages. Plasma cells appear in these areas, but antigen could not be demonstrated within these cells. In the cortex, antigen enters the circular sinus, is taken up by the macrophages which line this sinus, and then spreads to the lymphocytes. Antigen can be shown in contact with the processes of dendritic reticular cells and between lymphocytes. In preimmunized animals antigen localizes primarily in the dendritic macrophages of the cortex and becomes associated with antibody on the surface of these cells (Fig. 5-7). It will then be held, apparently not within these cells, but in contact with the dendritic processes. Thus, contact will be established with antigen target cells, apparently to stimulate the production of antibodies by these cells. It is evident that while antigen-processing by macrophages may be needed for a primary response, in the case of a preimmunized animal, antibody localized in dendritic macrophage processes may hold the antigen which can stimu-

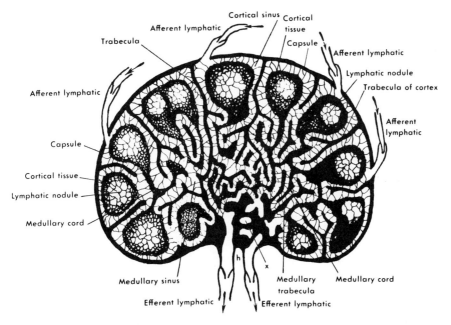

Fig. 5-4 Schematic diagram of the splenic architecture. From Bloom and Fawcett (8) with permission.

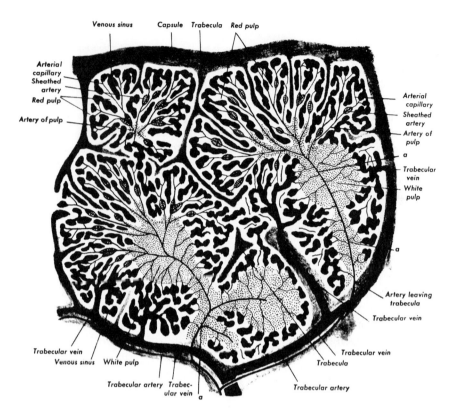

Fig. 5-5 A schematic representation of lymph node structure.
From Bloom and Fawcett (8) with permission.

late memory cells. This model is based on solid experimental evidence and proposes a somewhat different mechanism of induction of primary and secondary responses. It appears that in primary immunization antigen enters the macrophage and is preprocessed in order to stimulate the antigen target cell, while in secondary stimulation there may be no need of macrophage preprocessing. If this is the case, then it must be assumed that either antigen has a different role in stimulating cells for an anamnestic response or that the target cell for a secondary response is different from that found in nonimmunized animals.

Intracellular Localization of Antigen

Little direct evidence is available on the intracellular distribution of antigen. Studies using labeled antigens are complicated by the fact that many external labels, such as I^{131}, have short half-lives, and proteins internally labeled (biosynthetically) by radioactive S^{35}, H^3, or C^{14} amino acids are rapidly reutilized for the formation of new proteins after in vivo degradation. The most effective studies have involved the use of external labels consisting of artificial determinant groups containing radioactive labels such as S^{35}-azophenylsulfonate, H^3-azophenylarsonate, or other similar groups. In contrast to the internal labels, the external labels cannot be utilized for the biosynthesis of proteins. Using such labels, Roberts and

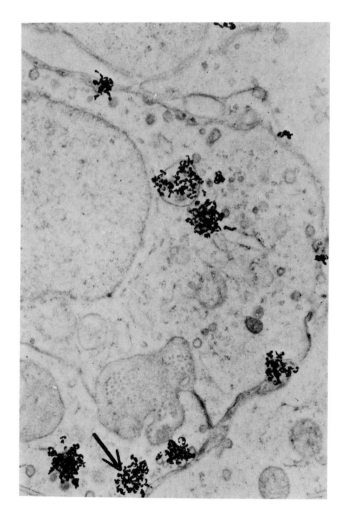

Fig. 5-6 Part of a littoral macrophage near the medullary sinus showing antigen at various stages of ingestion during a primary immune response. From Ada et al. (9) with permission.

Haurowitz (12) studied the intracellular localization of H³-aniline azo porcine gamma globulin following intravenous and subcutaneous injection into mice. They found intracytoplasmic localization of tritium in the phagocytic reticular cells of mesenteric lymph nodes, liver Kupffer cells, fixed macrophages of the splenic red pulp, and "septal cells," or fixed macrophages, of the lung. However, these autoradiographic techniques did not indicate any intranuclear localization of antigen. Similar observations

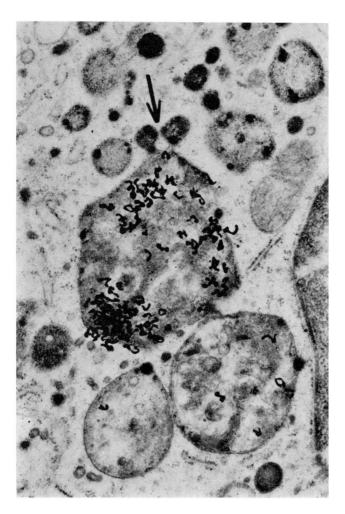

Fig. 5-7 Antigenic localization in the paranuclear region of a dendritic macrophage during a secondary response. From Ada et al. (9) with permission.

have been made by other investigators who also studied the localization of colored azo protein antigens during an immune response (13–15). These investigators reported no intranuclear localization of the colored azo proteins. Intranuclear localization of antigen in reticuloendothelial and hepatic parenchymal cells, detectable with fluorescence microscopy techniques, was reported by Coons et al. (16).

Further studies by Haurowitz et al. (17,18) revealed that the isotopically labeled azoproteins were found associated with the large and small cytoplasmic granules of spleen and liver homogenates. The large cytoplasmic granules consisted chiefly of mitochondria. Both Garvey and Campbell (19) and Hawkins and Haurowitz (20) have found S^{35}-azophenylsulfonated protein antigens in a bound or degraded form in association with RNA. However, ribosomes prepared from the organs of sensitized animals have been found to be free of antigen (21). In order to follow the fate of bacteriophages within the reticuloendothelial cells, Uhr and Weissmann (22) injected a mixture of ϕX174 and T2 bacteriophages into rabbits to determine the subcellular distribution of the phages and mitochondrial and lysosomal enzymes in liver fractions separated on sucrose density gradients. They found that the two phages and two lysosomal enzymes, β-glucuronidase and acid phosphatase, sedimented together; in contrast, the mitochondrial enzyme cytochrome oxidase sedimented separately (Fig. 5-8). These data indicate that phages are contained within lysosomes. Furthermore, a fraction of antigenic material can escape extensive digestion as long as 2 days after injection. This is evidenced by the finding that T2 plaque-forming units are detectable 48 hours after injection, although T2 is cleared from the circulation within several hours. These observations suggest that antigen must be taken up by macrophages and that some of it must remain relatively intact, since it is the tertiary structure of antigen and surface antigens to which specificity is usually directed (23). Uhr and Weissmann (22) suggest that the macrophages within lymphoid organs may have evolved special mechanisms for allowing a fraction of the antigenic molecules to escape the usual fate of degradation and to make their way to the surface of cells. Therefore, it is either antigen that has been endocytized by macrophages or antigen which escapes endocytosis that acts as immunogen.

Antigen Metabolism and "Immunogenic RNA"

An alternative possibility to the one described above is that antigen within macrophages may stimulate the formation of an RNA which is necessary for immunization. Either the RNA has all the information for the amino acid sequence, and hence the specificity of the antibody, or the RNA of

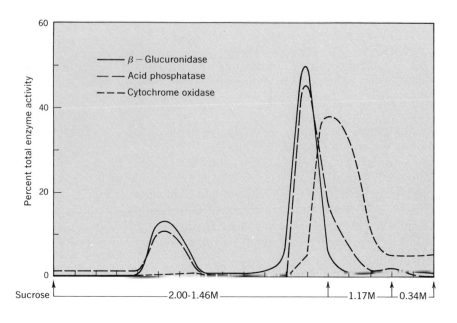

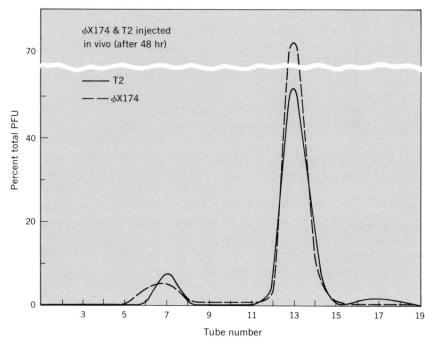

Fig. 5-8 Distribution of bacteriophages and lysosomal and mitochondrial enzymes in rabbit liver fractions separated on sucrose density gradients. From Uhr and Weissmann (22) with permission.

an antigen-RNA complex may be a mechanism for derepressing the potential antibody-forming cell after the RNA is guided to the right cell by antigen. A third possibility is that the macrophage RNA may act as a carrier of an immunogenic fragment of antigen and enhance cellular uptake of that fragment by antibody-forming cells.

In an attempt to define more specifically the role of macrophages in immune responses, macrophages have been isolated from the peritoneal cavity of experimental animals to study their metabolic processes after exposure to antigen in vitro. One of the earliest studies was that of Fishman and Adler (24), who reported that a nucleic acid obtained from rat macrophage cells, which had been incubated with antigen in vitro, was able to cause antibody synthesis in x-radiated animals which had received the RNA and normal lymph node placed in diffusion chambers. When nonradiated recipients were used, RNA alone was able to transfer the ability for specific antibody synthesis. Furthermore, the immunologic activity was found primarily in the top layer of a sucrose gradient which had been divided into three fractions. Such activity could be eliminated by treating the extract with RNase. In similar experiments, Friedman et al. (25) and Askonas and Rhodes (26) attributed the immunogenicity of RNA extracts from macrophage populations to antigen contamination. Complement fixation revealed T2 head, tail, and internal protein antigens in the RNA extract prepared by Friedman, an extract which had been obtained using techniques similar to those described by Fishman and Adler (24). Indeed, when Friedman et al. (25) examined an RNA extract obtained from Fishman and Adler, they were able to isolate T2 antigens. Not only were trace amounts of these antigens found, but in the case of tail antigen, they were present in sufficient concentration and with the proper molecular structure to ensure antigenicity. Askonas and Rhodes (26) studied the immunogenicity of mouse RNA extracts after stimulation with I^{131}-hemocyanin. They found that the activity of the extract was dependent upon the presence of the radioactive label which indicated antigen contamination.

Two basic questions emerge from this early work: (1) Is the immunogenicity of an RNA extract solely the function of antigen components? (2) Is the antigen merely a contaminant of the RNA extract, or is it bound in such a way as to form an immunologically essential complex of RNA and antigen? Subsequent reports tend to substantiate the fact that the immunogenicity of such extracts is due to the presence of antigenic fragments. Gottlieb et al. (27) found immunologic activity in the 28S fraction of a sucrose gradient of RNA extracted from rat macrophage cells. These animals had been stimulated with the antigen, T2 bacteriophage. Immunologic activity in the 28S fraction appeared to be relatively resistant to the action of RNase since a high enzyme-substrate ratio (30 μg RNA) was necessary to eliminate the activity. Pronase, however, did eliminate immunologic activity, indicating that protein was an essential component of the extract. Cesium sulfate gradients showed that the protein was complexed with the RNA in such a way as to cause a shift in the density of that RNA. Immunologic activity was localized in this minor band from the gradient. Because of such localization of activity, it appears that immunogenicity is the sole result of the antigenic fragment. The shift in the density of the RNA suggests that it is chemically bound to the protein.

This antigen-ribonucleoprotein, upon analysis, was shown to have a protein content of 28 percent and a molecular weight of approximately 12,000 (27a). This antigenic residue approximated a size of 30 to 35 amino acids and was a degradation product of the whole T2 protein in which the original tertiary structure had been destroyed. However, since this fragment did adsorb neutralizing antibody to the whole T2 antigen, tertiary structure was not necessary for the recognition of specific antibody in this instance (27b). The antigen fragments in the antigen-RNP complex also caused the synthesis of this specific antibody in previously unstimulated cells (27).

Although Bishop and Abramoff (28) isolated the immunologic activity in RNA from the 6 to 10S region of a sucrose gradient, they also found significant displacement of a portion of that RNA in a cesium gradient. By use of a radioactively labeled antigen (S^{35}-sulfanilic acid), the labeled antigenic fragments were localized in the minor band on the cesium gradient. Further evidence that the antigenic fragment is an essential component of RNA extracted from phagocytic cells is presented in the work of Roelants and Goodman (29). Labeled antigen was found in the 4 to 5S RNA fraction from a sucrose gradient, whether the antigen was tritiated poly-γ-D-glutamic acid or S^{35}-labeled T2 bacteriophage. Analysis of the antigen-RNA complex confirmed that the antigen was still in a polymer form and that the labeled polypeptide could not be dissociated from the complex by sucrose density centrifugation, adsorption chromatography, gel electrophoresis, cesium sulfate gradient centrifugation, or by competition with excesses of various unlabeled polypeptides. The RNA-polypeptide was eluted as a unit from cellulose columns, but the polypeptide alone was eluted in a different position. Similarly, the complex and the polypeptide alone separated in different positions in both cesium sulfate and sucrose gradients.

By employing an immunogenic copolymer of L-glutamic acid, L-alanine, and L-tyrosine, Gottlieb (30) has extended his observations of RNA-antigen complexes to include those formed with a soluble antigen. He again found the copolymer in association with the 28S fraction of the macrophage RNA from a sucrose gradient and with the RNP complex from a cesium sulfate gradient. Contrary to the results of Roelants and Goodman (29), Gottlieb was able to cause at least a partial dissociation of the complex by raising the ionic strength of the disk electrophoresis buffer.

From the results presented by these three groups of investigators (27–30) it would appear that an immunologic response will follow incubation of the RNA extract with a competent cell population only when the RNA extract carries antigenic fragments. Although the analysis of the RNA peptide complex by Roelants and Goodman (29) indicates that the complex may be formed as a result of "an active biologic process," the data of Gottlieb present a serious challenge to such a conclusion.

Somewhat more ambiguous are the studies of Adler et al. (31), who isolated two types of active RNA from the peritoneal exudate cells of rabbits. When recipient cells were incubated with an RNA extract from the peritoneal cells, antibody was produced in two waves which peaked at 4 to 5 days and 10 to 13 days, respectively. The antibody found in the early response was identified as IgM and carried the allotypic specificity of the donor cell. The antibody present on day 10, IgG, was allotypically identical to that of the recipient cell. In addition, the early response was highly sensitive to RNase treatment, while that occurring later was relatively insensitive. The RNA which was highly insensitive to RNase and which appeared to be responsible for the synthesis of IgG antibody was also precipitated by anti-T2 serum (specific for the antigen used). This would indicate that this RNA contained antigenic fragments and was comparable to the extracts of Gottlieb et al. (27), Bishop and Abramoff (28), and Roelants and Goodman (29). However, the delay in appearance of the antibody (10 to 13 days) in contrast with the early appearance of antibody reported by others (27,28) is unexplained. The existence of an RNA which stimulated synthesis of an IgM antibody with allotypic specificity of the macrophage cell is more puzzling. Since it is unlikely that the macrophage synthesizes antibody, it would seem improbable that it would make an RNA specific for such synthesis. This RNA may be a product of lymphoid cells present in the peritoneal exudate rather than of the phagocytic macrophage.

In an effort to provide additional data relevant to the role of antigen in RNA extracts, Chin and Silverman (32,33) attempted to transfer the ability to synthesize myeloma protein with an RNA extracted from the myeloma tumor. The myeloma protein has physicochemical, antigenic, and structural properties similar to normal 7S γ_2-globulin and does not appear to require the presence of antigen for its continued synthesis. Because of the lack of antigen, this system provided a model for an attempt to transfer globulin synthesis without the possibility of having antigen in the extract. Although the RNA extracted from mouse myeloma tumors was taken up by normal mouse lymphoid cells in an undegraded form, the cells did not synthesize a specific myeloma protein which could be identified by its antigenic determinants.

Although these negative data do not preclude the possibility that synthesis can be transferred by RNA free of antigenic components, they serve as a basis for further discussion of the apparent difficulty of such a possibility. Evidence has been presented that the heavy and light chains of the immunoglobulin molecule are synthesized on separate polysome structures. Such data allow the conclusion that synthesis of the two chains does not involve a single polycistronic mRNA. Therefore, it becomes increasingly difficult to suppose that a significant number of cells would take up two messenger molecules, one for each chain, to allow synthesis of a complete immunoglobulin molecule. In addition, if such uptake were to take place, the RNA would have to maintain structural integrity in order to function as a messenger molecule. Although Chin and Silverman (32,33) indicated that the RNA was taken up as an undegraded molecule, from 36 to 48 percent of that RNA was degraded during the first 2 hours after uptake. The range in the amount of degradation was dependent upon the amount of RNA used and whether or not the recipient cells had been treated with protamine. As the amount of RNA was decreased, degradation was decreased. The use of protamine also decreased the amount of degradation.

Current information can be summarized as follows: (1) After primary stimulation, antigen is taken up by macrophages and interacts with these cells. The synthesis of a new RNA seems to be induced, and a complex of this RNA with the product secreted by the macrophage appears to be responsible for the immunogenic action. It therefore appears that RNA complexed with antigen by-products is necessary to stimulate immune responses. (2) In secondary responses, antigen interacts with phagocytic cells in the presence of antibody but is not phagocytosed, and only a small portion of the cell is in contact with antigen, which is localized around the dendritic processes on the cell surface. Interaction with the antigen target cells in proximity to these phagocytic cells takes place. This stimulates them and induces them to proliferate, differentiate, and produce antibody.

While at least the first part of this model is constructed on data acquired by experiments carried out in vitro, evidence has been presented showing cytoplasmic bridges between macrophages and antibody-forming cells. The significance of this observation with respect to transfer of immunogenic materials is not clear (34). Antigen has only twice been found within antibody-forming cells. Antigen has been shown to be localized within the nucleus of some of the antibody-forming cells (35) and has also been seen within the antibody-forming cells (36). It is suggested, however, that this may be an artifactual occurrence caused by experimental manipulations. Existing evidence indicates that it would be extremely difficult to identify antigen within antigen target cells, since they are few in number (37). If it is assumed that there are 10^8 immunocompetent cells in the spleen, it can be calculated, on the basis of experimental data, that only 150 of these cells may be immunocompetent for a given antigen. Finding 1 of these 150 cells among 10 million cells would be very difficult. However, the ultimate solution resides in determining whether antigen at any time becomes associated with an antigen target cell either in its intact form or in a modified form or whether a different product induced by antigen within a cell other than the antigen target cell is then capable of interacting with the latter to stimulate it to produce antibody.

Persistence of Antigen

Regardless of what role the macrophage plays in the processing of antigenic materials, there is substantial evidence that antigen or antigenic fragments persist for long periods of time in vivo. There is little doubt that the long-lasting immunity which results following some viral infections (e.g., yellow fever) is due to the persistence of latent virus in the tissues. It has long been recognized that pneumococcal polysaccharides persist in mouse tissues for at least 1 year and possibly longer (38,39). Heidelberger (40) has shown the persistence of pneumococcal polysaccharides in humans for years following a single dose of antigen. Furthermore, this persisting antigen produces a maximal antibody response for the same period. It has been suggested that this long persistence is due to a lack of enzymes in man and the mouse which would be able to digest the bacterial polysaccharide.

Analogous persistence of protein antigens was considered improbable, since most tissues contain proteolytic enzymes. However, studies with isotopically labeled antigens are suggestive that antigenic determinants can indeed persist intracellularly for some time. Dixon et al. (2) followed the retention of iodinated bovine gamma globulin (I*BGG) in the tissues of rabbits and found localization of antigen in the plasma, liver, and spleen following a primary injection of the antigen (Fig. 5-9). The levels of I*BGG dropped sharply after the eighth day, after which time antibody appeared in the circulation. The rate of loss of I^{131} was then much slower, and tissue-bound BGG that was still antigenic for rabbits was found up to 2 weeks after injection. A BGG-like material that was capable of initiating anaphylactic shock in mice but was not antigenic in rabbits was detectable in the rabbit tissues for as long as 6 weeks. Using proteins coupled by diazo linkages and labeled with S[35] or C[14], Haurowitz et al. (41) found that although these antigens disappeared rapidly from the circulation, they persisted in organs, particularly spleen, liver, and bone marrow, for many months. Campbell and Garvey (42) have found that S[35]-labeled hemocyanin or BSA is detectable in the liver of rabbits for as long as 12 months after intravenous injection. The rate at which such antigenic material disappears is so slow after about 3 weeks that it seems reasonable to assume that some of it must persist for the life of the animal. The total amount of radioactive material found in the spleen or liver after 8 to 10 months may be only a few micrograms or less, but the number of molecules is as great as, if not greater than, the total number of cells in the liver. Haurowitz (43) has estimated that the radioactivity found in the rabbit liver 6 to 7 months after an intravenous injection of 30 mg ovalbumin-C[14]-o-azobenzoate per kg body weight corresponds to only 0.12 μg of antigen

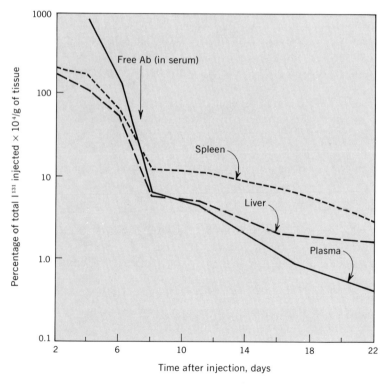

Fig. 5-9 Retention of I[131] in tissues after a primary injection of iodinated bovine serum albumin. From Dixon (2) with permission.

per g spleen, or a few hundred molecules per cell. Since some of the cells are free of antigen, others may contain several thousand molecules of antigen or antigenic fragments containing determinant groups.

The presence of antigenic molecules or fragments in a cell does prove that their presence is essential for antibody formation. The studies of Uhr and Weissmann (22) described above suggest that the continued presence of immunogen, protected by some intracellular mechanism from enzymatic attack, is necessary for an immune response. However, pigments used in tattooing persist in the cells of the skin for many years and yet it has not been demonstrated that they induce antibody formation. Furthermore, it is not possible to prove or disprove the suggestion that antibody formation can go on in an organism without the continued persistence of antigenic molecules or fragments.

ANTIBODY METABOLISM

Induction Period

The first contact of antigen with antigen target cell is followed by an interval called the induction period or the lag period of antibody production. The induction period, usually a few hours to a few days long, is observed with all antigens that have been studied. The first measurable antibody does not appear until the end of this period. From studies of the induction period, it is apparent that RNA synthesis takes place and that ribosomes accumulate in lymphoid cells which differentiate (see Chap. 6). Cohen and Raska (44) have shown that new species of RNA can be detected and indicated that these may represent mRNA. Little is known about the induction period; in fact, most of what is known seems to be of a negative nature. Whatever occurs during this period is necessary, however, for antibody production to start. Because of the largely negative data from studies of the induction period, it was assumed that this lag phase may not have been a real entity, but that it was dependent upon the inability to measure antibody in the very low amounts which occur early after antigen administration (45). Most methods of measuring antibody are quite insensitive and require fairly large amounts of antibody to be present before any detection can be made (see Chap. 11). For this reason the idea developed that antibody was made much earlier than it could be detected and that the induction period could be an artifactual one. This would be reasonable, since protein synthesis is known to require only a short induction period. It thus appears unnecessary to need hours to days as a lag phase for the induction of antibody synthesis. Although it seems reasonable to think in these terms, the idea that the induction period was a real entity and not an artifact was discarded in light of the following experiments. If a rabbit is immunized and given labeled amino acids and the lymph node cells from this animal are then transferred 2 days after immunization into an x-radiated recipient, labeled antibody will not be found in the new rabbit. This indicates that during the first 2 days there is no synthesis of either antibody or a precursor of antibody. Otherwise some labeled material would be found in the antibody (46). Many other experiments show that the induction period is an important preparatory phase. Various agents, capable of inhibiting the immune response, work best if given during the induction period (see Chap. 10). The purine analog 6-mercaptopurine and the amino acid analog β-3-thienylalanine will depress antibody production almost completely if given during the induction period, but will not be very effective if given later (47,48). It is well known that 6-mercaptopurine inhibits the synthesis of RNA, and β-3-thienylalanine has also been shown to block this pathway. The data presented above are not unequivocal; however, what occurs during the induction period appears to be the synthesis of a new species of RNA which may be necessary for the manufacture of antibody. Depression of this RNA synthesis leads to the depression of later stages of antibody synthesis. Thus it appears that rather than reflecting inefficiency of our measurement methods, the induction period represents a period during which RNA synthesis occurs in preparation for the synthesis of new antibody. The induction period can be viewed as a time during which new species of messenger RNA and ribosomes are synthesized and during which some work preparatory to the synthesis of antibody is occurring. It should be added that after the first experience with antigen, the induction period is usually shortened. This might be explained by postulating that during an anamnestic response there are more ribosomes ready to be used for antibody production and that this would make the induction period shorter.

Synthetic Phase

The induction period of an immune response is followed by a three-part production phase. First there is a logarithmic increase in the amount of antibody in the serum, followed by a plateau phase which in some cases is transitory and in some cases almost nonexistent, and then there is a decline phase. The antibody titer rises logarithmically for about 5 to 10 days until it reaches a peak. This is followed by a plateau of 1 to 3 days and then a gradual decline (Fig. 5-10). During the log phase, production of antibody exceeds catabolism; during the plateau phase, they are equal;

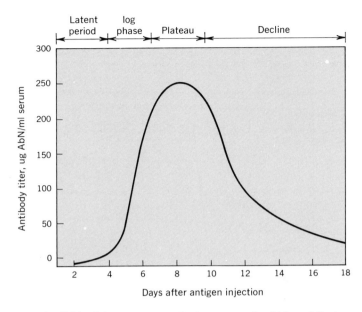

Fig. 5-10 Primary serum antibody response in chickens following a single intravenous injection of bovine serum albumin.

and during the decline, catabolism exceeds synthesis. This will vary from antigen to antigen and with the persistence of antigen.

In attempting to quantitate the antibody response, one must consider not only the antibody which appears after the elimination of antigen from the circulation but also the antibody which is utilized in the immune elimination phase of the induction period. The antibody which combines with antigen, thereby hastening its catabolism, is itself destroyed with the antigen. Thus, the antigen-bound antibody, which is not itself detectable as free antibody in the serum, may amount to somewhat less than one-half of the total antibody synthesized during the primary response. Dixon (1) has demonstrated that the amount of antibody formed during the first 1 to 2 days after a primary injection of I^{131}-BGG in rabbits is extremely small, as judged by the rate of antigen elimination. In 3 to 4 days after antigen injection, an increased rate of antigen elimination indicates the appearance of antibody. The rate of antibody production appears to increase logarithmically during the next few days, as indicated by the increasing rate of immune elimination of antigen and the subsequent rapid appearance of antibody in the blood (Fig. 5-11). Following a short plateau period the rate of antibody synthesis drops abruptly to levels slightly lower than the maximum rate some time before the maximum serum antibody concentration is reached. The interval by which the decrease in antibody synthesis precedes the maximum serum antibody level is equal to the

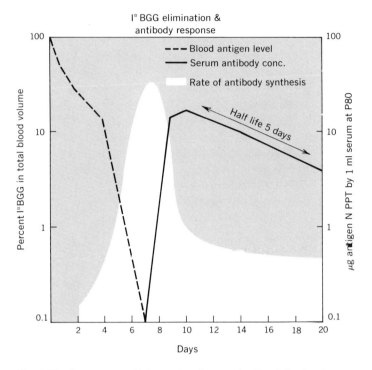

Fig. 5-11 Serum concentrations of antigen and estimated rate of antibody synthesis following a primary injection of bovine gamma globulin in rabbits. From Dixon (1) with permission.

time necessary for antibody to get from the antibody-producing cells to the bloodstream. Thus, in the primary immune response, there is a rapidly accelerating rate of antibody production during and perhaps for a short time after the period of antigen elimination, followed by an abrupt, almost complete cessation of antibody production at or shortly after the time when antigen can no longer be detected in the host.

The course of antibody production during a secondary response differs considerably from that seen during the primary response. Dixon (1) found in the rabbit that following a third bimonthly intravenous injection of BGG, the antigen elimination from the blood is completed within 4 days, and maximum serum antibody concentration is reached 3 to 4 days later (Fig. 5-12). Following this, the serum antibody level falls at a rapid rate with a half-life of approximately 5.7 for 20 days. Then the rate of decline of serum antibody slows considerably, finally approaching a logarithmic rate with a half-life of slightly more than 2 months. During the slow decline of serum antibody, the half-life of homologous antibody remained normal, 5 to 7 days, indicating that continued synthesis of anti-

158

body and not slowed catabolism was responsible for the slow antibody decline. For a more thorough discussion of the secondary response see Chap. 8.

Abramoff and Brien (49) have correlated the morphologic differentiation in the chicken spleen cell population and the appearance of humoral antibody with release of antibody by individual spleen cells by utilizing the Jerne plaque technique (49a). Following a single intravenous injection of sheep red blood cells, there was a 2 percent increase in the number of plasmacytic cells in the spleen by 13 hours after antigenic stimulation (Fig. 5-13). Morphologic differentiation continued so that plasmacytic cells comprised 9 percent of the spleen cell population at 2 days. At this point there was a significant increase in plaque formation. These data indicated that despite increasing numbers of plasmacytic cells during the previous 24 hours, significant numbers of plaque-forming cells were not present until 3 days after antigenic stimulation. Thus the rise in plaque formation occurred only when the cell population showed the greatest number of differentiated cells. These observations substantiate the fact that peak cellular synthesis of antibody precedes by several days the peak humoral antibody response in the circulating blood.

By using *Salmonella typhi* where antigen may be present for long periods of time, there is a prolonged plateau phase with a very late decline phase (50), indicating that production usually requires the presence of antigen. A

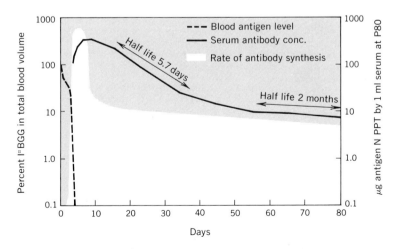

Fig. 5-12 Serum concentrations of antigen and estimated rate of antibody synthesis during an anamnestic response to bovine gamma globulin in rabbits. From Dixon (1) with permission.

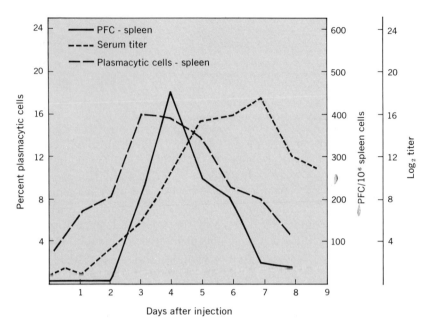

Fig. 5-13 Relationship of the cellular and humoral immune response of the chicken following a single intravenous injection of sheep red blood cells. From Abramoff and Brien (49) with permission.

definitive correlation between antigen persistence and prolonged plateau has not been established beyond doubt. The decline phase is also a function of synthesis and destruction, and it is apparent that during this phase, synthesis is less active than catabolism. This may be in varying degrees, and therefore, either a slower or faster decline of antibody can be observed. The doubling time of antibody during the log phase of increase has been studied and found to be 6.5 to 7 hours for both primary and secondary responses and for optimal antigen doses. The data obtained from measurement of antibody half-lives in various species are summarized in Table 5-2 (51).

Kinetics of Antibody Formation

In recent years it has been demonstrated that two molecular classes of antibody are formed in a characteristic sequence during the primary immune response. Depending upon the type of antigen, its mode of introduction, the dosage employed, and various other factors, the earliest detectable serum antibodies are of the 19S (IgM) type, while IgG (7S) antibodies appear somewhat later (52). The formation of IgM antibodies is generally transient, and within approximately 2 to 3 weeks of the antigenic challenge, IgG is the principal class of specific antibody produced (Fig. 5-14). A similar sequence of antibody formation has been observed in adult mammals (52), chickens (53), frogs and goldfish (54), and turtles (55).

The question of the significance of the heterogeneity of the immune response cannot be answered satisfactorily at present. However, during immunization, there is a progressive increase in binding affinity of 7S antibody molecules that appear in the circulation. Taliaferro et al. (56) studied the kinetics of change in avidity of antibody during the primary hemolysin response in rabbits and found that the avidity increased as the antibody titer rose and decreased after peak titer was achieved. During the secondary response there was a more rapid increase in avidity as serum antibody rose with a subsequent slight decrease after peak titer was achieved. Eisen and Siskind (57) have observed that the difference between early and late 7S antibodies to 2,4 dinitrophenyl may be as great as ten thousandfold. This increasing avidity of antibody with increasing time after immunization has been observed against a variety of antigens such as bacteriophage (52,58), sheep red blood cells (56), and BSA (59). Thus, during immunization there is a progressive change in the quality of 7S molecules produced resulting in an increased efficiency in their capacity to bind to specific antigen.

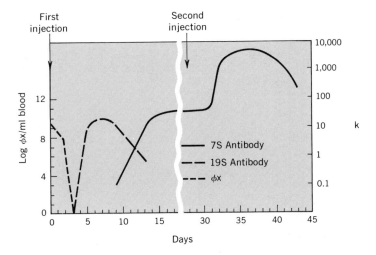

Fig. 5-14 Antibody response to ϕX in the guinea pig after two intravenous injections of 10^{11} PFU ϕX administered 1 month apart. From Uhr (63) with permission.

TABLE 5-2
Comparative Half-lives of Various Plasma Proteins in Different Species

Species	ALBUMIN Label	ALBUMIN T½‡ (days)	IgG-IMMUNOGLOBULIN Label	IgG-IMMUNOGLOBULIN T½ (days)	TRANSFERRIN Label	TRANSFERRIN T½ (days)	FIBRINOGEN Label	FIBRINOGEN T½ (days)
Cow (185,000 g) †	I131	20.7						
Man (65,000 g)	I131	10.5	I131	6.0	I131	8.7	I131	4.3
		15		13.1		7.6		5.1
		18		11.5–19.0		8.8		1.5–3.0
		12–13		10.6–16.6				
		16.3		8–17				
		15–25		21–26				
		14.3						
		18.0		16.5–31				
		14.8		16–26				
		19.5						
	N15	20.0						
	C14	28–39					S35	5.6
	S35	26–48	S35	22.4				11
		55–60		25.8				3.7
		17–26						
		26.5						
Baboon (20,000 g)	I131	16	I131	12				
Dog (13,000 g)	I131	8.2	I131	8.0			I131	2.4
	C14	13.9	C14	21.6				1.7–3.0
	C35	14.4	S35	20.4			S35	4.1

Animal[†]	Isotope				
Rhesus monkey (2500 g)	I^{131}		6.6		
Rabbit (2000 g)	I^{131}	5.7	5.3		2.8
		5.0	3.3		2.5
		8.0	6.3		
		8.4	6.3		
			7.0		
	C^{14}	8.3	5.3		2.9
		7.5	6.3		
		7.0	7.0		
		8.6			
	S^{35}	9.9	7.0		2.3
			7.0		
			5.4		
Guinea pig (730 g)	I^{131}	2.8	6.0		
Rat (250 g)	I^{131}	2.5	5.5	4.0	1.3
		2.7	2.4		
		3.3	7.0		
		1.9			
	S^{35}	3.15	5.3		
		2.9	5.4		
		3.6			
Mouse (25 g)	C^{14}	3.7	7.2		
	I^{131}	1.2	1.9		
		0.7–1.1	4.6		

† Average weight in parentheses.
‡ Half-life (in days) measured from the terminal slope of the plasma.
SOURCE: Adapted from Schultze and Heremans (51) with permission.

Furthermore, 19S antibody to SRBC (56), bacteria (60), and bacteriophage (58) can be extremely efficient in binding these particulate antigens and causing hemolysis and neutralization, respectively. Also, 19S in contrast to 7S diphtheria antitoxin does not neutralize diphtheria toxin in vivo (61). On the basis of these observations Uhr and Finkelstein (52) have suggested that the IgM system might be regarded as a first line of defense, capable of prompt production of large numbers of antibody molecules which can readily "coat" particulate antigens such as red blood cells, bacteria, and bacteriophage, but which are relatively inefficient in their capacity to bind to soluble antigens such as serum proteins and toxins, and in which the cells do not take part in long-lived synthesis, in the improvement in the quality of antibody produced, or in the development of immunologic memory. In contrast, the 7S system may be initially represented by a small population of cells not capable of an immediate vigorous response, but eventually able to synthesize more efficient antibody molecules for long periods of time and to participate in the development of a persisting immunologic memory.

Another clue to the possible significance of an immune system composed of different classes of immune globulins is provided by the observation that IgA immunoglobulins alone are selectively secreted by the parotid gland and that only this class of γ-globulins binds to skin, smooth muscle, and mucous membranes (62). "Bound" IgA antibody after interaction with antigen can cause release of histamine and other pharmacologic agents at the local site of interaction. The significance of histamine release is not yet known, but it is possible that these unusual biologic attributes of IgA antibody may play a role in defending exposed body cavities to surface penetration by infective agents. Thus, the varied challenges met by an organism may be met by a multicomponent immune system in which each component is specialized to perform a particular function at a particular time.

CONTROL OF ANTIBODY SYNTHESIS

Role of Antigen

What controls the synthesis of antibody and how the levels of immunoglobulins are regulated is not clear. However, much work has been directed to solving this question. The first question to be answered is: How does antigen induce the production of antibody? This question has been discussed at some length earlier in this chapter. The second problem is to know whether antigen is necessary for the production of antibody. Experiments of Campbell and Garvey (62) have shown that antigen can persist in liver cells for long periods in amounts capable of inducing continued production of antibody. On the other hand, experiments by La Via (50) have shown that while the antigens of S. *typhi*, which are proteins and therefore easily degradable, will induce prolonged production of antibody, the antigens of sheep erythrocytes, which are polysaccharide in nature and difficult to degrade enzymatically, will lead to antibody production characterized by a short plateau phase and a rapid decline with return to normal a few days after injection of antigen.

The short duration and abrupt cessation of 19S antibody formation following a primary injection of ϕX antigen have suggested that the depletion of antigen is responsible for this type of response (63). To test this possibility guinea pigs were injected with a second injection of ϕX at the time when 19S antibody synthesis had virtually ceased. It was found that a second injection on day 9 could again stimulate 19S antibody synthesis (Fig. 5-15). The prompt increase of circulating antibody after the second injection indicates synthesis by the same population of cells which had previously formed antibody. If a new population of cells had responded, there would have been a delay of approximately 1 week before antibody formation was sufficient to increase noticeably the existing level of serum antibody. Furthermore, the stimulation by the second antigen was immunologically specific, since no such effect occurred in the control group which received T2 phage on day 9. Similar results have been reported by Svehag and Mandel (64) using poliovirus in rabbits. These studies suggest that antigen must persist for the continued synthesis of 19S antibody and that depletion of antigen can terminate such synthesis.

In addition to the duration of 19S antibody synthesis, the dose of ϕX can affect several other aspects of the immune response. It appears that low concentrations of antigen will result primarily in 19S antibody production and as the concentration of antigen increases, first the relative rate of 19S antibody production increases, then 7S antibody production is initiated, and finally, at high antigen concentrations, immunologic unresponsiveness is induced. Thus there appears to be a delicate balance between stimulation and paralysis for every antigen, and this balance appears to be under genetic control. Gill et al. (65) have postulated that a poor antigen induces paralysis easily, whereas a good immunogen stimulates antibody production. Therefore, antigen metabolism may regulate antibody formation by controlling the amount of antigen left intact and capable of stimulating antibody formation. For example, poor antigens such as synthetic ᴅ-polypeptides and pneumococcal polysaccharides are poorly degraded, and thus the concentration of the intact antigens is high enough to induce immunologic paralysis.

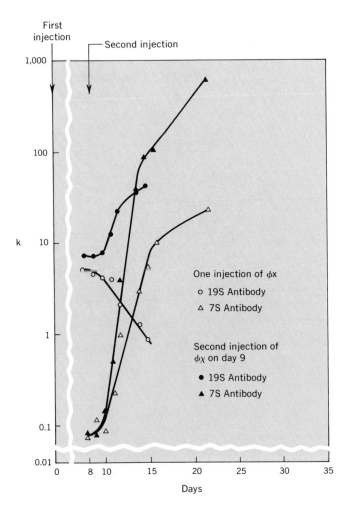

Fig. 5-15 Effect of a secondary injection of ϕX on day 9 on the primary 19S and 7S responses in the guinea pig. From Uhr (63) with permission.

Good antigens are rapidly degraded, so that over a wide range of doses, optimal amounts of antigen are available to stimulate antibody formation.

Role of Antibody

Although the synthesis of antibody requires the presence of antigen for its initiation, it is not known whether antigen has to persist for longer periods of time for antibody production to continue, or whether this function can be maintained by the induced cells in the absence of antigenic determinants. In view of this, it would be of interest to discuss the possible

166

mechanism or mechanisms which may regulate the rise and maintenance of immunoglobulin production and its fall after this initial antigenic stimulus. Antigen is the initiator of the synthesis of immunoglobulin. Once this interaction between antigen and antigen target cell has been started, how is the synthesis regulated so that it can be shut off when no more antibody is needed? This is particularly interesting in the case of long persisting antigen. It appears that a reasonable mechanism of control may be by feedback. In fact, a third component has been added to the system: antibody. It is possible that this now acts as a regulator of further synthesis by interacting with antigen and antigen target cells. Several lines of evidence exist which indicate that IgG antibodies affect the immunoglobulin sequence by a negative feedback mechanism.

X-radiation, methothrexate, and 6-mercaptopurine (6-MP) in low doses will not only inhibit IgG antibody synthesis but also produce a prolongation of 19S antibody formation. Sahiar and Schwartz (66) infused isologous IgG anti-BGG antibodies into either normal or 6-MP-treated rabbits and followed the production of IgM antibodies. Rabbits were injected with 2 mg of BGG, treated with 6-MP, and on the twelfth experimental day infused with 4.0 ml of hyperimmune serum containing 7S anti-BGG rabbit antibodies intravenously. There was a prompt cessation of IgM antibody synthesis (Fig. 5-16). Rabbit anti-EA antiserum

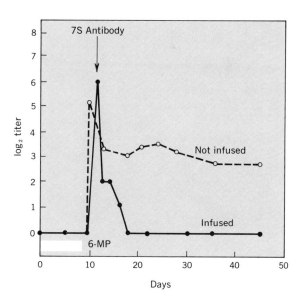

Fig. 5-16 Inhibition of 19S antibody synthesis in 6-MP-treated rabbits by passively infused 7S antibody. From Sahiar and Schwartz (66) with permission.

similarly administered had no effect on the synthesis of IgM antibodies (Fig. 5-17). Also, Ag-Ab complexes had no effect on IgM synthesis.

In another experiment Sahiar and Schwartz (66) injected rabbits with 2 mg BGG and, on the same day, began 6-MP treatment. On the thirteenth day a second injection of 2 mg BGG was given. They found that there was a rapid increase in antibody that was entirely due to 7S antibody (Fig. 5-18). At the same time, titers of 19S antibody fell sharply and within 1 week of the second dose of antigen there was essentially no 19S antibody.

This evidence suggests that IgG does indeed affect the immunoglobulin sequence by a negative feedback mechanism. Since the administration of hyperimmune serum containing a non-cross-reacting antibody (anti-EA) was without effect, the implication of possible anti-antibodies or other nonspecific factors can be ruled out. Furthermore, when the specific binding sites of the antibody were taken up by antigen (Ag-Ab complexes), its effect on 19S antibody formation was lost. This suggests that the 7S antibody acts by complexing with antigen in vivo and thus removes it from sites of antibody synthesis.

Another line of evidence for the homeostatic control of immunoglobulin production by antibodies has come from studies involving the administration of antibody together or shortly before or after antigen injection. [For a comprehensive review see Uhr and Möller (67).] Most of the experiments conducted to date have examined the suppression of

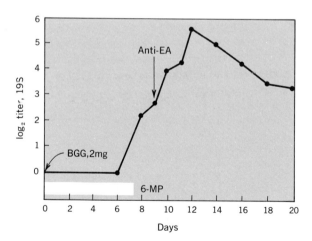

Fig. 5-17 Failure of rabbit anti-egg albumin antibodies to inhibit the synthesis of 19S bovine gamma globulin antibodies in 6-MP-treated rabbits. From Sahiar and Schwartz (66) with permission.

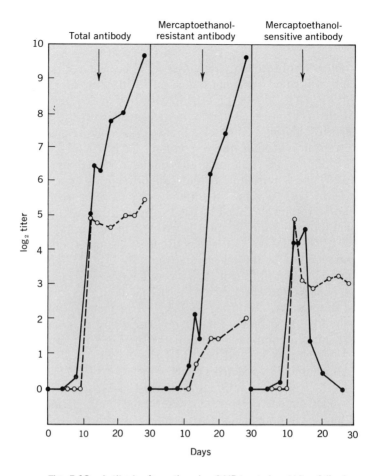

Fig. 5-18 Antibody formation in 6-MP-treated rabbits following a second injection of antigen (solid line), compared to antibody production in 6-MP-treated animals given only one injection of BGG (dashed line). From Sahiar and Schwartz (66) with permission.

antibody by whole serum, 19S and 7S immunoglobulins, and immunoglobulin fragments and have been directed to a study of the effects on primary response, "priming" of the animals, or secondary response. Uhr and Baumann (68,69) reported that the suppressive effect of immunoglobulin was specific, since horse diphtheria antitoxin suppressed, and nonspecific γ-globulin did not. These studies also showed that binding only some of the antigenic sites on the antigen will still permit the suppression to occur, since their preparations with ratios of one antigen molecule to three molecules of antibody suppressed as well as mixtures of one antigen to five antibody molecules. Antibody production to strong antigens was more difficult to suppress than to weak ones. The suppression of priming of

169

animals or of secondary responses could be achieved only with greater difficulty and could be demonstrated only with some special technical manipulations. The results of experiments by Rowley and Fitch (70,71) and Möller (72) were essentially in agreement with the original observations reported above. Using the localized hemolysis in gel technique, these investigators studied the response at the cell level in sheep erythrocytes. In addition to confirming the results obtained by Uhr and Baumann (68,69) they were able to show suppression of hemolytic plaque-forming cells by both 19S and 7S antibody. Moreover a secondary reaction could also be readily abolished by the treatment administered. For this suppression to occur antibody must be given soon after antigen administration.

The question of the effectiveness of suppression by 19S and 7S has been studied by several investigators (70–75). Whereas Möller (72) has found 7S to be efficient, Rowley and Fitch (70,71) demonstrated 19S to be suppressive. Pearlman (73) found both 19S and 7S to be effective in suppression. By using 5S (Fab')$_2$ fragments, Rowley and Fitch (74) were able to depress immune responses, thus demonstrating the need of the antigen combining piece of the antibody for suppression. The 3.5S Fab fragments showed only half the activity of 5S (Fab')$_2$. Fink and LoSpalluto (75) injected rabbits with IgG typhoid H antibody, two levels of IgM typhoid H antibody, or normal rabbit serum intravenously. Serum samples obtained from each were tested for agglutination titer 24 hours later. Each animal was then challenged with typhoid H antigen. It was found that the agglutinin titers in the control animals and low level IgM antibody recipients were similar, whereas those of the IgG recipients were considerably lower. It was also apparent that formation of IgG agglutinins was suppressed and delayed in those animals receiving IgG antibodies. Low levels of IgM appeared to have no appreciable effect on subsequent antibody formation, but some inhibitory effect in formation of 19S and 7S agglutinins was observed when higher levels were preinfused. It appears that the requirement of higher doses of IgM antibody to inhibit 19S and 7S antibody is due to the fact that IgM antibodies have shorter half-lives and less avidity than do the IgG antibodies.

The results obtained after intravenous injection of antibody are supported by those obtained after administration of Ag-Ab complexes. It was seen that antigen administered in the form of an IgG antibody excess complex induced no 7S agglutinins and low but significant levels of IgM agglutinins. On the other hand, IgM-antigen complexes induced formation of both 7S and 19S agglutinins in titers similar to those obtained with antigen alone. Since IgM antibodies appear to be less avid, and since they have a considerably shorter half-life than IgG antibodies, antigen may have been released in amounts sufficient to induce a normal immune response with IgM complexes and not with the IgG complexes.

The enhancement of tissue grafts observed in animals presensitized with antibodies against the graft has been described (76,77). Since much of the rejection phenomenon is part of the system of delayed hypersensitivity responses, this was the first indication that a humoral feedback mechanism regulates delayed hypersensitivity also. More recently, Axelrad and Rowley (77a) have shown that delayed hypersensitivity induced in rats by subcutaneous injection of sheep erythrocytes with Freund's adjuvant can be suppressed by intravenous administration of either sheep erythrocytes (which will induce an immune response of the humoral type) or rat antiserum to sheep erythrocytes. This suppressive effect of antibody upon delayed hypersensitivity has been confirmed by Stuart et al. (77b) in experiments in which renal homografts, transplanted against a major histocompatibility barrier in rats (Ag-B locus), were maintained for up to 231 days by treatment of recipients with antigen before transplantation and antiserum administered at various intervals after homografting. The best conclusion on the basis of existing data is that the production of both 19S and 7S antibody is regulated by a feedback mechanism in which the rise of one antibody beyond certain levels may eventually lead to the shutoff of the production of this antibody. The relationship between 19S and 7S in terms of their capacity to turn synthesis of each other off is not clear. Whether this is a phenomenon which is mediated through the binding of existing antigen so that it cannot stimulate further antibody production (67) or whether there is a feedback mechanism acting at the level of the producing cells (74) is also a debated question. It is apparent that at least a secondary mechanism of regulation of antibody in the serum of animals is by a feedback that is determined by increases in molecular species which will be capable of blocking further synthesis either by combining with antigen or by depressing the synthetic mechanism of cells.

Another complicating factor has been introduced by Henry and Jerne (78). These authors noted that while 7S antibody is capable of inhibiting the number of plaque-forming cells, 19S will enhance plaque-forming cell appearance as a result of immunization. This is observed only when small doses of antigen are used and can be interpreted as an enhancement of a suboptimally induced response.

The last point to be mentioned is the question of immunologic memory. (See Chap. 8 for a full review of this subject.) This is an important characteristic of the immune response, since it permits the organism to react more efficiently and strongly to a second attack by an antigen. Immunologic memory is a phenomenon which can be demonstrated upon reinjection of antigen into an animal that has already had a previous experience with that antigen. The second administration will usually lead to a shortening of the induction period, a faster rise of antibody to higher peak titers, and a more prolonged plateau and slower decline phase. Although the mechanism of this phenomenon is still unknown, it appears that this does not represent an increase in the amount of antibody synthesized by each individual cell but rather reflects the fact that there are more cells prepared for antibody production that are therefore synthesizing larger total amounts of antibody, even though each cell synthesizes the same amount (see Chap. 8). One possible interpretation is that if cells are present which have already been sensitized by antigen and have produced the ribosomal apparatus needed for the production of that specific antibody, these cells may now be capable of starting the synthetic process faster than before. For this reason one would expect the induction period to be shortened. Also, because these cells are now more numerous and, therefore, the precursor cells are in larger numbers, one would expect the titer to rise more rapidly to higher peak levels, be maintained for a longer period of time, and decline more slowly.

REFERENCES

1. Dixon, F. J.: *J. Allergy*, **25**:487, 1954.
2. Dixon, F. J.:*J. Cell. Comp. Physiol.*, **50**(Suppl. 1):27, 1957.
3. Weigle, W. O.: in "Mechanisms of Antibody Formation," M. Holub and L. Jaroskova (eds.), Czechoslovak Acad. Sciences, Prague, 1960.
4. Patterson, R., Weigle, W. O., and Dixon, F. J.: *Proc. Soc. Exp. Biol. Med.*, **105**:330, 1960.
5. La Via, M. F., Barker, P. A., and Wissler, R. W.: *J. Lab. Clin. Med.*, **48**:237, 1956.
6. Ada, G. L., Nossal, G. J. V., and Pye, J.: *Australian J. Exp. Biol. Med. Sci.* **42**:295, 1964.
7. Talmage, D. W., Dixon, F. J., Bukantz, S. C., and Dammin, G. J.: *J. Immunol.*, **67**:243, 1951.
8. Bloom, W., and Fawcett, D. W.: "A Textbook of Histology," 8th ed., W. B. Saunders Company, Philadelphia, 1962.
9. Ada, G. L., Parish, C. R., Nossal, G. J. V., and Abbot, A.: *Cold Spring Harbor Symp. Quant. Biol.*, **32**:381, 1967.
10. McDevitt, H. O.: *J. Reticuloendothel. Soc.*, **5**:256, 1968.
11. Ehrenreich, B. A., and Cohn, Z. A.: *J. Reticuloendothel. Soc.*, **5**:230, 1968.
12. Roberts, A. N., and Haurowitz, F.: *J. Exp. Med.*, **116**:407, 1962.
13. Gitlin, D.: *Proc. Soc. Exp. Biol. Med.*, **74**:138, 1950.
14. Gitlin, D., Landing, B. H., and Whipple, A.: *Proc. Soc. Exp. Biol. Med.*, **78**:631, 1951.
15. McMaster, P. D., and Kruse, H.: *J. Exp. Med.*, **94**:323, 1951.
16. Coons, A. H., Leduc, E. H., and Kaplan, M. H.: *J. Exp. Med.*, **93**:173, 1951.
17. Haurowitz, F., and Crampton, C. F.: *J. Immunol.*, **68**:73, 1952.

18. Crampton, C. F., Reller, H. H., and Haurowitz, F.: *J. Immunol.*, **71**:319, 1953.
19. Garvey, J. S., and Campbell, D. H.: *J. Immunol.*, **76**:36, 1956.
20. Hawkins, J. D., and Haurowitz, F.: *Biochem. J.*, **80**:200, 1961.
21. Manner, G., Gould, B. S., and Slayter, H. S.: *Biochim. Biophys. Acta,* **108**:659, 1965.
22. Uhr, J. W., and Weissmann, G.: *J. Reticuloendothel. Soc.*, **5**:243, 1968.
23. Scharff, M. D., Shatkin, A. J., Jr., and Levintow, L.: *Proc. Nat. Acad. Sci. U.S.*, **50**:686, 1963.
24. Fishman, M., and Adler, F. L.: *J. Exp. Med.*, **117**:595, 1963.
25. Friedman, H. P., Stavitsky, A. B., and Solomon, J. M.: *Science,* **149**:1106, 1965.
26. Askonas, B. A., and Rhodes, J. M.: *Nature (London)*, **205**:470, 1965.
27. Gottlieb, A. A., Glišin, V. R., and Doty, P.: *Proc. Nat. Acad. Sci. U.S.*, **57**:1849, 1967.
27a. Gottlieb, A. A., and Straus, D. S.: *J. Biol. Chem.*, **224**:3324, 1969.
27b. Gottlieb, A. A.: *Science,* **165**:592, 1969.
28. Bishop, D. C., and Abramoff, P.: *J. Reticuloendothel. Soc.*, **4**:441, 1967.
29. Roelants, G. E., and Goodman, J. W.: *Biochemistry (Wash.)*, **7**:1432, 1968.
30. Gottlieb, A. A.: *Biochemistry,* **8**:2111, 1969.
31. Adler, F. L., Fishman, M., and Dray, S.: *J. Immunol.*, **97**:554, 1966.
32. Chin, P. H., and Silverman, M. S.: *J. Immunol.*, **99**:476, 1967.
33. Chin, P. H., and Silverman, M. S.: *J. Immunol.*, **99**:489, 1967.
34. Schoenberg, M. D., Mumaw, V. R., Moore, R. D., and Weisberger, A. S.: *Science,* **143**:964, 1964.
35. Wellensiek, H. J., and Coons, A. H.: *J. Exp. Med.*, **119**:685, 1964.
36. Roberts, A. N.: *Amer. J. Pathol.*, **44**:411, 1964.
37. Makinodan, T., and Albright, J. F.: *Progr. Allergy*, **10**:1, 1967.
38. Felton, L. D.: *J. Immunol.*, **61**:107, 1949.
39. Stark, O. K.: *J. Immunol.*, **74**:130, 1955.
40. Heidelberger, M.: in "The Nature and Significance of the Antibody Response," A. M. Pappenheimer, Jr. (ed.), Columbia University Press, New York, 1953.
41. Haurowitz, F., Reller, H. H., and Walter, H.: *J. Immunol.*, **75**:417, 1955.
42. Campbell, D. H., and Garvey, J. S.: *Advan. Immunol.*, **3**:261, 1963.
43. Haurowitz, F.: "Immunochemistry and the Biosynthesis of Antibodies," Interscience-Wiley, New York, 1968.
44. Cohen, E. P., and Raska, K., Jr.: *Cold Spring Harbor Symp. Quant. Biol.*, **32**:349, 1967.
45. Uhr, J. W.: *Science,* **145**:457, 1964.
46. Taliaferro, W. H., and Talmage, D. W.: *J. Infect. Dis.*, **97**:88, 1955.
47. Šterzl, J.:*Nature (London)*, **185**:256, 1960.
48. La Via, M. F.: *Proc. Soc. Exp. Biol. Med.*, **114**:133, 1963.
49. Abramoff, P., and Brien, N. B.: *J. Immunol.*, **100**:1204, 1968.
49a. Jerne, N. K., and Nordin, A. A.: *Science,* **140**:405, 1963.

50. La Via, M. F.: *J. Immunol.*, **92**:252, 1964.
51. Schultze, H. E., and Heremans, J. F.: "Molecular Biology of Human Proteins," vol. 1, Elsevier Publishing Company, Amsterdam, 1966.
52. Uhr, J. W., and Finkelstein, M. S.: *Progr. Allergy*, **10**:37, 1967.
53. Benedict, A. A., Brown, R. J., and Hersh, R. T.: *J. Immunol.*, **90**:399, 1963.
54. Uhr, J. W., Finkelstein, M. S., and Franklin, E. C.: *Proc. Soc. Exp. Biol. Med.*, **111**:13, 1962.
55. Grey, H. M.: *J. Immunol.*, **91**:819, 1963.
56. Taliaferro, W. H., Taliaferro, L. G., and Pizzi, A. K.: *J. Infect. Dis.*, **105**:197, 1959.
57. Eisen, H. N., and Siskind, G. W.: *Biochemistry (Wash.)*, **3**:996, 1964.
58. Finkelstein, M. S., and Uhr, J. W.: *J. Immunol.*, **97**:565, 1966.
59. Grey, H. M.: *Immunology*, **7**:82, 1964.
60. Robbins, J. B., Kenny, K., and Suter, E.: *J. Exp. Med.*, **122**:385, 1965.
61. Jerne, N. K., and Avegno, P.: *J. Immunol.*, **76**:200, 1956.
62. Campbell, D. H., and Garvey, J. S.: *Advan. Immunol.*, **3**:261, 1963.
63. Uhr, J. W.: *Science*, **145**:457, 1964.
64. Svehag, S. E., and Mandel, B.: *J. Exp. Med.*, **119**:21, 1964.
65. Gill, T. J., III, Kunz, H. W., and Papermaster, D. S.: *J. Biol. Chem.*, **242**:3308, 1967.
66. Sahiar, K., and Schwartz, R. S.: *J. Immunol.*, **95**:345, 1965.
67. Uhr, J. W., and Möller, G.: *Advan. Immunol.*, **8**:81, 1968.
68. Uhr, J. W., and Baumann, J. B.: *J. Exp. Med.*, **113**:935, 1961.
69. Uhr, J. W., and Baumann, J. B.: *J. Exp. Med.*, **113**:959, 1961.
70. Rowley, D. A., and Fitch, F. W.: *J. Exp. Med.*, **121**:671, 1965.
71. Rowley, D. A., and Fitch, F. W.: *J. Exp. Med.*, **121**:683, 1965.
72. Möller, G.: in "Gamma Globulins," Nobel Symp. 3, J. Killander (ed.), Interscience-Wiley, New York, 1967.
73. Pearlman, D. S.: *J. Exp. Med.*, **126**:127, 1967.
74. Rowley, D. A., and Fitch, F. W.: in "Regulation of the Antibody Response," B. Cinader (ed.), Charles C Thomas, Springfield, Ill., 1968.
75. Fink, C. W., and LoSpalluto, J. J.: *Immunology*, **12**:259, 1967.
76. Kaliss, N.: *Cancer Res.*, **18**:992, 1958.
77. Möller, G.: *J. Immunol.*, **96**:430, 1966.
77a. Axelrad, M. A., and Rowley, D. A.: *Science*, **160**:1465, 1968.
77b. Stuart, F. P., Saitoh, T., and Fitch, F. W.: *Science*, **160**:1463, 1968.
78. Henry, C., and Jerne, N. K.: *J. Exp. Med.*, **128**:133, 1968.

6
Cellular Sites of Antibody Synthesis

An individual is made up of many cells, each with a specific function necessary for the functional integrity of the whole organism. Although it appears reasonable to assume that they could be pluripotential, since they all have the same amount of DNA and thus the same information, in actuality there is considerable division of labor in multicellular organisms. The immune response is a series of complex reactions and interactions leading to the synthesis of a unique protein endowed with a high degree of specificity. It is apparent that such a remarkable series of phenomena must have a cellular basis. This chapter will examine the cells, tissues, and organs which are endowed with the property of responding to antigenic stimuli with the production of specific antibodies. This ability to produce antibodies resides in the lymphoreticular system, a complex system of cells located in various parts of the body of vertebrates. Its development is paralleled by the development of immunologic responsiveness. For this reason, it is believed that the immune response is a function of the lymphoreticular cells (see Chap. 4).

LYMPHORETICULAR SYSTEM: MORPHOLOGY AND PHYSIOLOGY

Knowledge of the lymphoreticular system is still incomplete, since many of the complex interrelationships between cells of this system are not understood. The lymphoreticular system includes many diverse cells primarily located in close relationship to the reticulum of fibers which is prominent in lymphoid- and blood-forming organs (Fig. 6-1). In addition, a system of reticular fibers is present in other organs, such as the liver and lungs, and is distributed in varying amounts throughout the body. The small lymphocyte is the most characteristic cell of this system and the most numerous (Fig. 6-2). It usually measures up to 7 μ in diameter and consists of a nucleus surrounded by a thin rim of cytoplasm. Electron microscopic observations reveal that the nucleus has clumps of heterochromatin lying close to the nuclear membrane and separated by areas of less tightly arranged euchromatin. Heterochromatin can sometimes be found toward the center of the nucleus. The cytoplasm is a very thin layer containing a few polysomes and mitochondria. Usually no other subcellular organelles are seen in small lymphocytes. In addition, the family of lymphoid cells includes larger cells with nuclei of the appearance described above and with different cytoplasmic characters (Fig. 6-3). These cells include the medium and large lymphocytes, a classification dependent on their size and appearance as observed by light and electron microscopic examination. They are larger than small lymphocytes; their cytoplasm contains many polysomes, varying amounts of rough endoplasmic reticulum, a Golgi apparatus, and many mitochondria. They vary in size from 7 to 12 μ.

Another important component of the lymphorecticular system is the macrophage (Fig. 6-4). This is a large cell, usually 15 to 20 μ in diameter, irregularly shaped, with a large amount of cytoplasm and a medium-sized nucleus. The nucleus contains tightly packed heterochromatin distributed in a thin rim close to the nuclear membrane and in a few clumps throughout the remainder of the nucleus. The largest amount of chromatin is the finely divided, granular or filamentous, euchromatin type. The cytoplasm is characterized by the presence of numerous digestive vacuoles and lysosomes in various stages of development containing material which has been ingested by the cell. This cell has phagocytic properties and maintains a clean environment by removing foreign matter, which is ingested and digested. For this reason the lysosomes are highly developed and contain numerous hydrolytic enzymes which are necessary for digestion of foreign matter.

The reticular cell is morphologically similar to the macrophage (Fig. 6-5). It is usually an elongated cell with an elongate nucleus occupying

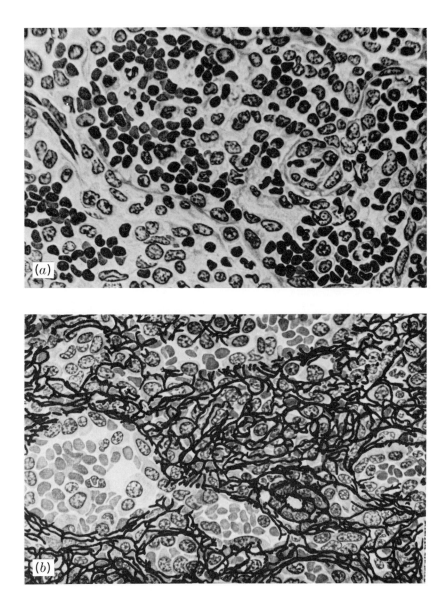

Fig. 6-1 Human spleen sections stained with H and E (a) and with H and E after Bielschowsky impregnation for reticular fibers (b) × 600. From Bloom and Fawcett (1) with permission.

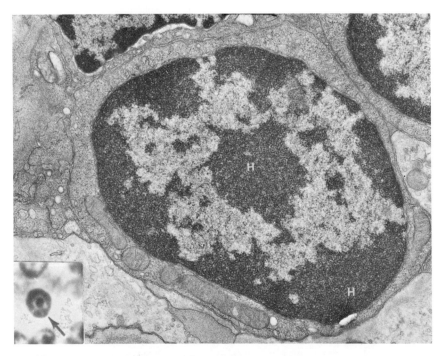

Fig. 6-2 Typical small lymphocyte of the rat spleen. As observed with the electron microscope, this cell shows the characteristic nucleus with clumps of heterochromatin (H) fibers packed close to the nuclear envelope and in the center. A thin cytoplasmic rim with a few ribosomes and mitochondria surrounds the nucleus. The insert shows the same cell viewed with the light microscope.

the central portion of the cell and a fairly abundant cytoplasm surrounding the nucleus. It is a nondescript cell, since it does not assume any of the commonly used histologic stains in any degree. The nucleus has finely divided granular and filamentous chromatin with a few clumps of scattered heterochromatin and a thin layer of heterochromatin adjacent to the nuclear membrane. Usually no nucleoli are present. The cell cytoplasm is devoid of organelles, contains only a few ribosomes, a few polyribosomes, and an occasional mitochondrion. Sometimes a Golgi region is apparent.

The plasma cell, the fifth member of the lymphoreticular family of cells, has a characteristic appearance and is easily recognized by light and electron microscopy (Fig. 6-6). It is an elongated cell, about 2 to 3 times the size of a small lymphocyte, with an oval-shaped nucleus with its major axis perpendicular to the major axis of the cell. Light microscopy reveals a clear area near the nucleus which, under electron microscopy, appears to be a highly developed Golgi apparatus. The cytoplasm of this cell is characteristically filled by widely dilated cisternae of endoplasmic reticulum, which usually contain protein synthesized by the cell (Fig. 6-7). The Golgi region is highly developed. The nucleus is typically lymphoid, with large clumps of heterochromatin dispersed around the nuclear membrane. One or more prominent nucleoli are usually present within the nucleus (1-3).

It is apparent that these cells are related to each other, since they are often found close together; it appears that they transform into one another easily. Our present understanding of the interrelationships of these cells is meager, since the methods available for an investigative approach to this problem have not been sufficiently precise to be conclusive. Apparently the reticular cell is a multipotential blast cell; that is, it will differentiate

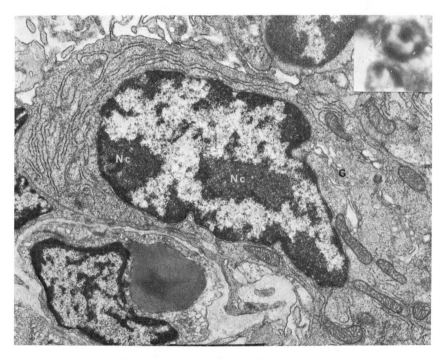

Fig. 6-3 An "intermediate cell" observed during antibody response is shown. The nucleus has the characteristics seen in lymphocytes and in addition exhibits prominent nucleoli (Nc). The cytoplasm is greatly expanded and cisternae of granular endoplasmic reticulum are apparent. The Golgi region (G) is well developed. In the insert, the same cell is seen by light microscopy.

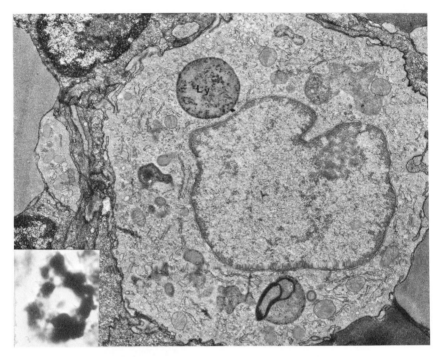

Fig. 6-4 The macrophage of the rat spleen has a small nucleus with a thin rim of marginated heterochromatin. The cytoplasm contains granular endoplasmic reticulum, several mitochondria, and lysosomes (Ly) in various stages of development. In the insert, a macrophage is observed by light microscopy.

in any one of a number of directions according to the stimulus received (1). It appears that the small lymphocyte is derived by division and transformation of reticular cells under thymic control (4). The lymphocyte seems to exist as a multipotential antigen target cell. Thus, the small lymphocyte appears to be an immunocompetent cell which, upon stimulation with the appropriate antigen, may divide, differentiate, and ultimately give rise to plasma cells (5). Furthermore, the plasma cell may be capable of transformation back to a small lymphocyte by shedding its cytoplasm and reforming a lymphocyte-like cytoplasm (6). On the other hand, observations exist which indicate that a small lymphocyte may become a macrophage by direct transformation and ingestion of phagocytosable material (7). The reticular cell also appears capable of giving rise to macrophages (1). Studies of the physiology and kinetics of lymphoid cells have indicated that two distinct populations of lymphocytes exist with a different life-span, different functions, and perhaps somewhat different morphology (8).

ARCHITECTURE OF LYMPHOID ORGANS

Thymus

The thymus is a small organ usually located behind the upper margin of the sternum within the thoracic cavity (Fig. 6-8). In most animals it is made up of several lobes, enveloped by a capsule from which trabeculae originate and form a network which subdivides the organ into a regular series of interconnected "chambers." The arrangement of cells within these saclike areas is such that a cortical and a medullary area can be distinguished. They differ in the arrangement of small lymphocytes which are densely packed in the cortical area but loose in the medullary area. The medullary area also contains several reticular cells. This area is much

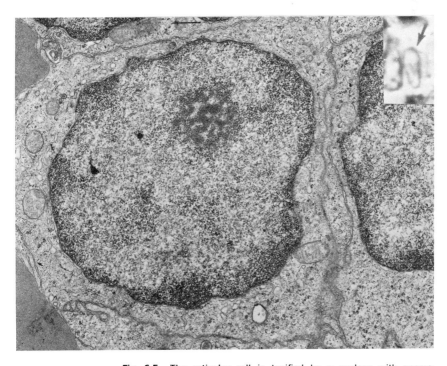

Fig. 6-5 The reticular cell is typified by a nucleus with sparse euchromatin and a few clumps of heterochromatin close to the nuclear envelope. The cytoplasm contains a few ribosomes, mitochondria, and an occasional cisterna of granular endoplasmic reticulum. The insert shows a reticular cell as seen with the light microscope.

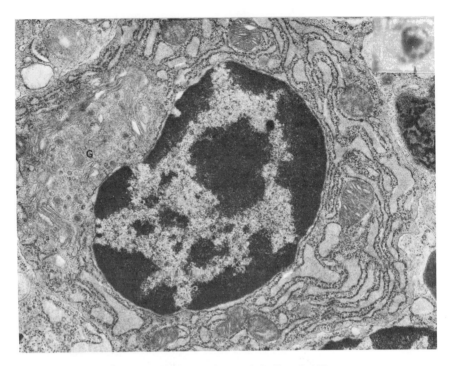

Fig. 6-6 Plasma cells still maintain the characteristic "lymphoid" nucleus. The abundant cytoplasm is packed with granular endoplasmic reticulum cisternae. Mitochondria are tightly bound by the endoplasmic reticulum. The Golgi region (G) is highly developed. The insert shows many of these features as seen with the light microscope.

paler staining and appears lighter than the cortical area. Although no precise line of demarcation can be distinguished between these two areas, they can be identified by the staining properties and arrangement of the cells. In addition to small lymphocytes the thymus has a number of larger lymphocytes and a large number of cells in mitotic division. Located within the medulla are the so-called Hassall's bodies, which consist of cells arranged in a concentrical manner and giving rise to a structure which, in many cases, is partially hyalinized.

Lymph Node

The structure of the lymph node is similar to the thymus (Fig. 6-9). A capsule sends trabeculae into the node, with the formation of saclike areas in which lymphocytes are arranged in a cortical and medullary pattern. The lymph nodes have a hilus through which both lymphatic and blood vessels enter and leave the node. These vessels are distributed throughout the lymph node and ultimately form an open sinusoidal network so that cells can move freely in and out of the vascular spaces. Lymph nodes are primarily composed of small lymphocytes as well as some plasma and reticular cells. Generally speaking, the same cell types are found within the lymph nodes as in the thymus.

Spleen

The spleen is the largest single lymphoid organ, and its structure is similar to that of the thymus and lymph nodes (Fig. 6-10). The capsule is collagenous in nature, like most other organs, and sends trabeculae into the splenic parenchyma. The trabeculae are pierced by trabecular veins that course within them. The arteries of the spleen subdivide as they leave the hilus and eventually become surrounded by a sheath of small lymphocytes to form the Malpighian follicle. In many cases a number of larger lympho-

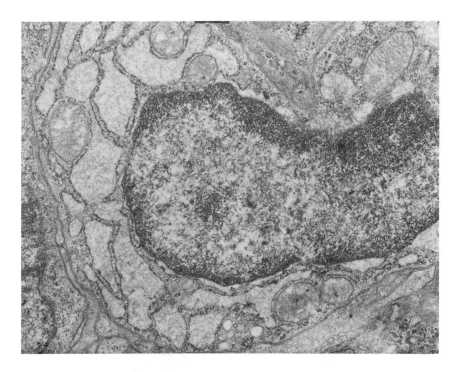

Fig. 6-7 A plasma cell from the rat splenic red pulp. Note the filamentous and granular material filling the cisternae and the ribosomes lined on the cisternal membranes.

cytes with mitotic figures are found in the center of the follicle. This is called the germinal center, since it appears that new lymphocytes may arise from this area. The follicles make up the white pulp of the spleen. The remainder of the spleen, the so-called red pulp, contains a network of sinusoids surrounded by varied cell types. Erythrocytes are abundant, since the spleen is endowed with the function of destruction of old erythrocytes. The spleen also contains macrophages, reticular cells, lymphocytes, fibroblasts, and other cells of the lymphoreticular system. The red pulp tissue merges gradually with the white pulp tissue at the marginal zone, an area surrounding the white pulp nodules and composed primarily of lymphocytes.

Other accumulations of lymphoid tissue occur along the gastrointestinal tract. These are the Peyer's patches and the appendix. They are generally organized like other lymphoid organs and consist of a cortical area with tightly packed small lymphocytes and a medullary area with more loosely packed cells. The medullary area contains a larger number of

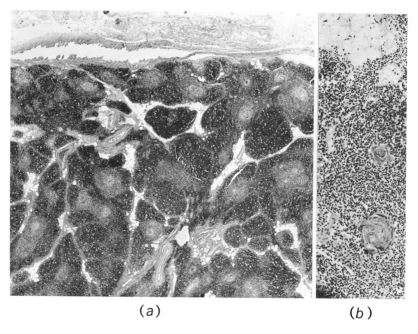

(a)   (b)

Fig. 6-8 Low-power views of the human thymus to show the architecture of this organ. In (a) the capsule can be seen subdividing the lobes of the thymus. Lighter areas are the medullary portion and the darker stains are the cortical areas. In (b) two Hassall's corpuscles are illustrated. Photograph courtesy of R. P. Morehead.

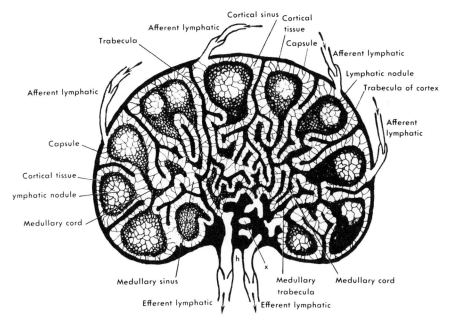

Fig. 6-9 A schematic representation of the lymph node structure. From Bloom and Fawcett (1) with permisssion.

less mature or less differentiated lymphocytes and sometimes a germinal center.

HISTOLOGY AND CYTOLOGY OF THE IMMUNE RESPONSE

Chapter 5 examined our present knowledge of the events that accompany antigen entry into cells and the mechanisms by which antigenic stimuli may reach the antigen target cells. To summarize, it appears that antigen may be stimulating antigen target cells in one of several ways: (1) antigen may be taken up by the antigen target cell; (2) antigen may act by associating with antigen target cells and stimulating them without penetrating the cell by a series of membrane phenomena; (3) antigen may be picked up by a phagocytic cell and a stimulus transmitted from the phagocytic cell to the antigen target cell. The third instance may involve one of three possible mechanisms: (*a*) release of informational RNA which may stimulate the cell to produce antibody; (*b*) release of some by-product of antigenic material which will enter the antigen target cell and stimulate it to initiate synthesis; (*c*) release of RNA in combination with antigenic material. It appears that antigen or some carrier of antigenic information

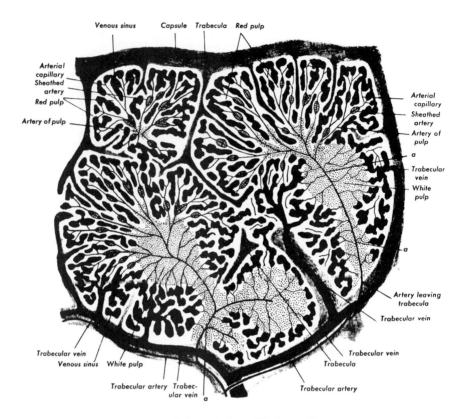

Venous sinus   Capsule   Trabecula   Red pulp

Arterial
capillary
Sheathed
artery
Red pulp
Artery of pulp

Arterial
capillary
Sheathed
artery
Artery of
pulp
a
Trabecular
vein
White
pulp

a

Artery leaving
trabecula
Trabecular vein

Trabecular vein
Venous sinus   White pulp

Trabecular vein
Trabecula

Trabecular artery   Trabecular vein
a

Trabecular artery

Fig. 6-10 Schematic diagram of the splenic architecture. From Bloom and Fawcett (1) with permission.

must interact with antigen target cells to stimulate them to produce antibody.

The spleen, lymph nodes, the lymphoid portion of the bone marrow, and other nodules of lymphoid tissue throughout the body, such as the Peyer's patches, appendix, etc., are the primary areas where antibody production occurs. Under special conditions small nodules of lymphoid tissue can arise in other locations and antibody may be produced there. Antibody production has occurred in alum granulomas (9), lung (10), and various other organs where lymphoid tissues are found [reviewed by McMaster (11)].

The initial events which follow injection of antigen into an immunocompetent experimental animal are not understood at present. The introduction of antigen is followed by a lag phase, which is interpreted as being a preparatory phase (12). Some workers have denied the existence of such a phase, ascribing the inability to detect antibodies during this time to our insensitive methods of measuring immune responses (see Chap. 5).

Baker and Landy (13) have shown that the response to Vi antigen of
E. coli and to type I pneumococcal capsular polysaccharide is characterized
by the appearance of "antigen reactive cells (ARC)" as early as 4 hours
after immunization. Their demonstration is based on the specific attachment of bentonite particles coated with antigen to lymphoid cells of the
primarily immunized animals. The response appears to be similar to that
observed in hyperimmunized animals and could be characteristic of a
secondary, rather than a primary, response. Considerable evidence suggests that this lag phase or induction period is a real occurrence. An
experimental demonstration has been offered by Taliaferro and Talmage
(12) (see Chap. 5). Immunized rabbits were injected with S^{35}-labeled
amino acids and their minced spleens transferred to irradiated recipients
soon after immunization. The antibody produced in the recipients did not
appear to be radioactive. It was concluded that no antibody was synthesized in the time that elapsed before lymph node transfer. The same question has been extensively examined by Sterzl (14), who has shown that
antigen administered to adult pigs did not change the number of antibody-
forming cells for the first 24 hours after immunization. Furthermore, if
antigen was given to newborn sterile pigs in a dose capable of inducing an
immune response, 36 hours had to elapse before antibody-forming cells
were detected. This occurred in the presence of a massive dose of antigen
(20 ml of a concentrated sheep erythrocyte suspension). It seems logical
that such an induction period should exist, since a finite amount of time
is necessary to synthesize the essential ribosomal and messenger RNA.
Several experiments have shown that during the first 24 to 48 hours after
immunization: (1) active RNA synthesis takes place; (2) both mRNA and
rRNA are synthesized; (3) agents which inhibit antibody synthesis are
particularly active because they interfere with the synthesis of RNA (see
Chaps. 5 and 10). These events can also be followed by morphological
studies, which have shown an accumulation of ribosomal aggregates in
lymphoid cells with enlargement of the cytoplasm and hypertrophy of the
nucleolus (15). Functional studies, on the other hand, have shown that
no antibody-forming cells can be detected until the second day after
immunization by means of the localized hemolysis in gel technique (16).
It can be concluded that antigen injection is followed by a short period
characterized by active RNA synthesis and beginning of differentiation of
lymphoid cells without any demonstrable antibody synthesis (see Chap. 5).

The first cellular changes seen in lymph nodes and spleen occur in
the lymphoid follicle. Antigenic materials percolate through the follicles
(see Chap. 5) and are distributed to some of the follicular cells (17).
However, most of the antigen moves into the sinusoid surrounding the
follicle and spreads into the medullary areas of the lymph nodes and the

red pulp of the spleen (17). Shortly after injection of antigen and antigen trapping in these areas, cell division occurs. Numerous mitotic figures are observed in the areas where antigen has localized, and immunofluorescent staining methods reveal that these dividing cells contain antibody (18) (Fig. 6-11). Cells in division have also been observed by microcinematography in the middle of hemolytic plaques (19) (Fig. 6-12). The dividing time of these cells is estimated to be 40 minutes. Recently, plasma cells in division with apparent granular endoplasmic reticulum have been observed by electron microscopy (20) (Fig. 6-13). Soon after antigen injection and uptake, mitoses are abundant. As outlined in Chap. 10, several studies, primarily with x-radiation and other treatments known to inhibit the immune response, have shown that the proliferation of cells is absent when antibody production is inhibited. This has provided another link between the processes of cell division and antibody formation. Nossal (21) and Makinodan and Albright (22) have also provided experimental

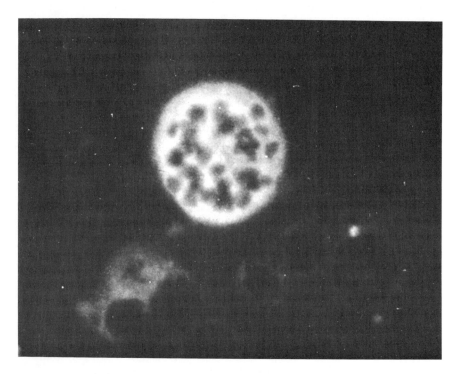

Fig. 6-11 A cell in mitosis, as indicated by the free chromosomal masses, stained by immunofluorescent methods to demonstrate its antibody content. Photograph courtesy of J. J. Vazquez.

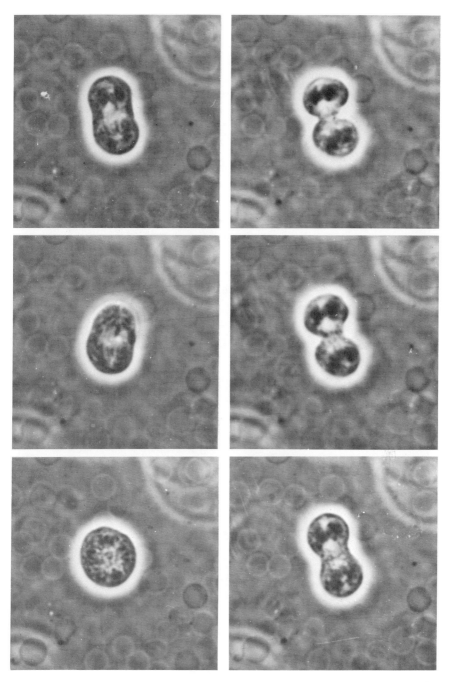

Fig. 6-12 The mitosis of a cell in the center of a hemolytic plaque viewed by time-lapse photography. From Claflin and Smithies (19) with permission.

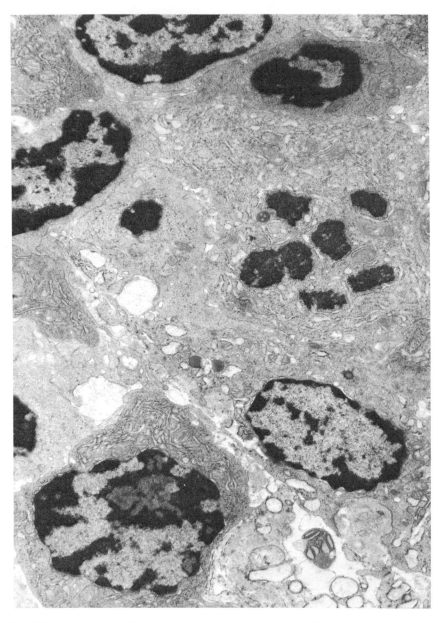

Fig. 6-13 A cluster of plasma cells in mouse splenic fragment with a dividing plasma cell in the center.

evidence of the cellular proliferation accompanying antibody formation. Nossal, studying rats immunized with *S. typhi* antigens, showed that antibody-forming cells take up tritiated thymidine and divide to give rise to more antibody-forming cells. Makinodan and Albright (22), on the other hand, used mice immunized with sheep erythrocytes and studied spleen cells explanted into irradiated recipients. They were also able to show an increase in antibody-forming cell members by actual counts of cells maintained in semipermeable chambers in the peritoneal cavity of x-radiated mice. It is apparent that cellular proliferation is a necessary factor for the initiation of the cellular events leading to antibody production.

The next series of events to follow is the differentiation of the products of this cell division. The histologic pattern of response to immunization has been described by several authors. The first observations can be traced to the work of Bjørneboe and Gormsen (23), who described the accumulation of very high numbers of plasma cells in lymphoid tissue of hyperimmunized animals. Typical plasma cells also accumulated in such areas as the perirenal fat after immunization had been continued for months with daily injections of horse serum. Fagraeus (24), in a classic monograph, next described the cellular proliferation which follows injection of antigen, demonstrating by tissue culture techniques that the areas of the spleen involved in the production of antibody are in the red pulp. With the aid of a microscope, the spleen was dissected into red and white pulp pieces and cultured. It was found that cellular proliferation occurred primarily in the red pulp and that the antibody activity was higher in tissue culture fluid from red pulp cultures. This work was carried out in hyperimmunized rabbits. Ehrich et al. (25) and Harris and Harris (26) also showed that rabbits immunized with various antigens accumulated lymphoid cells in the medullary areas of the lymph node. This proliferation was always present after antigen injection and during the production of antibodies. These two groups extended their observations to include chemical analysis of the nodes, thus showing that there was an increase in both RNA and DNA, as would be expected as a result of cell division and accumulation of mRNA and ribosomes. Makinodan et al. (27,38) described the same type of cellular reaction in the spleen of chickens immunized with BSA. The results were interpreted as showing that the red pulp of the spleen of these animals had the major role in supporting the proliferation of plasma cells leading to the production of antibody. La Via et al. (29) and Wissler et al. (30) also demonstrated an increase in lymphoid cells in the splenic red pulp after immunization with *S. typhi*. The cells were pyroninophilic, and the pyroninophilia increased with time, thus indicating a progressive accumulation of RNA. This reaction took place entirely in the red pulp of the spleen. Mitosis was very prominent in the splenic red pulp and preceded cell differentiation. Ward et al. (31) injected rabbits with BGG and found that the cellular proliferation observed was primarily in the follicular areas of the spleen. Langevoort (32) tried to determine the site of the histologic reaction that follows immunization and related the cells which proliferate in response to antigen to the areas of the spleen in the vicinity of the follicles. It appeared from this work that antibody-forming cells arise primarily in the periarteriolar sheath present in the vicinity of the follicle. Hanna (33) recently made similar observations, implicating the follicular portion of the spleen as the area where the primary reaction in response to antigens occurs.

In summary, it appears that following the introduction of antigen, there is a sizable increase in the number of cells in the red or white pulp of the spleen and in the medullary or cortical areas or lymph nodes. The cells are characterized by increasingly pyroninophilic cytoplasm and a large nucleus with blocked chromatin. The bulk of the evidence favors this type of reaction, although disagreement exists as to whether the reaction occurs primarily in the red pulp of the spleen and the medullary area of the lymph node or primarily in the white pulp of the spleen and the cortical area of the lymph node. These differences could be interpreted as being due to different antigens, different animal species, or different modes of injection. It is clear, however, that the production of antibody induces, at the histologic level, a series of reactions which lead to an increase in the number of cells with a high content of RNA. These cells are apparently responsible for antibody production (Fig. 6-14).

The next step in the study of the morphology of immune responses came with the demonstration by Coons et al. (34,35) that the newly proliferated cells contain antibody. This was accomplished by conjugating the antibody to a fluorescent dye, fluorescein. The tissue section was then treated with the appropriate antigen. This antigen combined with the antibody present in cells. The section was treated again with the fluorescein-labeled antibody and combined with the antigen. This resulted in a layering of antibody in the cells, antigen on top of it, and fluorescein-labeled antibody on top of this antigen layer (sandwich technique) (Fig. 6-15). When the preparation was exposed to ultraviolet light, the fluorescence of fluorescein was excited and became visible wherever the labeled antibody had reacted with antigen, which in turn was combined with cellular antibody (Fig. 6-16). It was thus demonstrated that antibody was present in cells in the areas of proliferation. The ultrastructural studies of dePetris and Karlsbad (36) and of Leduc et al. (37) have been helpful in elucidating the type of cellular response observed in

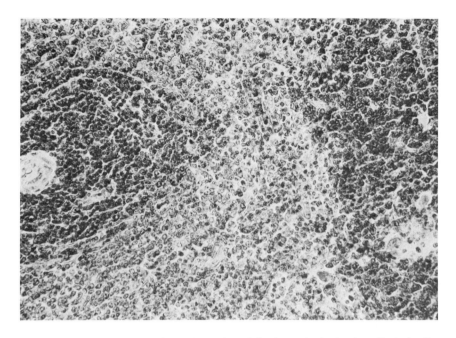

Fig. 6-14 This section of the immunized rat spleen illustrates the accumulation of pyronin-staining cells in the red pulp on the fourth day after antigen injection.

immunized animals. The former authors used ferritin as antigen. They demonstrated the presence of antiferritin antibody by reacting ferritin with the antibody in tissue sections. Electron microscopic observation disclosed the presence of the antibody in the cisternae of the endoplasmic reticulum. Leduc used rabbits hyperimmunized with the enzyme horseradish peroxidase and localized the antibody by reacting antigen (horse-

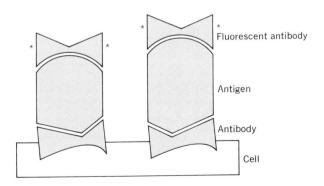

Fig. 6-15 Schematic representation of the "sandwich" method used to detect antibody in cells by immunofluorescence techniques.

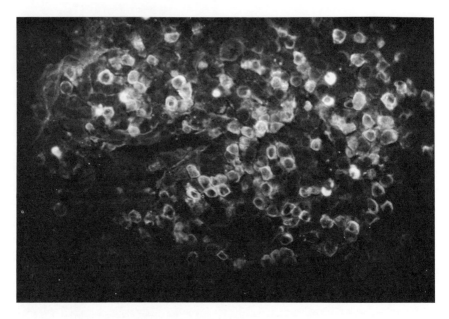

Fig. 6-16 Antibody containing cells of the rabbit popliteal lymph node 4 days after a secondary stimulation with bovine serum albumin. The cells were stained with unlabeled antigen followed by labeled antibody. Photograph courtesy of A. H. Coons.

radish peroxidase) with it in tissue sections. Carrying out the enzymatic reaction for the peroxidase yielded an electron opaque product. Under electron microscopy this opaque product was apparent in the nuclear cisternae of cells still devoid of other endoplasmic reticulum and successively in the cisternae of the granular endoplasmic reticulum (Fig. 6-17).

In summary, it can be stated that antibody production is dependent on cell differentiation and that antibody can be demonstrated in the cells which differentiate by immunohistochemical methods. This differentiation is preceded and accompanied by abundant mitotic activity which is inhibited by treatments which depress antibody production. The process of cellular response to antigen injection is then one of differentiation which is preceded by active cell division. The mitotic figures observed have also been shown to contain antibody, and in fact, cells in division during antibody production have been observed by microcinematography. The event accompanying this massive cellular proliferation and differentiation is a considerable increase in the size of lymphoid organs during the immune response. However, in most cases, by the end of the first week after the primary immunization, the active proliferation subsides and the organ involved returns to a close to normal size.

CELLULAR EVENTS

It would be useful to review some of the cells observed during antibody production and to correlate them with one another. As an introduction let us trace the development of ideas about the cells involved in an immune response. The macrophage played an important role, since numerous studies purported to show that this cell was solely responsible for the production of antibodies (9,38). While some experimental facts are still difficult to reconcile, the general belief today is that macrophages do not have any antibody-synthesizing activity and that their role in antibody production is to somehow manipulate antigens so as to render them available for the antigen target cells (see Chap. 5). The lymphocyte and the plasma cell were strongly propounded by two separate groups, each proposing one or the other as the sole manufacturer of antibody (25,26).

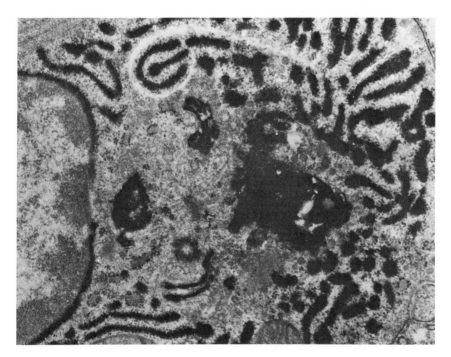

Fig. 6-17 Electron micrograph of a plasma cell from an animal immunized with horseradish peroxidase. The cell was treated with the enzyme and then reacted with a substrate to form a precipitate where the substrate reacted with antibody-bound enzyme. Photograph courtesy of E. H. Leduc.

Thus, three cells of the lymphoreticular system were connected with the immune response.

The process by which the reticular cell gives rise to lymphocytes is somehow controlled by the thymus (see Chap. 4). This may occur by a mitotic process which, at least in some cases, must be asymmetric. Thus one blast cell may give rise to a lymphocyte and to another lymphocyte and another blast cell (39). This mechanism is similar to the one involved in the differentiation of primitive blood-forming cells (40). It must operate in this manner if one is to account for the maintenance of a population of stem cells capable of giving rise to more lymphocytes as time goes on (Fig. 6-18). Thus four members of the lymphoreticular family of cells have been implicated in antibody production. Although ideas as to their respective roles have changed, it appears true that they are all active participants in immune responses.

The role of the macrophage as a possible antigen processor has already been discussed (see Chaps. 5 and 11). The lymphocyte appears to be the most likely candidate for the role of antigen target cell (41). It has traditionally been regarded as a terminal, or end-stage, cell, incapable of further division or transformation. However, recent experiments have modified our ideas on small lymphocytes (42) by revealing that the lymphocyte is indeed capable of dividing and differentiating into a medium and large lymphocyte and ultimately into a plasma cell producing immunoglobulin. Both in vitro and in vivo studies substantiate this idea, and it is commonly accepted that the lymphocyte can give rise to less differentiated cells with protein-synthesizing capabilities. Thus, a small lymphocyte may be an antigen target cell, and it may divide upon antigenic stimulation to produce two cells capable of further division and differentiation into

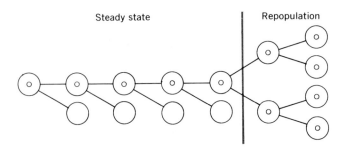

Fig. 6-18 A schematic representation of steady-state maintenance of cell population by asymmetric division and repopulation by symmetric division. From Talmage and Claman (39) with permission.

antibody-forming cells. Some experimental evidence of this role of the lymphocyte has recently been provided by Nossal et al. (41), who have succeeded in concentrating small lymphocytes from thoracic duct effluent. They have shown that the whole population of thoracic duct cells will respond to both sheep erythrocyte and *S. typhi* antigens. However, if small lymphocytes only are exposed to these antigens, the response to sheep erythrocytes is good but the response to *S. typhi* is absent. Although sheep erythrocyte antigens appear to be very active in stimulating small lymphocytes to produce antibody, the antigens of *S. typhosa* use as their antigen target cell both small and large lymphocytes. It is conceivable that these larger lymphocytes could have already initiated differentiation in the direction of plasma cells. Once a lymphocyte divides and differentiation starts, free polyribosomes begin to increase rapidly in the daughter cells (15) (Fig. 6-19). These polysomes are needed to support the active protein synthesis taking place in these cells. It has also been shown that new species of RNA are formed to code for the new protein to be made

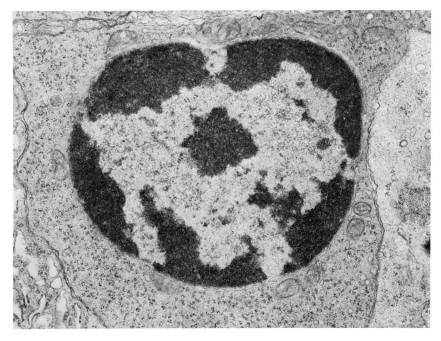

Fig. 6-19 A "large lymphocyte" as seen with the electron microscope. Note the large cytoplasm with numerous clusters of ribosomes.

(see Chaps. 5 and 7). Further differentiation leads to the appearance of a granular endoplasmic reticulum (Fig. 6-20), the cisternae of which are at first flat and devoid of content but soon begin to swell and to show large amounts of antibody within their cavities (15,37). Polysomes on the outside of the cisternae (Fig. 6-21) can be demonstrated to be fairly long, usually assuming a spiral shape (43). The nucleolus in these cells is extremely active because of the active RNA synthesis which takes place. A few days after antigen injection, the predominant cell type observed is a large lymphoid cell with a typical lymphoid nucleus, a large nucleolus, and a cytoplasm packed with dilated cisternae of endoplasmic reticulum containing antibody (Fig. 6-22). The Golgi apparatus is highly developed and in a position near the nucleus. This cell has been classically termed *the plasma cell*. It appears that it is not long-lived. Its life, estimated on the basis of experimental evidence, is approximately 2 to 3 days (44). The fate of these cells is not well understood, and it appears that some of them may shed their cytoplasm and resynthesize a cell membrane and a cytoplasm similar to that of small lymphocytes (6) (Fig. 6-23).

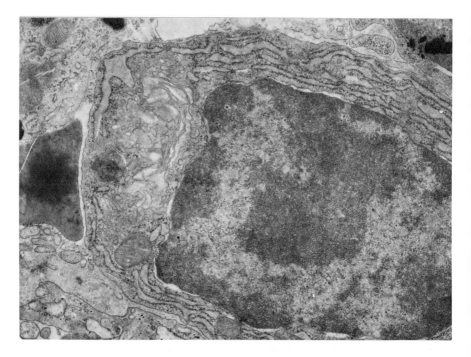

Fig. 6-20 The granular endoplasmic reticulum in this lymphocyte is seen as flattened cisternae with some electron opaque material.

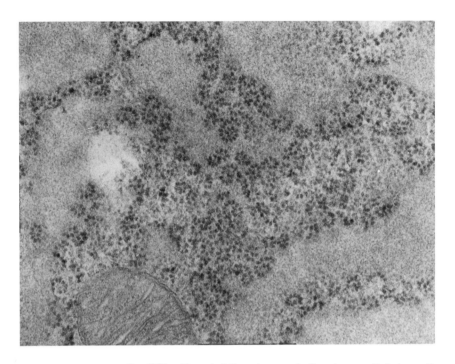

Fig. 6-21 Characteristic polysomes in the plasma cell during antibody response. Note the long arrays of polysomes arranged in a spiral fashion.

The existence of memory cells has been postulated to provide continuity between the primary and subsequent immune response in the cellular reactions accompanying antibody production. This cell should have the properties of a reasonably long life-span, previous experience with antigen, and perhaps (although not necessarily) previous antibody-synthesizing activity. The memory cell has not been identified precisely yet, but it is thought to be a lymphocyte. Experiments reveal that small lymphocytes are indeed capable of carrying immunologic memory (45). It appears that the lymphocyte might fit this role, since it is a cell burdened by a minimum amount of cytoplasm and which contains a large amount of DNA to carry information. A plasma cell may, by shedding its cytoplasm, turn into a lymphocyte. This hypothesis would provide the link between the antibody-synthesizing cell and the memory cell. The memory cell is supposedly a cell containing all the necessary information to synthesize antibody and one which has already synthesized antibody.

The relative roles of lymphoreticular cells in antibody production can be summarized as follows: The macrophage takes up antigen, digests it, and passes a stimulus on to another cell called an *antigen target cell*. This

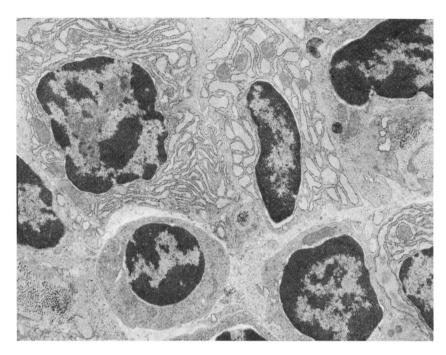

Fig. 6-22 A cluster of antibody-forming cells in the splenic red pulp of a rat hyperimmunized with S. typhi.

cell has been tentatively identified as a small lymphocyte which differentiated from a blast (reticular) cell under thymic influence. This antigen target cell is capable of active division and differentiation in the direction of antibody-forming cells. When mature, they resemble a plasma cell (Fig. 6-24). Alternate schematic representations of the cellular transformations which follow antigenic stimulation may be devised. It might be that the lymphocyte, which is capable of transforming into a phagocytic cell after antigen phagocytosis and digestion, may then turn back into a small lymphocyte and proceed to synthesize antibody. On the other hand, it is quite possible that the macrophage takes up antigen only as an incidental phenomenon and that the antigen taken up by the macrophage is not important in the production of antibody. The small fraction of antigen which comes in contact with lymphocytes might then be considered the stimulating fraction and may, through a series of membrane phenomena, turn on the appropriate genes which then provide the messenger RNA necessary for the synthesis of protein. However, present experimental data suggest that the scheme originally outlined in this chapter most closely reflects the cellular events occurring during the synthesis of antibody.

HOMEOSTASIS OF LYMPHOID CELL POPULATIONS

The lymphocyte population is divided between a circulating and a stationary compartment contained within lymphoid organs and the bone marrow. A constant exchange occurs between these two compartments (46). The regulation of lymphocyte proliferation during ontogenesis appears to reside in the thymus (see Chap. 4). Whether this organ regulates the lymphoid tissues by introducing new cells into the circulation, by a secreted humoral thymic factor, or by a combination of both is not yet clear (47). The most likely possibility is that both a humoral thymic factor and thymus cells participate in the regulation of lymphoid homeostasis. The lymphocyte population is made up of about 90 percent small lymphocytes and 10 percent larger lymphocytes. The small lymphocytes seem to consist of two populations, each with a distinct circulating life-span, origin, and perhaps function (46). A report by Ruhenstroth-Bauer and Lucke-Hühle (48) has provided evidence that the functional

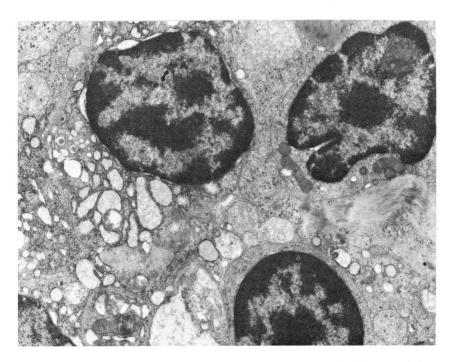

Fig. 6-23 The "free nucleus" of a plasma cell still surrounded by cytoplasmic remnants is seen here together with two small lymphocytes which may have "reformed" a cytoplasm.

properties of the two populations of small lymphocytes are indeed different as far as their immunologic competence is concerned. By electrophoretic mobility and volume measurements, the small thoracic duct lymphocytes of the rats were separated into two populations. Of the cells 77 percent had a faster and 23 percent a slower mobility; 79 percent had a volume of 141 μ^3 (6.5 μ diameter) and 21 percent a volume of 196 μ^3 (7.2 μ diameter). Irradiation of the donors (800 r of x-ray) led to the almost complete disappearance of the slower lymphocyte population, with most of the remaining lymphocytes falling into the small-volume category, thus indicating a correspondence between size and mobility. When lymphocytes were tested for their antibody-forming ability, only 0.02 percent of the faster, smaller lymphocytes were capable of producing antibody, whereas there was a direct correlation between slower, larger lymphocytes and antibody producers. Up to 1 in approximately 300 circulating lymphocytes was capable of giving an antibody response.

Lymphocyte differentiation is thymus-dependent, and unless the thymus is present, no lymphocyte differentiation will occur, as shown by thymectomy experiments (47). (See Chaps. 4 and 10.) Furthermore, no

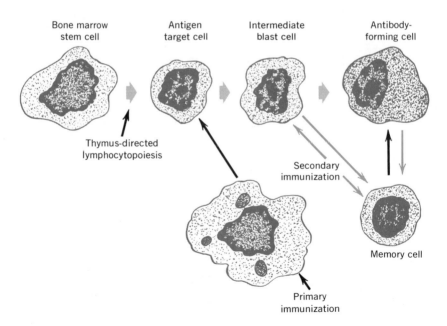

Fig. 6-24 Schematic representation of the changes observed at the cellular level in antibody formation.

antibody production will occur if the thymus has been removed during the embryonic or neonatal periods (47). (See Chap. 11.) Observations on the ontogenesis of the immune response have clearly shown that at least the thymus and one or two lymph nodes are needed for the production of antibody (49). (See Chap. 4.) Experiments in which thymic antibody production was studied with negative results substantiate the fact that the thymus alone is not capable of supporting antibody production. This would support the statement that two populations of lymphocytes exist. It seems reasonable to conclude that of these two populations, the one residing in the thymus is not capable of producing antibodies, while the other is. Confusion exists about the role of the thymus in lymphocytic homeostasis, since it is difficult to visualize how the migration from the thymus of lymphocytes, which are not capable of supporting an immune response while in the thymus, would make them immunocompetent when they move to other organs.

The cat is a notable exception to the scheme of lymphocyte differentiation, since lymphoid tissue appears in the form of lymph nodes before the thymus has developed (50). This is in disagreement with our present ideas of lymphocyte homeostasis. The role of bone marrow lymphocytes in this scheme is hard to visualize, particularly in view of recent experiments demonstrating a definite role for these lymphocytes in immune responses (51,52). It has been shown that bone marrow and thymus cell mixtures could restore the immunologic competence of a heavily irradiated animal, while bone marrow or thymic cells alone would not (52). Furthermore, it was observed that the restorative capacity lay with the bone marrow cells rather than the thymus (53). To complicate matters further, it must be remembered that in the lymphoreticular system, the precursor cell is multipotential and capable of moving in a number of directions according to the stimulus received. Therefore, we may be dealing not only with bone marrow lymphocytes but with cells of a different nature which, under ordinary circumstances, might be considered as precursors for the formation of circulating blood cells. Present data suggest that the lymphocyte is the antigen target cell residing in the lymph node or spleen from where, at the end of the primary response, it may move to settle in the bone marrow. It may then leave the bone marrow under some sort of thymic control to participate in a secondary response after having resettled in lymph nodes or spleen. This scheme, supported by several experiments, indicates a well-established fact that lymphocytes are in constant movement.

The heterogeneity of the cells participating in immune responses has been stressed by a series of experiments. Mosier (54) reported that induction of antibody synthesis by sheep erythrocytes in vitro requires two types of splenic cells: one that adheres to glass surfaces and one that does not. In later experiments in which the cell interactions were extrapolated from available data, Mosier (55) obtained tentative evidence showing that a three-cell interaction may be needed for the induction of this immune response. Plotz and Talal (56) have reported that immunized spleen cells can be separated by their property to adhere or not to adhere to a glass surface. There were a lower number of antibody-forming cells among nonadherent cells than among cells that adhered to glass. Raidt et al. (57) demonstrated that spleen cells from immunized animals can be separated by albumin gradients. The antibody-forming cells were found in different fractions at various times after immunization. Finally, Claman et al. (52) and Mitchell and Miller (53) have demonstrated that there is an interaction between cells obtained from the thymus and the bone marrow in immune systems. Bone marrow or thymus cells alone will not support immune responses in irradiated recipients, but mixtures of the two will. These experiments show that ideas on antibody diversity will have to include some concepts of the diversity of cells stimulated by antigen to produce a specific immunoglobulin. We can no longer think in terms of a simple one-cell system, for cell interactions between two or three different cell types may be involved in the response to antigens. Thus it is apparent that the diversity of antibodies and the heterogeneity of immunoglobulins are not only genetically determined factors expressed in chemical structure but properties which start at the level of the immunocompetent cell. Different antigen target cells have been observed; different cell populations have been isolated from active antibody-producing tissue with different properties; the thymus, bone marrow, and lymph node lymphocytes appear to be divided into two populations with considerably different physiological properties. All of these observations point to great heterogeneity.

KINETICS OF IMMUNOLOGICALLY RESPONSIVE CELLS

A brief review will be made of some of the known facts on the kinetics of antibody-forming cells, particularly as they relate to possible theoretical schemes of antibody production. Many experiments devised to test the clonal selection hypothesis of antibody production stated that one cell could make, after its selection by antigen, only one type of antibody or, at best, a limited number of antibodies (see Chap. 11). Although not all experiments were successful in achieving proof for the clonal selection theory, many facts about the kinetic behavior of antibody-forming cells have been gathered, some of which have a bearing on this hypothesis.

At the beginning of a primary response, the number of cells capable of responding to a given antigen are limited (22). Figures given by various authors place the number of antigen target or precursor cells present in the spleen of an unimmunized mouse between 150 and 2000 (4,22). However, in the 6 to 7 days before peak antibody titer is reached, as many as 150,000 to 400,000 antibody-forming cells accumulate in a mouse spleen (4,22). The first question to be asked is: How is this increase in cell number achieved? Is it by division of preexisting precursor cells, by recruitment of more cells, or by a combination of both? Other important questions concern the mechanism of maintenance of the population of precursor cells, the stimulation of these cells and the kinetics of this transformation into antibody-forming cells, and of antibody-forming cell proliferation. Most studies have suggested that antibody-forming cells increase by stimulation of precursor cells which then divide to give rise to antibody-forming cells. However, there continues to be a "recruitment" of other cells into the population of antibody-forming cells rather than only a division of cells which had been stimulated at time zero (58). It has been established that antibody-forming cells divide rapidly during their differentiation, as shown by experiments in which cells in mitotic division contained antibody (18). In other experiments, cells found in the center of a hemolytic plaque which had synthesized antibody were followed by microcinematography and were shown to divide (19). Plasma cells in division have also been found in foci of plaque-forming cells (20). The mitotic time of antibody-forming cells has been found to be 40 minutes. Thus the existence of cell division during antibody production is well established.

A recent paper by Saunders (58a) provided further clarification of some of the differentiating events occurring during the first 32 hours after antigenic stimulation. His studies employed a system in which spleen cells were cultured on an agar bed containing sheep erythrocytes which provide both the inducing and detecting antigen. This work pointed out that antibody-forming cells are already present 4 hours after antigenic stimulation and before any cell division has occurred. The replication of antibody-forming cells will not occur until 18 hours after immunization, at which point a first doubling of the antibody-forming cell population is seen. This is then followed by a second doubling between 20 and 22 hours after antigenic stimulation and by a third doubling occurring between 28 and 30 hours. Thus it appears that in this system inductive events are very short, that antibody synthesis begins before cell division can be measured, and that cell division will proceed synchronously for at least three cell doublings.

The manner in which the population of precursor cells can be maintained was discussed earlier. Experiments to substantiate this or other possible mechanisms are still lacking, but it is reasonable to assume that asymmetric division may be the most likely way this is achieved. A demonstration of this pathway has been provided for erythropoietic tissue. Some ideas about the differentiation of precursor cells into antibody-forming cells were provided by the work of Papermaster (4) and of Till et al. (59). As the antigen dose increased, the number of precursor cells stimulated also increased. This was achieved by experiments in which cells from normal, unimmunized donor mice were transferred into x-radiated recipients. The recipients were then given an injection of sheep erythrocytes and the sites in the spleen containing foci of hemolytic cells were analyzed by plating spleen pieces, maintained in the original arrangement in which they were cut out of the intact spleen, on agar containing sheep erythrocytes. Hemolytic foci appeared under some areas of the spleen. These were interpreted as indicating the localization in that area of one or a unit number of precursor cells which had then given origin to a clone of antibody-forming cells (Fig. 6-25). A direct relationship between number of foci and thus of precursor cells and antigen dose was established. These experiments were expanded by Kind and Campbell (60) to show that precursor cells are not stimulated equally in all areas of the spleen by the same dose of antigen. In fact, when the same experiment was carried out, but in addition the positive and negative areas were analyzed for plaque-forming cells and precursor cells, the positive areas contained higher ratios of precursor to plaque-forming cells than the negative areas, indicating that precursor cells in the negative areas were not stimulated equally. The rate of proliferation of plaque-forming cells and precursor cells was also measured. It was found that both types of cells increase after antigen injection, the increase being greater with higher antigen doses (61). The doubling times of the populations of plaque-forming cells and of precursor cells were also shown to decrease every time the antigen dose was increased. These data confirmed and extended the work of Papermaster (4) and of Till et al. (59).

The series of experiments reported by Makinodan and Albright (22) have elucidated the kinetics of differentiation and proliferation of antibody-forming cells. They employed heavily irradiated mice into which spleen cells from normal donors had been injected or had been transferred inside peritoneal chambers which were not permeable to cells but were permeable to humoral factors. Thus, a study could be made of either the humoral antibody response or the cells within the peritoneal chambers to get direct counts of cells remaining or of cell increases in the case of proliferation. These experiments revealed that the number of progenitor cells

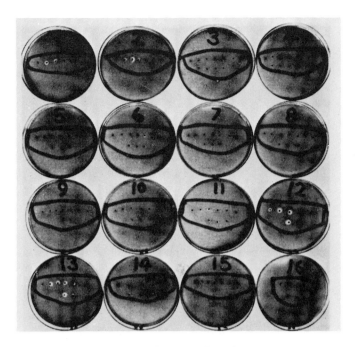

Fig. 6-25 An example of the three-dimensional assay system involving live spleen pieces. The photograph shows 16 petri dishes containing sheep erythrocytes in agar and pieces of a single spleen from a recipient which was injected with 10^6 unstimulated donor spleen cells. Three separate areas of activity can be seen: one in plates 1 and 2, a weak area in plates 6 and 7, and a strong area in plates 11 to 13. From Papermaster (4) with permission.

existing in an unimmunized spleen is approximately 170. In the 4 days it takes to reach the maximum number of antibody-forming cells after primary immunization, each one of these progenitor cells gives rise to approximately 1000 antibody-forming cells. Calculations proved that the number of progenitors in the same amount of time increased approximately one hundredfold so that there were 100 times as many cells ready for a secondary response. From these data the generation time of the antibody-forming cells was calculated to be 8 to 9 hours. This work also showed that most of the cells observed during the early lag phase are antibody-producing cells and that most of the functional cells during the late period of the lag phase are descendants of antibody-producing cells not in active division. It was concluded that the progenitor cells will divide as many as 10 times. These data agree reasonably well with Papermaster's (4) estimation that there are about 2000 antigen target cells in the lymphoid population of the spleen and that these give rise to approximately 200,000 plaque-forming cells by the end of the fourth day after immunization. The studies of Papermaster also provided figures for numbers of target cells in bone marrow and thymus. While the former had about 1 cell per 10^6, the thymus showed about $\frac{1}{5}$ cell per 10^6.

One question remains concerning the number of antibodies a given cell is capable of producing. Current theories to explain antibody specificity and their mode of production by cells have been outlined in Chap. 11. Many experiments conducted in the last few years to investigate the mode of response of antibody-forming cells to antigen have strongly supported the theory proposed originally by Jerne (62) and in modified form by Talmage (63) and by Burnet (64). This theory states that the antigen target cell, once contacted by the antigen, is locked into a synthetic pattern and cannot be influenced to form antibodies to antigens other than the one which stimulated the cell or a closely cross-reacting one. Nossal and Mäkelä (65) demonstrated that in rats immunized with *S. typhi*, which contained non-cross-reacting flagellar type antigens, only one type of antibody was produced to one of the antigens by each of a number of single cells. These cells had been isolated by micromanipulation and were tested with the specific antigens and other antigens. Mäkelä (66) has recently reported a series of experiments by a similar technique with results in agreement with those of his previous experiments with Nossal (65). His work was carried out to confirm or deny the observations of Attardi et al. (67) that single cells producing antibodies to two different antigens could be found in animals immunized with a bacteriophage. Mäkelä's work showed that this is not the case. The question is still open, however, as to whether a cell can make only one antibody or whether certain cells are capable of responding to a limited number of antigens.

By immunofluorescence techniques Chiappino and Pernis (68) were also able to show that in human spleens 19S macroglobulins and 7S gamma globulins are synthesized in different cells. Experiments of Dutton and Mishell (69), further clarifying these questions, have presented the best evidence to date that one cell population appears to respond to only one antigen. A technique was used which provided a way of selectively killing dividing cells during a definite period of time. Cells were cultured in the presence of antigen, and tritiated thymidine of very high specific activity was added to the cell suspensions at various times (Fig. 6-26). The cells in division at the time of addition of thymidine incorporated the isotope and were killed by irradiation. It appeared from these experiments that when cells were irradiated no plaque-forming cells were obtained and, therefore, that all cells that became capable of producing antibody were derived from progenitor cells by division. This argued against continued

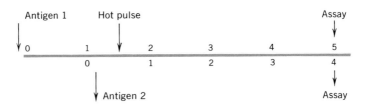

Fig. 6-26 Spleen cell suspensions from normal mice were incubated with antigen 1 added on day 0. Antigen was added on day 1, and all cultures were hot pulsed from 2 day 1 to 2 (i.e., in the 24-to-48-hour period with respect to antigen 1 and the 0-to-24-hour period with respect to antigen 2). Cultures were assayed on day 5 with respect to antigen 1 (day 4 with respect to antigen 2). From Dutton and Mishell (69) with permission.

recruitment of cells into the antibody-forming cell pool, but indicated that they were derived from precursor cells by mitotic division. In addition, inhibition began at 24 hours, indicating that a phase exists during which some preparatory events take place not related to cell division as such. This lag period demonstrated that antigen target cells involved in the response to two non-cross-reacting antigens are different. The antigens used were the erythrocytes from sheep and burros. From these results it appears that the cells which respond to one antigen are a completely different population from those responding to a second antigen.

Thus, the theoretical reasons presented in favor of clonal selection theories by the proponents have been strengthened by this large body of experimental evidence. Although no single experiment or group of experiments has proven beyond reasonable doubt that one cell makes only one or a limited number of antibodies, it appears that this may indeed be the most tenable hypothesis at present.

Albright and Makinodan (70) recently studied the effect of senescence of immunologic responsiveness and of the immunologically competent cell population. They examined the question of whether the animal shows any change in his capability to respond to antigen as it ages. This question is of great interest in the general area of the phenomenon of aging. The unquestionable fact which has emerged from these experiments is that as the animal reaches maturity and begins to advance into old age, its immunologic responses become less capable of protecting it from the attacks of noxious antigenic material. In other words, the immunologic responsiveness becomes less alert. Whether this is a phenomenon which reflects merely a change in homeostasis or in other factors which may relate to immunologic responsiveness is not clear. Undoubtedly, however, it also affects the immunologic responsiveness of animals in a negative way in that these animals are less capable of defending themselves.

209

REFERENCES

1. Bloom, W., and Fawcett, D.: "A Textbook of Histology" 8th ed., W. B. Saunders Company, Philadelphia, 1962.
2. Rhodin, J. A. G.: "An Atlas of Ultrastructure," W. B. Saunders Company, Philadelphia, 1963.
3. Kurtz, S. M. (ed.): "Electron Microscopic Anatomy," Academic Press, Inc., New York, 1964.
4. Papermaster, B. W.: Cold Spring Harbor Symp. Quant. Biol., **32**:447, 1967.
5. Ellis, S. T., Gowans, J. L., and Howard, J. C.: Cold Spring Harbor Symp. Quant. Biol., **32**:395, 1967.
6. La Via, M. F., and Vatter, A. E.: J. Reticuloendothel. Soc., **6**:221, 1969.
7. Chapman, J. A., Gough, J., and Elves, M. W.: J. Cell Sci., **2**:371, 1967.
8. Everett, N. B., Caffrey, R. W., and Rieke, W. O.: Ann. N.Y. Acad. Sci., **113**:887, 1964.
9. Hartley, G., Jr.: J. Infect. Dis., **66**:44, 1940.
10. Askonas, B. A., and Humphrey, J. H.: Biochem. J., **70**:212, 1958.
11. McMaster, P. D.: in "The Nature and Significance of the Antibody Response," A. M. Pappenheimer, Jr. (ed.), Columbia University Press, New York, 1953.
12. Taliaferro, W. H., and Talmage, D. W.: J. Infect. Dis., **97**:88, 1955.
13. Baker, P. J., and Landy, M.: J. Immunol., **99**:687, 1967.
14. Šterzl, J.: Cold Spring Harbor Symp. Quant. Biol., **32**:493, 1967.
15. Moore, R. D., Mumaw, V. R., and Schoenberg, M. D.: Exp. Mol. Pathol., **4**:370, 1965.
16. Jerne, N. K., Nordin, A. A., and Henry, C.: in "Cell-bound Antibodies," B. Amos and H. Koprowski, (eds.), Wistar Institute Press, Philadelphia, 1963.
17. Ada, G. L., Parish, C. R., Nossal, G. J. V., and Abbot, A.: Cold Spring Harbor Symp. Quant. Biol., **32**:381, 1967.
18. Baney, R. N., Vazquez, J. J., and Dixon, F. J.: Proc. Soc. Exp. Biol. Med., **109**:1, 1962.
19. Claflin, A. J., and Smithies, O.: Science, **157**:1561, 1967.
20. La Via, M. F., and Vatter, A. E.: In preparation.
21. Nossal, G. J. V.: Advan. Immunol., **2**:163, 1962.
22. Makinodan, T., and Albright, J. F.:Progr. Allergy, **10**:1, 1967.
23. Bjørneboe, M., and Gormsen, H.: Acta Pathol. Microbiol. Scand., **20**:649, 1943.
24. Fagraeus, A.: Acta Med. Scand., **130**(Suppl. 204): 1948.
25. Ehrich, W. E., Drabkin, D. L., and Forman, C.: J. Exp. Med., **90**:157, 1949.
26. Harris, T. N., and Harris, S.: J. Exp. Med., **90**:169, 1949.
27. Makinodan, T., Ruth, R. F., and Wolfe, H. R.: J. Immunol., **72**:39, 1954.

28. Makinodan, T., Ruth, R. F., and Wolfe, H. R.: *J. Immunol.*, **72**:45, 1954.

29. La Via, M. F., Fitch, F. W., Gunderson, C. H., and Wissler, R. W.: *RES Bull.*, **3**:15, 1957.

30. Wissler, R. W., Fitch, F. W., La Via, M. F., and Gunderson, C. H.: *J. Cell. Comp. Physiol.*, **50**(Suppl. 1) :265, 1957.

31. Ward, P. A., Johnson, A. G., and Abell, M. R.: *Lab. Invest.*, **12**:180, 1963.

32. Langevoort, H. L.: *Lab. Invest.*, **12**:106, 1963.

33. Hanna, M. G., Jr.: *Int. Arch. Allergy*, **26**:230, 1965.

34. Coons, A. H., Leduc, E. H., and Connolly, J. M.: *J. Exp. Med.*, **102**:49, 1955.

35. Leduc, E. H., Coons, A. H., and Connolly, J. M.: *J. Exp. Med.*, **102**:61, 1955.

36. De Petris, S., and Karlsbad, G.: *J. Cell Biol.*, **26**:759, 1965.

37. Leduc, E. H., Avrameas, S., and Bouteille, M.: *J. Exp. Med.*, **127**:109, 1968.

38. Roberts, J. C., Jr., Dixon, F. J., and Weigle, W. O.: *Arch. Pathol.*, **64**:324, 1957.

39. Talmage, D. W., and Claman, H. N.: in "The Thymus in Immunobiology," R. A. Good and A. E. Gabrielsen (eds.), Harper & Row, New York, 1964.

40. Lajtha, L. G.: *J. Cell. Physiol.*, **67**(Suppl. 1):133, 1966.

41. Nossal, G. J. V., Shortman, K. D., Miller, J. F. A. P., Mitchell, G. F., and Haskill, J. S.: *Cold Spring Harbor Symp. Quant. Biol.*, **32**:369, 1967.

42. Gowans, J. L.: *Int. Rev. Exp. Pathol.*, **5**:1, 1966.

43. La Via, M. F., and Vatter, A. E.: Unpublished observations.

44. Vazquez, J. J.: in "The Thymus in Immunobiology," R. A. Good and A. E. Gabrielsen (eds.), Harper & Row, New York, 1964.

45. Gowans, J. L., and Uhr, J. W.: *J. Exp. Med.*, **124**:1017, 1966.

46. Caffrey, R. W., Rieke, W. O., and Everett, N. B.: *Acta Haematol.*, **28**:145, 1962.

47. Metcalf, D.: "The Thymus," Springer-Verlag, New York, 1966.

48. Ruhenstroth-Bauer, G., and Lucke-Hühle, C.: *J. Cell Biol.*, **37**:196, 1968.

49. La Via, M. F., Rowlands, D. T., Jr., and Block, M.: *Science*, **140**:1219, 1963.

50. Ackerman, G. A.: *Anat. Rec.*, **158**:387, 1967.

51. Claman, H. N., Chaperon, E. A., and Triplett, R. F.: *Proc. Soc. Exp. Biol. Med.*, **122**:1167, 1966.

52. Claman, H. N., Chaperon, E. A., and Triplett, R. F.: *J. Immunol.*, **97**:828, 1966.

53. Mitchell, G. F., and Miller, J. F. A. P.: *Proc. Nat. Acad. Sci. U.S.*, **59**:296, 1968.

54. Mosier, D. E.: *Science*, **158**:1573, 1967.

55. Mosier, D. E., and Coppleson, L. W.: *Proc. Nat. Acad. Sci. U.S.*, **61**:542, 1968.
56. Plotz, P. H., and Talal, N.: *J. Immunol.*, **99**:1236, 1967.
57. Raidt, D. J., Mishell, R. I., and Dutton, R. W.: *J. Exp. Med.*, **128**:681, 1968.
58. Tannenberg, W. J. K.: *Nature (London)*, **214**:293, 1967.
58a. Saunders, G.: *J. Exper. Med.*, **130**:543, 1969.
59. Till, J. E., McCulloch, E. A., Phillips, R. A., and Siminovitch, L.: *Cold Spring Harbor Symp. Quant. Biol.*, **32**:461, 1967.
60. Kind, P., and Campbell, P. A.: *J. Immunol.*, **100**:55, 1968.
61. Campbell, P. A., and Kind, P. D.: *J. Immunol.*, **102**:1084, 1969.
62. Jerne, N. K.: *Proc. Nat. Acad. Sci. U.S.*, **41**:849, 1955.
63. Talmage, D. W.: *Ann. Rev. Med.*, **8**:239, 1957.
64. Burnet, F. M.: *Australian J. Sci.*, **20**:67, 1957.
65. Nossal, G. J. V., and Mäkelä, O.: *Annu. Rev. Microbiol.*, **16**:53, 1962.
66. Mäkelä, O.: *Cold Spring Harbor Symp. Quant. Biol.*, **32**:423, 1967.
67. Attardi, G., Cohn, M., Horibata, K., and Lennox, E. S.: *J. Immunol.*, **93**:94, 1964.
68. Chiappino, G., and Pernis, B.: *Pathol. Microbiol.*, **27**:8, 1964.
69. Dutton, R. W., and Mishell, R. I.: *Cold Spring Harbor Symp. Quant. Biol.*, **32**:407, 1967.
70. Albright, J. F., and Makinodan, T.: *J. Cell. Physiol.*, **67**(Suppl. 1): 185, 1966.

7
Subcellular Sites of Antibody Synthesis

The early studies of subcellular events during antibody production sought to determine if specific antibody was synthesized de novo and established that radioactively labeled amino acids were incorporated into antibody protein (1–4). This synthesis would be expected to follow the established pattern of protein synthesis: transcription of DNA-encoded information into RNA, translation of such information into polypeptide chains, and assembly and release of the complete antibody molecules. With the introduction of the messenger RNA hypothesis of Jacob and Monod (5), immunologists accelerated their attempts to describe the subcellular events of antibody synthesis, particularly in regard to the possibility of isolating specific mRNA involved in immune responses.

More recently, attention has been directed toward the ribosomal sites of antibody assembly and the subsequent cellular release of such antibody. Again the impetus for such studies came from immunologic investigations, but more importantly it came from areas of molecular biology not directly concerned with immunologic problems.

213

This chapter will discuss the subcellular events associated with transcription, translation, and peptide assembly in immunologically active cell populations. It will also examine studies dealing with the secretion of antibody molecules and with some of the terminal events in antibody synthesis, such as carbohydrate attachment.

NUCLEIC ACID METABOLISM

DNA Metabolism

A period of cellular proliferation accompanied by differentiation is the usual situation in any developmental process. Studies on the cellular kinetics of the immune response indicate that antigen stimulates mitotic activity, which allows proliferation of cells eventually capable of synthesizing antibody (see Chap. 6). Dutton (6) was the first to critically examine DNA synthesis in cultures of spleen cells stimulated with antigen. He was able to show that H^3-thymidine uptake was increased after antigenic stimulation and that it began early after antigen addition to cultures. Cohen and Talmage (7) have also studied the relationship between antibody synthesis, as judged by immunofluorescence, and DNA synthesis, as seen by autoradiography, in spleen cells of mice given a secondary injection of antigen. Spleen cell suspensions were prepared at various times after immunization, incubated in medium containing H^3-thymidine, and injected into irradiated mice. Spleens from the irradiated recipients were examined and donor cells identified by immunofluorescence and autoradiography. Only cells positive by both methods were scored. None of the cells taken from donor mice 2 hours after antigen injection was labeled with H^3-thymidine. Of those taken 3 hours after antigen injection, only 8.0 percent were synthesizing DNA. However, 38 percent of the cells from donor mice given antigen 6 hours before sacrifice was labeled. The percentage decreased thereafter, until cells removed from donor mice 48 hours after exposure to antigen were found to contain no label. These results suggest that 3 to 6 hours after exposure to BGG antigen, precursors of antibody-forming cells began to synthesize DNA, and by 6 hours such synthesis had reached a maximum level.

Similar data were obtained by Mach and Vassalli (8) in studies with rats injected with an antigenic mixture of killed *H. pertussis* and sheep erythrocytes. Following a primary injection, DNA synthesis in spleen and lymph node cell populations increased dramatically until approximately 5 hours after injection. In the secondary response, the peak DNA synthesis occurred about 1 hour earlier.

Since increased synthesis of DNA depletes existing pools of nucleo-tides, the specific activity of enzymes involved in nucleotide metabolism might be expected to increase following the synthetic period. An increase in the specific activity of thymidine kinase was found to occur within 4.5 hours after a primary injection of SRBC in mice (9). This activity con-tinued to rise until 48 hours after stimulation, with the range of increase being from 1 μM TMP/mg protein at time zero to 3.5 μM TMP/mg protein at 48 hours.

RNA Metabolism

The cellular proliferation and differentiation which lead to synthesis of a specific protein would be a process expected to include increased RNA synthesis. Specific information regarding the amount and type of RNA synthesis during the immune process would add considerably to our knowledge of the mechanism of the immune response. The major diffi-culty is in differentiating between RNA specifically involved in antibody synthesis (mRNA) and that made to produce cellular proteins in rapidly dividing cells.

In the same studies reporting increased DNA synthesis in cells of immunized rabbit spleen and lymph nodes, Mach and Vassalli (8) found similar increases in RNA and protein synthesis. The relative increase in the RNA paralleled that of DNA, although peak incorporation of radio-active label was about 75 percent of that reported for DNA. Base com-position studies identified much of the newly synthesized RNA to be ribosomal, suggesting that synthesis of that species of RNA occurred at a rapid rate. However, by sucrose gradient centrifugation, a rapidly labeled RNA with a sedimentation coefficient of less than 12S was also isolated. Salt precipitation removed part of this RNA, but the specific activity of the remaining RNA was still high. In addition to having a high specific activity (indicating new synthesis), this fraction of RNA did not maintain its high activity with longer labeling periods, thus suggesting a rapid turn-over. Finally, RNA was isolated from six regions of the sedimentation gradient corresponding to the following fractions: >34S, 26 to 34S, 20 to 26S, 12 to 20S, 6 to 12S, and <6S. In each instance, the fraction was able to stimulate incorporation of amino acids into protein in an *E. coli* cell-free system, although the activity in the 6 to 12S region appeared to be double that of any of the other areas. This same RNA was the first to be isolated on microsomes and was found to have a base composition close to that of DNA. These last two points, along with rapid turnover rate and high template activity, indicate that such RNA had the molecular and biologic characteristics of mRNA. Although very suggestive, this information does not prove that this RNA carries a message specific for the synthesis of antibody protein.

Recently, Lazda et al. (10,11) have studied the kinetics of RNA synthesis in spleen cells of rats immunized 24 hours earlier with flagella antigens. In agreement with Mach and Vassalli, they observed an increased synthesis of a ribosomal RNA for 16 hours after injection of P³². Increased synthesis also occurred in the RNA fraction sedimenting from 6 to 12S. Although a rapid turnover occurred in at least a portion of this RNA, evidence was presented which indicated that a portion of this RNA did accumulate and represented a fraction of RNA similar to stable mRNA (12). These investigators suggested that the unstable portion of the 6 to 12S RNA might be involved with the synthesis of structural protein, while the more stable fraction carried the code for antibody synthesis.

Following preliminary experimentation to determine the specificity of and optimal conditions for molecular hybridization of DNA and RNA strands, Cohen (13) employed this technique to analyze the "proportion of the genome" involved in the immunologic process. Results showed that, following immunization of mice with SRBC, hybrid formation increased beginning at day 1 and continued for 4 days after immunization. Specifically, if RNA was extracted 2 days after immunization, 0.48 percent of that RNA was found to hybridize with isologous DNA, while 0.38 percent of the RNA from nonimmunized mice formed hybrids. The increased hybridization appeared to occur with RNA isolated from two regions of a sedimentation gradient, the 18S and 8 to 12S fractions. The base ratios of the RNA from these two areas of the gradient were different from the RNA obtained from nonimmunized animals. This suggested that immunization did not merely cause an increased synthesis of the normal RNA, but also the production of a different RNA as determined by base composition studies. Whether this RNA is specific for the assembly of immunoglobulin polypeptide chains or more generally related to cellular protein synthesis remains an unsolved question. It has been reported that mitogenic agents such as phytohemagglutinin induce increased synthesis of rRNA and of an RNA which is polydisperse in sedimentation analysis (14). Although the function of the polydisperse RNA remains a matter of conjecture, it has been suggested that it is a polycistronic message (15), the precursor of a cytoplasmic messenger RNA (16), or unrelated to cytoplasmic messenger RNA (17).

These studies of the role of RNA and DNA in the synthesis of immunoglobulin suggest that antibiotics, particularly actinomycin D and streptomycin, which inhibit the synthesis of protein by interaction at the transcriptional and translational levels, respectively, could be expected to influence antibody synthesis in a similar manner. Uhr (18) has demonstrated that actinomycin D inhibited in vitro synthesis of both RNA and specific antibody protein, although the lymph node cells were able to synthesize another protein if new RNA was provided. Krueger (19) also presented data suggesting that streptomycin caused a translational error which changed an antibody so that it had a reduced ability to neutralize its respective phage antigen.

Another RNA associated in a still unclear manner with immune responses has been extensively studied in isolated macrophage populations. This RNA, which is synthesized after antigenic stimulation, seems to be of low molecular weight, to have antigen fragments associated with it, and to be important in the initiation of immune responses. A comprehensive discussion of the work on this subject is found in Chap. 5. It was shown that an extract of macrophages exposed to antigen is capable of inducing an immune response (20). This was demonstrated by preparing peritoneal macrophages of rats and linking them in vitro with a preparation of T2 bacteriophage. Lymph node cell cultures were set up, and the macrophage extract was capable of stimulating the production of phage-neutralizing antibodies in these cultures. Additional experiments showed that the material responsible for immune induction in this system is ribonuclease-sensitive. This latter finding led to further experiments in which phenol-extracted RNA derived from macrophages exposed to T2 phage was used to stimulate antibody production. Immunogenic activity was demonstrated by mixing RNA and lymph node cells in cell-impermeable peritoneal chambers, which were then implanted into x-radiated recipients (21). This, then, appeared to be an interesting, simple system for antibody induction. Further studies, however, demonstrated that in extracting RNA from antigen-treated macrophages, a certain amount of antigenic material is also carried through (22, 23). This may be responsible for the immune induction in conjunction with the RNA, and the complex may be considered a "superantigen" (22). Recent additional evidence indicates that the RNA is newly synthesized, at least in part, and is contained in the low-molecular-weight fraction of RNA (24). This would add one important feature to the superantigen idea by suggesting that it may consist of an informational RNA needed to convey some information from the macrophage to the antigen target cell in combination with some antigenic material. The idea that this might be a species of messenger RNA which can induce antibody production is also a suggestive one. It appears, however, that this RNA is of a molecular weight too low to code for the synthesis of antibody polypeptide chains (25). It is not clear whether this is an artifact of an in vitro system or whether it occurs in vivo in the same fashion. Unless such proof is given, it cannot be stated categorically that this mechanism operates in vivo.

Much interest has been directed to a study of RNA derived from lymphoid organs of immunized animals (26). RNA extracted from spleen or lymph nodes has been used to induce specific antibody synthesis in normal spleen and lymph node populations (27–33). Cohen and Parks (27) reported that an RNA extract from spleens of immunized mice converted a small percentage of isologous nonimmune spleen cells to antibody-forming cells. Friedman (28) demonstrated an immune response in recipient nonimmune mouse spleen cells after exposure to a ribonuclease-sensitive extract from mice immunized with sheep erythrocytes.

Abramoff and Brien (33) reported that the immunologic activity of an RNA extract affected by RNase at a high enzyme-substrate ratio. However, the effect of the enzyme treatment was evidenced only in a delay of antibody formation by the recipient chick spleen cell population. There was no decrease in the number of antibody plaque-forming cells formed at the time of maximum antibody synthesis. These results are contrary to those of Cohen et al. (32), who reported an inhibition of antibody formation following such treatment of the RNA extract. It must be pointed out that in Cohen's experiments, the recipient cell population was exposed to the treated RNA for no longer than 30 minutes, while Abramoff and Brien found no evidence of antibody synthesis until 48 hours after initiation of the incubation period. Such results suggest that in Abramoff's experiment, the RNA may act as a carrier of the immunogenic fragment and enhance cellular uptake of that fragment.

Conclusion

Since cell proliferation has been shown to be an essential process in the immune response, studies showing increased DNA and RNA synthesis merely confirm the necessity of these processes at the molecular level. The studies of Mach and Vassalli (8) and Cohen (13) indicate that the RNA which they describe might be mRNA specific for directing the synthesis of antibody. This is strongly suggested by several lines of evidence and particularly by its unique base composition. As will be discussed later, it has been found that the polysomes on which each chain is synthesized are of sufficient size to account for an mRNA with the necessary number of nucleotides to code for the entire L or H chain (34). It has been determined, also, that the mRNA associated with polysomes on which the L chain is assembled sediments at 9 to 11S, while that associated with polysomes on which the H chain is assembled sediments at 14 to 16S (35). Such data correlate well with those of Cohen which identified immunologically active RNAs with similar sedimentation coefficients (13).

No conclusive statement can be made concerning the immunogenic activity of RNA extracts. This subject has been reviewed extensively in Chap. 5. Extracts from peritoneal exudate cells appear to depend upon an antigen-RNA complex for activity. The complex appears to occur as a result of a biologic process rather than contamination of the extract by antigen. Whether antigen is a necessary component of whole organ extracts is not known; Abramoff and Brien (33) indicate that it may be; the data of Cohen et al. (32) suggest the contrary.

ASSEMBLY OF THE ANTIBODY MOLECULE

The final question in the study of subcellular mechanisms of immunoglobulin synthesis relates to the actual assembly of the protein molecule. The transfer of information from DNA to protein involves the action of RNA which directs the sequence of component amino acids in that protein. This final transfer of information to the product is referred to as the translation process which occurs at the ribosomal level.

Biology of the Ribosome

Electron microscopy has revealed the ribosome of *E. coli* to be a particle composed of two unequal subunits (36). This particle has a sedimentation coefficient of 70S, a molecular weight of 2.8×10^6, contains 60 percent protein and 40 percent RNA by weight, and is stable in a magnesium concentration of the order of 1 mM. Upon lowering the Mg concentration (0.1 mM), a reversible dissociation of the ribosomal particle results in the release of the two subunits, which have sedimentation coefficients of 30S and 50S and molecular weights of 0.85 and 1.8×10^6, respectively.

Shelton and Kuff (37) have recently studied the substructure of mammalian ribosomes from mouse plasma cell tumors and rabbit reticulocytes. The same two-unit structure was found to be present in these ribosomes, with the large subunit being of uniform shape and size and measuring 180×220 Å. The small subunit had a variable shape; its average size was 100×260 Å. The whole ribosome had a height of 300 Å. These authors described the structure of small polyribosomes as rosettelike, of polysomes larger than pentamers as an attempt at spiral formation, and of still larger polysomes as definite spirals. The attachment of ribosomes to endoplasmic reticulum membranes occurred by means of the large subunit, thus confirming the observations of Sabatini et al. (38). Sedimentation coefficients for rat liver ribosomes have indicated an 80S value for mammalian ribosomes, as opposed to 70S for bacterial ribosomes.

Although Huxley and Zubay (36) and Shelton and Kuff (37) were able to isolate individual ribosomes for structural analysis, functional activity appeared to be associated with ribosomal aggregates rather than with the individual particle. In mammalian systems, the rabbit reticulocyte, in which synthesis of hemoglobin is a primary activity, provided a system for analysis of both the structural and functional activity of ribosomes and ribosomal aggregates. Electron microscopy of gradient fractions from the rabbit reticulocyte revealed that individual ribosomes were closely packed to form polyribosomes, and the polysomes, themselves, appeared in clusters or strands (39). The ribosomes, measuring 230 Å in diameter, were sometimes separated along the strand; in such instances, a single 10 Å thread, perhaps a strand of RNA, could be seen connecting the particles. When the cells had been subjected to osmotic shock or freezing and thawing, sucrose gradient centrifugation of the cytoplasmic extracts showed that the ribosomes existed as single particles with a sedimentation coefficient of 76S (40). If the cells had been incubated with radioactive amino acids prior to treatment, the radioactivity was found to be associated with the monosomes. However, if, after similar exposure to the radioactive amino acids, the cells were disrupted by a less drastic method, such as by lowering the ionic strength of the incubation medium, the sedimentation profile of the extract was quite different (41). Radioactivity was associated with gradient fractions sedimented in the 170S region. Electron micrographs of these fractions showed that the aggregates were composed of ribosomal tetramers and pentamers (42).

Having found newly synthesized protein associated with the polyribosomal fraction of cytoplasmic extracts, two additional questions were asked. Does synthesis proceed in an orderly manner from one end of the peptide chain to the other, or can it begin at any position and proceed in either or both directions? Secondly, is there a relationship between the length of the polypeptide chain and the size of the ribosomal aggregate upon which it is synthesized? By separating and examining various portions of the α-hemoglobin chain at short intervals after exposure to a radioactive amino acid, Dintzis (43,44) was able to determine the direction of synthesis. If the peptide is synthesized linearly, then an analysis of the distribution of radioactivity in the peptide should confirm such a mechanism. Those amino acids incorporated into the growing peptide chain nearer the end of the incubation period would be progressively "hotter." The experiments were conducted at 15°C in order to retard the rate of synthesis and to allow for analysis of samples in the early stages of that synthesis. After a 4-minute pulse, only four peptides at the carboxyl end of the peptide chain were labeled, while by 7 minutes the entire chain was labeled. Labeling increased from the carboxyl toward the amino terminal end as the incubation period lengthened. This would indicate that a linear pattern of synthesis proceeded from the amino terminal to the carboxyl terminal amino acid. In addition, the "hottest" amino acid was positioned at the C-terminus.

Based upon the evidence for sequential synthesis of peptide chains, a model has been proposed which predicts that each ribosome aligned on a monocistronic strand of RNA will carry a nascent polypeptide chain proportionate in size to the length of RNA the ribosome has traveled. Kuff and Roberts (45) have followed the distribution of radioactive labeling of peptide chains on various sized free polyribosomes from plasma cell tumors after short in vivo labeling. They predicted that if the ribosomes were evenly spaced along a monocistronic strand of RNA—the space being equal to the increment (w) of weight increase of the peptide chain per ribosome—then, the cumulative weight of the aggregate peptides on a polysome (N ribosome) would be $w(N^2 + N/2)$. The cumulative average peptide weight would equal $w(N + 1)/2$ (Fig. 7-1).

According to the proposed model, if the radioactivity was proportional to w, then there would be a linear relationship between polyribosomal size and specific activity. Kuff and Roberts (45) found that such a relationship did hold for polysome aggregates having from 2 to 15 component

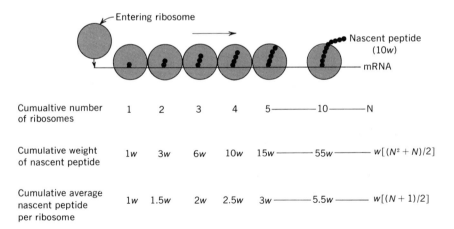

Cumualtive number of ribosomes	1	2	3	4	5————10————N	
Cumulative weight of nascent peptide	1w	3w	6w	10w	15w————55w———— $w[(N^2 + N)/2]$	
Cumulative average nascent peptide per ribosome	1w	1.5w	2w	2.5w	3w————5.5w———— $w[(N + 1)/2]$	

Fig. 7-1 Schematic representation of the increment in nascent peptide with increasing number of ribosomes in a polyribosomal chain. The ribosomes are spaced evenly along the mRNA strand with the active sites separated by a distance of approximately one ribosome diameter. In moving this distance along the mRNA, each ribosome is assumed to acquire an increment of nascent peptide w, represented diagrammatically as •. From Kuff and Roberts (45) with permission.

ribosomes. Although these workers derived their polysome preparations from plasma cell tumors, including the RPC-20 tumor in which λ-type light chains are the secretory product of the cell, their labeled peptides were not specifically identified as immunoglobulin molecules. However, their success in determining a positive correlation between polysomal size and the assembled product has provided an experimental basis for studies of the biosynthesis of immunoglobulin molecules.

Biosynthesis of Immunoglobulins

IgG is a multichain protein which, upon partial reduction, yields two heavy and two light chains, with molecular weights of 20,000 and 50,000 respectively (46,47). Structural studies indicate that within a given class of immunoglobulins, each chain is composed of a segment with a constant amino acid sequence and a segment with a variable sequence (see Chap. 3). The amino terminal portion of the chain has the variable sequence. In considering the control of biosynthesis of immunoglobulins at the molecular level, certain questions arise, such as, how many cistrons are involved in the synthesis of a single four-chain IgG molecule, and, are the variable and constant segments of both the heavy and light chains synthesized separately or as a single unit? If the type of experiments performed by Kuff and Roberts (45) are valid, then examination of polysomal units involved in immunoglobulin synthesis should reveal a correlation between polysome size and size of the heavy or light immunoglobulin chain. In addition, an experiment of the sort conducted by Dintzis (43,44) should allow for the determination of the rate of synthesis of different portions of the immunoglobulin chain relative to the total time for synthesis of the whole chain, thereby determining if continuous synthesis occurs.

Early reports suggested that radioactively labeled nascent immunoglobulin chains were associated with single ribosomes or dimers in the lymphoid tissue of immunized animals (48,49). However, Norton et al. (49) reported isolation of radioactivity in the polysome region as well as in the monosome region. Scharff and Uhr (50) demonstrated the extreme lability of polysomes during certain extraction procedures. They diminished excessive breakdown of polysomes by homogenizing labeled lymph node cells in the presence of a large excess of unlabeled HeLa cells. The latter probably bound excess degradative enzymes. After such treatment, the radioactivity was located in regions of the gradient having sedimentation coefficients from 100 to 350S. The greatest concentration of radioactive protein occurred at 200S.

More recently Williamson and Askonas (34,51,52) have employed the ascitic form of the murine plasmacytoma 5563 as a model system. The plasma cells of this mouse tumor produce considerable amounts of IgG myeloma protein; 15 to 35 percent of the total cellular protein synthesized is myeloma protein. By using antisera specific for the two types of immunoglobulin chains, the growing peptide chains still bound to polyribosomes were isolated. Because a 2-minute labeling period was sufficient to allow maximum incorporation of the labeled amino acids into the myeloma protein, while still maintaining reduced levels of specific activity in soluble protein (release globulin), the cells were exposed to H^3-leucine for 2 minutes, washed and suspended in a sucrose solution with deoxycholate, and subsequently layered over a sucrose gradient. The radioactive material was associated primarily with the polysome fraction. By using rabbit reticulocyte ribosomes as markers, it was obvious that the H^3-leucine was located on polysomes larger than the reticulocyte pentamers or hexamers.

To characterize the class of polysomes carrying the heavy chain, antisera specific for the Fc fragment (C-terminal parts of the heavy chain joined by disulfide bonds) of the immunoglobulin molecule were used. Maximum specific precipitation occurred with nascent chains on polyribosomes having sedimentation coefficients of 250S and greater. If the polyribosomes were fractionated on a sucrose gradient for 2.5 hours rather than for 3.0 hours, the specific activity was associated with heavier ribosomal aggregates corresponding to 300S. Isolation of polysomes associated with nascent light chains proved to be more difficult. In addition to being smaller, light chains contained only one-third the amount of H^3-leucine and appeared to undergo immediate release from the polyribosomes. This latter characteristic will be considered in more detail later. It was found that the anti-light-chain sera precipitated very little radioactive material in any portion of the gradient. The small amount which was precipitated could very well have been bound to heavy chains on the polysomes. Since rabbit anti-mouse-light-chain serum was used to precipitate the nascent light chains, goat anti-rabbit IgG was added to the gradient fractions after anti-light-chain serum had been added. The anti-IgG serum would precipitate any antigen-antibody complex which did not specifically precipitate upon addition of the anti-light-chain serum. Although only small amounts of radioactivity were precipitated, increased precipitation occurred in the region of the 120 to 180S polysomes.

These results confirm that de novo synthesis of immunoglobulin chains occurs in a manner similar to that observed in the synthesis of other proteins. The actual significance of the work lies, however, in the extrapolations the data allowed. To determine if the polyribosomes isolated were, in fact, of sufficient size to accommodate the synthesis of entire light or heavy peptide chains, the number of ribosomes per polyribosome was estimated. On the basis of previous reports concerning the reticulocyte system of Warner et al. (42), in which 5 ribosomes (170S polyribosomes) were found on an mRNA of 450 nucleotides, Williamson and Askonas (34) calculated that the polyribosomes (270S) associated with the heavy chain contained about 15 ribosomes. An RNA of approximately 1350 nucleotides would be associated with this size polysome, and an RNA molecule of this size would contain information sufficient for the synthesis of a protein of 450 amino acid residues. This corresponds with the size of the heavy chain of IgG. Similarly, the polysomes associated with the light chain contained about 7 ribosomes, a number sufficient to support the synthesis of a light chain containing 200 amino acid residues.

Similar results have been reported by Shapiro et al. (35,53) utilizing a different experimental model and varied techniques. Comparing the polyribosomal profiles of different mouse plasma cell tumors it was found that MPC_{11} tumor cells synthesize both H and L chains, while Bence-Jones tumor cells make only light chains. The distribution of radioactively incorporated amino acids varied in the different cell types. Relatively more radioactivity was associated with the larger polysomes (250 to 290S) in extracts from MPC_{11} cells, while in the gradient profile from Bence-Jones tumor cells the labeled amino acids segregated with the 170 to 210S fractions. Electropherograms of the fractions showed that the peptides associated with the larger polyribosomes were H chains, while nascent L chains were associated with both the larger and smaller (170 to 210S) polysomes. Thus the L chains appear to have been assembled on the lighter polysomes, were released, and then were attached to the H chain peptide still on the heavier polyribosome.

In addition to identification of the polyribosomal site of synthesis for the individual immunoglobulin chains, Shapiro et al. (35,53) sought to identify the size of the newly synthesized RNA or mRNA associated with the polysomes. In order to avoid labeling 28S or 16S rRNA, the tumor cells were exposed to a 10 to 15 minute pulse of H^3-uridine. Polysomes from the 190S and 270S areas of the gradient were subsequently concentrated by centrifugation and the RNA extracted from each fraction. The rapidly labeled RNA, associated with 190S polysomes, sedimented at a peak of 9 to 11S, and the RNA from the 270S fraction peaked between 14 and 16S. RNA of these sizes would contain sufficient message to code for polypeptide chains with molecular weight of 24,000 and 50,000, respectively.

While the two groups of workers cited agreed on the sizes of the polysomal aggregates which support synthesis of the peptide chains, and that these polysomes were of sufficient size to accommodate synthesis of an entire chain, whether a heavy or light chain, La Via et al. (54) have questioned the latter suggestion. Although they agreed that, in spleen cells from hyperimmunized rats, synthesis of immunoglobulin chains also occurred on 190 to 200S and 270S or heavier polysomes, they did not agree that these fractions contained the number of ribosomes suggested by Askonas and Williamson (51,52). Rather, La Via et al. (54) found from electron microscopy that the lighter fractions were composed of trimers and tetramers, while the heavier fractions contained octamers and decamers. These results were contrary to those obtained by de Petris (55) who, in examining the polysomes in the 300S fraction by electron micros-copy, found the clusters to be composed of 16 to 18 ribosomes. Similarly, the fraction from the 120 to 180S region contained clusters of seven to eight ribosomes. The question of whether linear and complete synthesis of each heavy or light chain can occur on polyribosomes with these sedimentation coefficients can only be answered by pulse-labeling experiments that demonstrate the sequential growth of each complete chain. Results of such experiments are reported by Knopf et al. (56,57). Portions of the IgG heavy chain from mouse plasma cell tumors were examined at various times after exposure to radioactive amino acids. The rate at which the specific activity of the Fc (C-terminal) and Fd (N-terminal) fragments of the heavy chain approached equilibrium indicated whether they were synthesized as separate units or as a contiguous unit. Models were constructed to fit the experimental possibilities. Theoretical curves for the specific activity ratio, Fd/Fc, as a function of time are illustrated in Fig. 7-2. These models assumed that every amino acid position in the heavy chain was labeled with equal specific activity and that the rate of synthesis from the N-terminal amino acid to the C-terminus was constant.

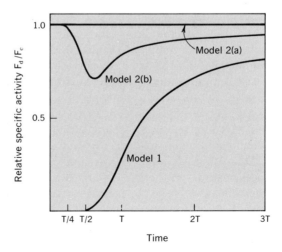

Fig. 7-2 Theoretical curves of the relative specific activity ratio, $(Fd/Fc)_{Rel}$, as a function of time. From Knopf et al. (56) with permission.

Since papain cleaves the heavy chain into approximately equal fragments, Fd and Fc were assumed to be of equal length. Model 1 presumed that a single strand of mRNA directed the synthesis of the peptide chain as a single unit, and model 2 presumed the fusion of the products from two mRNA molecules according to alternative means. If the data had conformed to model 2a, then the two RNA molecules would have been of equal length, coding for the Fd and Fc fragments. If, instead, the data had supported model 2b, then the RNAs would have been unequal, with one mRNA coding for the amino terminal portion of the Fd segment (the variable portion of the chain) while the remaining three-fourths of the heavy chain would have been coded by the second mRNA. The experimental data supported the first model and, in so doing, presented strong evidence that the heavy chain of the IgG immunoglobulin was synthesized as an entire single unit. Similar data allow a similar conclusion regarding synthesis of the light chain (57). However, none of the data to date precludes the possibility of a sharing of subunits by a fusion of the RNA or possibly even the DNA (fusion of the genes, polycistron) prior to synthesis of the chain at the polyribosomal level. In other words, the RNA need not be monocistronic in the strictest sense of the word. But the fact that the heavy and light chains are synthesized on separate polysomes indicates that the RNA is not polycistronic as it relates to the two chains.

Mechanism of Assembly of Immunoglobulin Chains

Because of the conclusions arrived at thus far concerning the size of the polysome structure on which antibody synthesis occurs, additional questions arise. If the heavy and light chains are synthesized on separate polysomes, the problem of the means of assembly of the completed immunoglobulins must be considered.

The possible mechanisms of assembly must correlate with the independent synthesis of each type of immunoglobulin chain. Each chain could be independently released from its respective polysome and assembled by a process separate from that of synthesis, or the release of either chain might influence the process of assembly or at least the release of the other chain. Askonas and Williamson (51,52), in addition to localizing the synthetic sites for each chain, also followed the release of these molecules from the polysomes. Following disruption of the myeloma cells, the intracellular soluble proteins were layered on sucrose gradients. Specific antisera were used to precipitate the various parts of the labeled globulin molecule following gradient separation. Only two peaks were found which could be precipitated by antisera, one being precipitable with either light-chain antisera or antisera against the Fc fragment (carboxyl portion of the heavy chain). The material in the second peak, in addition to precipitating only with antibody to light chain, was located in the same position on the gradient as isolated alkylated light chain. That the second peak was indeed composed of light-chain determinants is evidenced by the inability of Fab antisera, which had been absorbed with light chain, to cause precipitation. Fc antisera did not precipitate free heavy chains; using these techniques there were no indications that free heavy chains existed intracellularly. Radioautography of the precipitin bands after immunoelectrophoresis of the soluble proteins and specific antisera confirmed the data from sucrose density analysis.

The time course of labeling in free light chains and whole myeloma protein is illustrated in Fig. 7-3. According to these results, the free light-chain pool would be expected to be undergoing rapid turnover. That such turnover did occur was substantiated by a pulse-chase experiment conducted by these workers. Light chains and whole globulin were about equally labeled after a 5-minute pulse. However, following a 5-minute chase with nonradioactive amino acids, the amount of label in the whole globulin had increased, while that in the free light chains decreased markedly. Such a turnover would be expected if the free light chain was in an intermediate state prior to assembly into the whole molecule. The possibility that light chains were lost through secretion could not be substantiated experimentally.

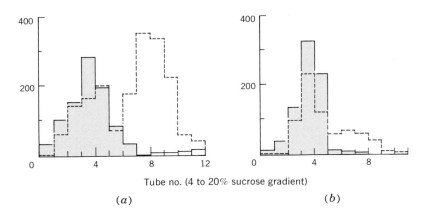

Tube no. (4 to 20% sucrose gradient)

(*a*) (*b*)

Fig. 7-3 Time course of labeling of free chain and myeloma protein. Plasma cells (5563 tumor) were incubated with H³-leucine for (a) 5 minutes, (b) 10 minutes. The soluble proteins after lysis of cells and sedimentation of the particulate components were fractionated on a sucrose gradient. Aliquots of each gradient fraction were reacted with antibody to light chain or Fc fragment in the presence of carrier antigen. The radioactivity of control precipitates of rabbit IgG with its antibody was subtracted from the values presented. ——— = Anti-Fc fragment; – – – – = anti-light chain. From Askonas and Williamson (51) with permission.

Somewhat similar conclusions can be drawn from the work of Shapiro et al. (35) with MPC_{11} tumor. After the characterization of the 190S and 270S polyribosomes as the sites for the synthesis of the light and heavy chains, the kinetics of release of these polypeptide chains from the polysomes were studied. In order to determine the patterns of assembly and release, these investigators pulse-chased for 15 and 30 seconds following a labeling period of 90 seconds. The labeled L chain was present in the 190S fraction after a 15-second chase, but had already disappeared by 30 seconds. H chains were found with the 270S polysomes until 60 seconds, after which time they disappeared. However, the L chain was also present in the 270S fraction for as long as 90 seconds. The ratio of radioactivity between light and heavy chains was compared in the completed and released chains following a 1½ minute pulse with C^{14}-amino acids. The isolated 7S globulin was treated to separate the two types of chains which were analyzed for radioactivity following 60-, 90-, and 120-minute chases. As shown in Fig. 7-4, the initial high activity in L chains compared to H chains reflected the earlier release of complete L chains. By 60 seconds the ratio had dropped considerably as more heavy chains were completed. The subsequent small rise at 90 seconds is most likely explained in terms of the first experiment. Labeled residual L chains from a pool of free light chains were bound to unlabeled heavy chains. The apparent steady state ratio of 2:1 radioactivity in L and H chains was expected from preliminary data obtained by these workers. They found that 4 times as many L chains were synthesized as H chains, but each H chain carried twice the number of counts as an L chain.

Some evidence exists that there also may be a small, rapidly turning over pool of heavy chains. The continued assembly of light-heavy chain dimers after exposure of cells to cycloheximide, which prevents release of nascent polypeptide chains, suggested that, in some instances, the disulfide bond may have been formed after release from the polysomes (53). The apparent lag in the labeling of the IgG molecule also indicated that in addition to a free pool of light chains, a small pool of heavy chains may also have existed.

The evidence that the light-chain component is synthesized and released into an intracellular pool appears conclusive. That this pool is rapidly turning over because of the incorporation of the L chains into the globulin molecule is also apparent. On the other hand, although no free H chains have been detected, evidence suggests that such a pool might exist. There is also evidence that light chains bind to heavy chains still on the polysomes. So, although the light chains may cause the release of the heavy chains, either by binding to them or by other mechanisms, such a proposal has not yet been proved.

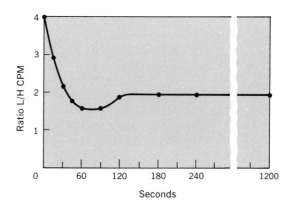

Fig. 7-4 Ratio of radioactivity in completed L and H chains after chasing. From Shapiro et al. (35) with permission.

Intracellular Site of Immunoglobulin Synthesis

Although the experimental data cited above establish that synthesis of antibody does occur on polyribosomes, the intracellular distribution of the polysomes remains to be identified. Kern et al. (58) first implicated the microsomal fraction of a lymph node extract as a site of antibody activity. Antigen (2,4 dinitrophenyl bovine γ-globulin) was selectively bound to the microsomes in a manner which suggested that a microsome-antibody complex existed. Antibody was released to the soluble phase of the microsomal extract by lowering the pH of the solution or exposing to urea.

The extraction procedure used by Kern et al. (58) does convert the endoplasmic reticulum (ER) to the closed vesicles which characterize a microsomal fraction. Since secreted proteins are generally thought to be synthesized on the membrane-bound ribosomes of the ER, a similar site would be expected for antibody synthesis. Indeed, Swenson and Kern (59) found that as much as 99 percent of the H^3-protein isolated in the microsomal fraction was γ-globulin. Although the amount of H^3-protein isolated in the cell sap was 5 to 20 times that found in the microsomal fraction, only 2 to 11 percent was γ-globulin. Therefore, although the bulk of the total H^3-protein was found in the cell sap, approximately 99 percent of the γ-globulin was located in the microsomal fraction. Contrary to the localization of antibody, a secreted protein in the microsomes, aldolase, also present in these cells but not as a secreted protein, was concentrated in the cell sap.

Additional evidence that antibody synthesis occurs on the membrane-bound ribosomes of the ER lies in the work of De Petris and Karlsbad (60), Vassalli (61), and La Via et al. (62). De Petris and Karlsbad, using electron microscopy, detected antiferritin antibodies on the cisternae of the

229

ER. Vassalli (61) was able to prepare a cell-free system for specific anti-body synthesis from lymph node microsomal vesicles. La Via et al. (62) separated the free and membrane-associated polyribosomes and precipi-tated the polysome-associated, newly synthesized peptide with anti-Fab antibody. Almost all of the precipitable radioactivity was associated with the bound polysomes, indicating that at least that portion of the antibody precipitated by anti-Fab was synthesized on bound polysomes.

Cellular Secretion of Immunoglobulins

The compartmentalization of the gamma globulin molecule in the micro-somal fraction of antibody-synthesizing cells has prompted further studies in an effort to correlate such a localization with the secretory process. Swenson and Kern (63), although continuing to find most of the globulin molecules in microsomal fraction, also demonstrated a second intracellular pool of γ-globulin. By labeling the γ-globulin with radioactive mono-saccharides, they isolated antibody molecules according to their specific carbohydrate moiety. In doing so, it was found that 98 percent of the H^3-galactose-labeled molecules were in the cell sap rather than the microsomal compartment. In these same experiments, labeling with H^3-leucine showed that only 6 percent of the total cellular γ-globulin was in the cell sap. This correlates with the observation that the radioactivity in the total γ-globulin when H^3-galactose was employed was only 3 percent of that found when H^3-leucine was used as a marker. Such information indicates that a small pool of antibody molecules was located outside of the microsomal fraction and that this pool was preferentially labeled by a monosaccharide isotope.

As early as 1961 evidence was presented suggesting that, following completion of intracellular synthesis of the globulin molecule, a lag period preceded the extracellular appearance of that molecule (64). The initial work on the rat lymph node cells indicated that such a lag phase might span a 20-minute period. Later reports on the plasma cell tumors of BALB/c mice suggested that as long as 60 minutes might lapse between synthesis and secretion. With the findings of Swenson and Kern (63) on the varied compartmentalization of globulins with and without carbo-hydrate moieties, attention was focused on the possibility that the addition of the carbohydrate portion of the molecule might account for the delayed secretion. Reports from three laboratories (63,65,66) confirmed that the biosynthesis of the carbohydrate portion did occur during the lag period and that subunits of that moiety were added progressively throughout the period. Melchers and Knopf (65) and Moroz and Uhr (66) confirmed that the glucosamine, which forms the aspartylcarbohydrate linkage, was added to the protein while the latter was still attached to the polysomes. However, neither group has yet identified the protein as gamma globulin rather than another cellular polypeptide chain. However, Swenson and Kern (67) showed that both glucosamine and galactose were incorporated specifically into the globulin molecule early in the lag phase, while sialic acid, a terminal residue of the carbohydrate chain, was added just prior to secretion. The intracellular and extracellular appearances of sialic acid occurred simultaneously, confirming the late addition of that residue. Similarly, Melchers and Knopf (65) found that chromatographic and electrophoretic analysis of intracellular and extracellular γ-globulin showed structural nonidentity between the globulins in the two locations. The analysis indicated that the incomplete carbohydrate moiety on the intracellular globulin, upon completion, was involved in the immediate release of the globulin from the cell.

REFERENCES

1. Green, H., and Anker, H. S.: *J. Gen. Physiol.*, **38**:283, 1955.
2. Taliaferro, W. H., and Talmage, D. W.: *J. Infect. Dis.*, **97**:88, 1955.
3. Taliaferro, W. H., and Taliaferro, L. G.: *J. Infect. Dis.*, **101**:252, 1957.
4. Kern, M., Helmreich, E., and Eisen, H. N.: *Proc. Nat. Acad. Sci. U.S.*, **45**:862, 1959.
5. Jacob, F., and Monod, J.: *J. Mol. Biol.*, **3**:318, 1961.
6. Dutton, R. W.: *Advan. Immunol.*, **6**:253, 1967.
7. Cohen, E. P., and Talmage, D. W.: *J. Exp. Med.*, **121**:125, 1965.
8. Mach, B., and Vassalli, P.: *Proc. Nat. Acad. Sci. U.S.*, **54**:975, 1965.
9. Raška, K., and Cohen, E. P.: *Clin. Exp. Immunol.*, **2**:559, 1967.
10. Lazda, V. A., Starr, J. L., and Rachmeler, M.: *J. Immunol.*, **101**:349, 1968.
11. Lazda, V. A., Starr, J. L., and Rachmeler, M.: *J. Immunol.*, **101**:359, 1968.
12. Lazda, V., and Starr, J. L.: *J. Immunol.*, **95**:254, 1965.
13. Cohen, E. P.: *Proc. Nat. Acad. Sci. U.S.*, **57**:673, 1967.
14. Cooper, H. L.: *J. Biol. Chem.*, **243**:34, 1968.
15. Scherrer, K., Marcaud, L., Zajdela, F., London, I., and Gros, F.: *Proc. Nat. Acad. Sci. U.S.*, **56**:1571, 1966.
16. Soeiro, R., Birnboim, H. C., and Darnell, J. E.: *J. Mol. Biol.*, **19**:362, 1966.
17. Attardi, G., Parnas, H., Hwang, M-I. H., and Attardi, B.: *J. Mol. Biol.*, **20**:145, 1966.
18. Uhr, J. W., Scharff, M. D., and Tawde, S.: in "Molecular and Cellular Basis of Antibody Formation," J. Šterzl (ed.), Academic Press, Inc., New York, 1965.

19. Krueger, R. G.: *Proc. Nat. Acad. Sci. U.S.*, **55**:1206, 1966.
20. Fishman, M.: *J. Exp. Med.*, **114**:837, 1961.
21. Fishman, M., and Adler, F. L.: *J. Exp. Med.*, **117**:595, 1963.
22. Askonas, B. A., and Rhodes, J. M.: in "Molecular and Cellular Basis of Antibody Formation," J. Šterzl (ed.), Academic Press, Inc., New York, 1965.
23. Friedman, H. P., Stavitsky, A. B., and Solomon, J. M., *Science* **149**:1106, 1965.
24. Bishop, D. C., Pisciotta, A. V., and Abramoff, P.: *J. Immunol.*, **99**:751, 1967.
25. Gottlieb, A. A.: *J. Reticuloendothel. Soc.*, **5**:270, 1968.
26. Cohen, E. P.: *Annu. Rev. Microbiol.*, **22**:283, 1968.
27. Cohen, E. P., and Parks, J. J.: *Science*, **144**:1012, 1964.
28. Friedman, H.: *Science*, **146**:934, 1964.
29. Friedman, H. P., Stavitsky, A. B., and Solomon, J. M.: *Science*, **149**:1106, 1965.
30. Askonas, B. A., and Rhodes, J. M.: *Nature (London)*, **205**:470, 1965.
31. Adler, F. L., Fishman, M., and Dray, S.: *J. Immunol.*, **97**:554, 1966.
32. Cohen, E. P., Newcomb, R. W., and Crosby, L. K.: *J. Immunol.*, **95**:583, 1965.
33. Abramoff, P., and Brien, N. B.: *J. Immunol.*, **100**:1210, 1968.
34. Williamson, A. R., and Askonas, B. A.: *J. Mol. Biol.*, **23**:201, 1967.
35. Shapiro, A. L., Scharff, M. D., Maizel, J. V., Jr., and Uhr, J. W.: *Proc. Nat. Acad. Sci. U.S.*, **56**:216, 1966.
36. Huxley, H. E., and Zubay, G.: *J. Mol. Biol.*, **2**:10, 1960.
37. Shelton, E., and Kuff, E. L.: *J. Mol. Biol.*, **22**:23, 1966.
38. Sabatini, D., Tashiro, Y., and Palade, G. E.: *J. Mol. Biol.*, **19**:503, 1966.
39. Slayter, H. S., Warner, J. R., Rich, A., and Hall, C. E.: *J. Mol. Biol.*, **7**:652, 1963.
40. Marks, P. A., Burka, E. R., and Schlessinger, D.: *Proc. Nat. Acad. Sci. U.S.*, **48**:2163, 1962.
41. Warner, J. R., Knopf, P. M., and Rich, A.: *Proc. Nat. Acad. Sci. U.S.*, **49**:122, 1963.
42. Warner, J. R., Rich, A., and Hall, C. E.: *Science*, **138**:1399, 1962.
43. Dintzis, H. M.: *Proc. Nat. Acad. Sci. U.S.*, **47**:247, 1961.
44. Naughton, M. A., and Dintzis, H. M.: *Proc. Nat. Acad. Sci. U.S.*, **48**:1822, 1962.
45. Kuff, E. L., and Roberts, N. E.: *J. Mol. Biol.*, **26**:211, 1967.
46. Edelman, G. M., and Poulik, M. D.: *J. Exp. Med.*, **113**:861, 1961.
47. Fleischman, J. B., Pain, R. H., and Porter, R. R.: *Arch. Biochem.*, *Suppl.* **1**:174, 1962.
48. Stenzel, K. H., Phillips, W. D., Thompson, D. D., and Rubin, A. L.: *Proc. Nat. Acad. Sci. U.S.*, **51**:636, 1964.
49. Norton, W. L., Lewis, D., and Ziff, M.: *Proc. Nat. Acad. Sci. U.S.*, **54**:851, 1965.
50. Scharff, M., and Uhr, J. W.: *Science*, **148**:646, 1965.

51. Askonas, B. A., and Williamson, A. R.: *Proc. Roy. Soc. (Biol.)*, **166**:232, 1966.
52. Askonas, B. A., and Williamson, A. R.: *Cold Spring Harbor Symp. Quant. Biol.*, **32**:223, 1967.
53. Scharff, M. D., Shapiro, A. L., and Ginsberg, B.: *Cold Spring Harbor Symp. Quant. Biol.*, **32**:235, 1967.
54. La Via, M. F., Vatter, A. E., Hammond, W. S., and Northup, P. V.: *Proc. Nat. Acad. Sci. U.S.*, **57**:79, 1967.
55. De Petris, S.: *J. Mol. Biol.*, **23**:217, 1967.
56. Knopf, P. M., Parkhouse, R. M. E., and Lennox, E. S.: *Proc. Nat. Acad. Sci. U.S.*, **58**:2288, 1967.
57. Lennox, E. S., Knopf, P. M., Munro, A. J., and Parkhouse, R. M. E.: *Cold Spring Harbor Symp. Quant. Biol.*, **32**:249, 1967.
58. Kern, M., Helmreich, E., and Eisen, H. N.: *Proc. Nat. Acad. Sci. U.S.*, **45**:862, 1959.
59. Swenson, R. M., and Kern, M.: *Proc. Nat. Acad. Sci. U.S.*, **57**:417, 1967.
60. De Petris, S., and Karlsbad, G.: *J. Cell Biol.*, **26**:759, 1965.
61. Vassalli, P.: *Proc. Nat. Acad. Sci. U.S.*, **58**:2117, 1967.
62. La Via, M. F., Vatter, A. E., and Northup, P. V.: *Federation Proc.*, **27**:318, 1968.
63. Swenson, R. M., and Kern, M.: *J. Biol. Chem.*, **242**:3242, 1967.
64. Helmreich, E., Kern, M., and Eisen, H. N.: *J. Biol. Chem.*, **236**:464, 1961.
65. Melchers F., and Knopf, P. M.: *Cold Spring Harbor Symp. Quant. Biol.*, **32**:255, 1967.
66. Moroz, C., and Uhr, J. W.: *Cold Spring Harbor Symp. Quant. Biol.*, **32**:263, 1967.
67. Swenson, R. M., and Kern, M.: *Proc. Nat. Acad. Sci. U.S.*, **59**:546, 1968.

8
Immunologic Memory

Memory and specificity constitute two outstanding characteristics of the immune response. If a memory phenomenon can be demonstrated in a particular biologic system, this is evidence for an immunologic mechanism. The failure to demonstrate memory is not conclusive evidence that the reaction is not an immunologic one, since under certain restricted conditions (see below), memory may not be demonstrable.

Immunologic memory may be described as the altered immune reaction of an organism to an immunologic stimulus as a result of having met that stimulus before. This description includes the restriction that the memory is specific for antigenic determinants and, therefore, excludes altered reactivity associated with generalized changes in immunologic responsiveness (see Chaps. 9 and 10).

Immunologic memory exists in two forms: positive immunologic memory and negative immunologic memory. With positive memory, the organism produces a greater immunologic response to the second antigenic stimulus than it did to the first. With negative memory, the organism generally fails to react at all to either the first or subsequent antigenic stimuli.

For reasons of simplicity we will discuss positive immunologic memory first, including circulating antibody production and cellular immunity.

POSITIVE IMMUNOLOGIC MEMORY—THE PRIMARY AND SECONDARY ("ANAMNESTIC") RESPONSES

General Features of the Primary and Secondary Responses in Serum

If an animal has never encountered an antigen, the first injection of this antigen is generally followed by the appearance of specific serum antibody. The kinetics of this appearance usually include a "latent period" of several days during which no antibody is detectable, followed by a moderate rise to a peak titer, with a subsequent leveling off and a decline of titer. This is a "primary" response. A second injection of the same dose of this antigen produces a response which includes the following features: the latent period is shorter, the rise steeper, and the peak higher than in the primary response. This second response is called an "anamnestic," or "secondary," response. The animal "remembers" having met the antigen before, and his positive immunologic memory is demonstrated by a faster and more powerful antibody response to the second stimulus. The general features are shown in Fig. 8-1. Tertiary responses usually do not differ greatly from secondary responses.

Many experiments have been done over the last 50 years in which a number of variables related to memory have been discussed. One variable is the effect of age on memory. Wolfe et al. (1) have shown that the age at which chickens were given a primary injection of bovine serum albumin (BSA) determined whether or not a secondary response could be evoked. For example, chickens given a primary antigenic stimulus at 20 days of age gave no anamnestic response if stimulated at 6, 12, or 22 weeks of age. Chickens first immunized at 6 weeks gave variable anamnestic responses at 12 and 22 weeks. Chickens first immunized at 12 weeks of age all gave good secondary responses at 22 weeks. These experiments were done using the precipitin test to measure serum antibody. This raises two questions: Could antibody have been detected in younger chickens if a more sensitive technique were used, and were the younger chickens partially tolerant?

Makinodan and Peterson (2) also studied the effect of age on the anamnestic response to sheep erythrocytes (SRBC) in mice. When there was a fixed interval between the primary and secondary stimulus, younger

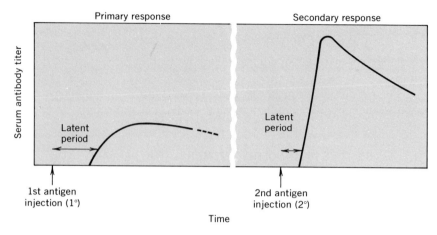

Fig. 8-1 Kinetics of appearance of serum antibody in primary and secondary responses.

mice gave the poorest anamnestic responses, adult mice, the best, and older mice (64 weeks old) showed intermediate responses. These studies indicate that immunologic memory, as a function of age, develops, matures, and wanes with senescence.

Other studies have looked at the relation between size of antigenic load and degree of response. Jílek and Šterzl (3) studied the response of mice to SRBC in terms of serum agglutinins and hemolysins. To summarize their results: In the primary response larger doses of SRBC produced greater hemagglutinin and hemolysin responses than did smaller amounts of antigen. In the anamnestic response, a standard secondary dose of SRBC produced greater agglutinin titers if it followed a large, rather than a small, primary stimulus. The hemolysin response behaved in contrary fashion, since the anamnestic response to a standard secondary dose was smaller if it followed a large rather than a small primary stimulus. These are interesting findings but are difficult to interpret because of the complex nature of the antigens, the multiple antibodies detected in the antibody assays, and the presence of feedback regulatory mechanisms in intact animals.

Antigens are often more efficient in producing a secondary than a primary response. In general, if a small dose of antigen is used to evoke a primary respose of moderate magnitude, the same dose injected into an animal which had already mounted a primary response to that antigen (a "primed" animal) will produce a far greater secondary antibody response. The increased effectiveness of antigens (particularly soluble antigens) in producing a secondary response may be accounted for by an increased number of available antigen-sensitive cells and by the presence of circulating antibody remaining from the primary response. This cir-

236

culating antibody will complex with reintroduced antigen, rendering it more immunogenic, since antigen-antibody complexes formed in antigen excess are highly immunogenic (4).

Positive immunologic memory may last a very long time. Early experiments in guinea pigs indicated that a typical anamnestic response was obtained over a year after a single primary injection of diphtheria toxoid (5). In humans, an anamnestic response to a booster injection of tetanus toxoid was seen over 10 years after the primary immunization procedure. Extrapolation of these data suggests that the memory is present for life, at least in this system (6).

The anamnestic response is specific for antigenic determinants. If the second antigen is unrelated to the first, the antibodies produced after the second antigenic stimulation will be directed only against antigenic determinants present on the second antigen. An animal immunized with one antigen will have an anamnestic response to a later injection of a second antigen only if the second antigen has determinants in common with the first (i.e., the second cross-reacts with the first) (7).

When the antigen consists of a hapten conjugated with a protein carrier, the early anamnestic response shows "carrier specificity." For instance, when the dinitrophenyl (DNP) hapten is conjugated to a carrier protein such as bovine gamma globulin (BGG) the DNP-BGG complex evokes an adequate secondary response of anti-DNP antibodies in rabbits 2 months after the primary stimulus with DNP-BGG. The same hapten complexed to a protein carrier which does not cross-react with BGG [e.g., egg albumin (OVA)] will not elicit a secondary response 2 months after primary immunization with DNP-BGG (8). The carrier specificity of the secondary response suggests that the antibody is directed to portions of both DNP and BGG. If, however, the hapten–heterologous-protein booster (DNP-OVA) is given later (i.e., 5 months after the DNP-BGG primary stimulus), there is a weak but definite anamnestic response of anti-DNP antibodies. This phenomenon is interpreted to represent cell selection and is discussed below under the changes in avidity occurring during the antibody response.

A similar phenomenon has been called "the doctrine of original antigenic sin" (9). In this case a second antigenic challenge will produce an antibody response directed mainly against a cross-reacting primary antigenic stimulus to which the animal had responded earlier. This was first noted in studies with influenza in which booster immunization with influenza vaccines produced antibodies which were mainly directed against strains of influenza to which the subjects had responded earlier. The response to the last vaccine itself was comparatively weak. This phenomenon has been explored by Eisen (10). His results are also most easily explained on a cell selection basis (see below under changes in avidity occurring during the antibody response).

This general distinction between primary and secondary antibody responses has been known for many years. Recent advances in immunology have shown that this distinction is not always clear and its demonstration may depend on variables such as the type, form, and route of introduction of antigen; the species in which the antibody is produced; and the methods of antibody measurement.

The general shape of the antibody responses may vary according to the type of antibody detected. For instance, Fig. 8-2 shows that the primary antibody response to BSA in rabbits as measured by a precipitin technique (solid line) reaches an early peak and quickly diminishes thereafter (11). On the other hand, if one uses a very similar experimental situation but measures the response by the antigen-binding capacity of the serum (dashed line), the shape of the primary antibody response is quite

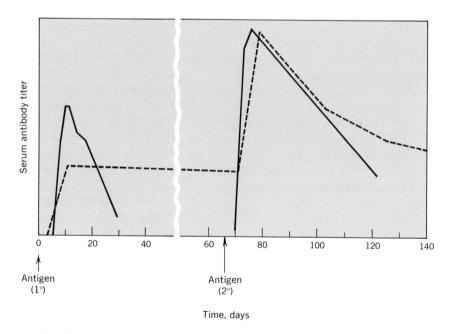

Fig. 8-2 Primary and secondary antibody responses measured by different methods. Rabbits given 15 mg/kg BSA intravenously. ———— Antibody titers measured by precipitation of I*BSA. Adapted from Dixon et al. (11). – – – – Antibody titers measured by serum antigen-binding capacity (ammonium sulfate precipitation technique). Adapted from Claman (12).

different (12). In this case the serum antibody activity rises to a plateau and remains level for several months without subsequent antigenic stimulation. Since the half-life of rabbit antibody is 5 to 6 days, the shape of this curve implies that antibody production continues for months. The shapes of the anamnestic responses measured by the two methods in Fig. 8-2 are quite similar.

The type of antigen may be important. In man, a first injection of purified pneumococcal polysaccharides is followed by the appearance of circulating antibodies. The titer remains high and level for many months. A second injection of antigen does not produce an anamnestic response (13). The reasons for this are not clear, but may be related to persistence of the original antigen (polysaccharides are difficult to degrade in humans) or to partial immunologic paralysis (see section on "negative" memory below). Another possibility is that the subjects had in fact previously encountered the antigen, even though no circulating antibody was detectable before immunization. In this case, what was considered to be a primary antigenic stimulus may have been in fact a secondary one, and the entire observed response may have been a secondary response. This situation occurs in mice stimulated with sheep erythrocytes (SRBC). The antibody response to a first injection of SRBC resembles a secondary response in its kinetics. The crucial point is that although no hemolytic antibody against SRBC can be demonstrated in the serum prior to injection of SRBC, the spleens of these "normal" animals contain a small number of cells synthesizing anti-SRBC (14), indicating that in fact the animal had responded previously to some SRBC antigens and the "primary" response, as observed in the laboratory, is indeed a secondary response. These "background" plaque-forming cells probably represent results of inapparent immunization from the natural environment. Data of this sort make it appear that if an anamnestic response is not generated upon reintroduction of antigen, the "primary" response observed may actually have been a "secondary" response.

Cellular Aspects of Immunologic Memory for Circulating Antibody

Historically, the distinction between primary and secondary responses was made by measurements of circulating antibody. Some of the problems raised by this distinction can be clarified by investigating the cells which produce these antibodies. Details of the cellular events following antigenic stimulation have been presented in Chap. 6. As applied to the distinction between the primary and secondary response, these events occur as follows. A small number of "precursor" cells are somehow stimulated by the first exposure to antigen so that they divide and differentiate (both processes overlapping) into a moderate number of antibody-producing cells. Following a secondary stimulus, the events appear qualitatively similar, but the quantity of antibody-forming cells is much greater (15,16). One is led to assume that the number of antigen-sensitive precursor cells existing prior to the secondary stimulus is greater than that existing prior to the primary stimulus. The first dose of antigen thus causes an increase in both producers and in precursors. The second dose of antigen reacts with the enlarged pool of antigen-sensitive precursors to form a secondary pool of producers larger than that seen in the primary response and accounting for the increased amount of antibody formed in the anamnestic response. This scheme is outlined in Fig. 8-3.

Radiosensitivity of Primary and Secondary Responses

The production of circulating antibody during the primary response appears to be more radiosensitive than the process of antibody production during the secondary response. The subject of inhibition of antibody synthesis by x-ray and related modalities is discussed at length in Chap. 10. That is, a dose of x-ray which inhibits the primary response in an intact animal will not inhibit the secondary response. This distinction is more apparent than real because the magnitude of decrease in antibody formation (produced by a given dose of x-ray) during a primary response is not different from the decrease produced by the same dose of x-ray during a secondary response. Thus the apparent difference is due to the larger number of antibody-forming cells active in the secondary response (17). It is unfortunate that this study was done in the mouse-SRBC system in which the distinction between primary and secondary response is blurred.

Changes in Antibody Avidity During the Antibody Response

Jerne and Avegno (18) showed that antibody produced late in the primary response or in the anamnestic response had higher avidity for antigen than did antibody formed early in the primary response. Antibody avidity is a measure of the tightness of the antigen-antibody bond. It may be measured by the association constant between antigen and antibody (see Chap. 12). Recent work has shown that the antibody populations produced in response even to purified haptenic antigens (e.g., DNP) exhibited a wide heterogeneity of binding affinities for the antigen (19). The anti-DNP antibodies synthesized early reacted weakly with a small

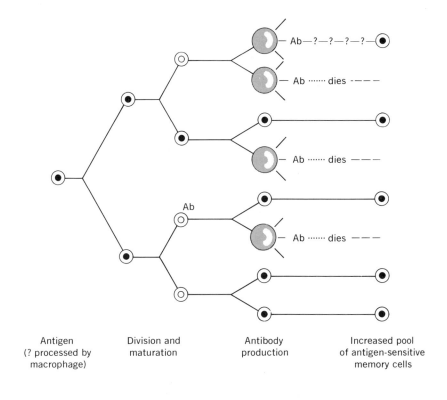

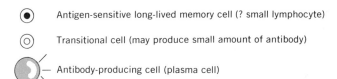

| Antigen (? processed by macrophage) | Division and maturation | Antibody production | Increased pool of antigen-sensitive memory cells |

⦿   Antigen-sensitive long-lived memory cell (? small lymphocyte)

◎   Transitional cell (may produce small amount of antibody)

   Antibody-producing cell (plasma cell)

Fig. 8-3 The effects of antigen on immunologically competent antigen-sensitive precursor cells.

portion of the DNP antigenic determinant, while the late high-affinity antibodies were more tightly bound to larger parts of the DNP determinant. The basis for this change in antibody avidity may lie at the cellular level, since experiments by Steiner and Eisen (20) have shown that lymphoid cells isolated early in the immune response synthesize antibodies of low average affinity, while lymphoid cells isolated late in the immune response synthesize antibodies of high average affinity.

Thus the average affinity of the antibodies in a particular serum sample taken at a particular time after immunization reflects the combined contribution of at least two populations of cells, with one making low-affinity antibody and the other making high-affinity antibody. The change (increase) in average antibody affinity during the course of immunization would reflect an increase in the number of antibody molecules made by high-affinity producers and a decrease in the number of molecules made by low-affinity producers. This change, according to Eisen, might be mediated by the presence of "sentinel" antibody molecules on the surface of the immunocompetent cells (10). These sentinel molecules are able to capture circulating antigen and then trigger antibody production. According to this theory, low-affinity producers have sentinel antibody sites triggered by high doses of antigen, but high-affinity producers are saturated and inhibited by high doses of antigen. Thus, early in the immune response when antigen is plentiful, antibody will be mainly produced by low-affinity producers. Later in the immune response, when the level of antigen declines, the high-affinity producers will be more successful in competing for the limited supply of antigen and will be selectively stimulated, leading to the production of serum antibody of high average avidity.

This same sort of "cell selection" may explain the lack of carrier specificity seen with some hapten-protein antigens. As mentioned earlier, a rabbit primed with DNP-BGG will give a booster response specific for DNP if the secondary stimulus is early and consists of DNP-BGG. If the early booster consists of DNP-OVA, no increase in anti-DNP antibodies will occur. On the other hand, if 5 months elapse between the primary injection of DNP-BGG and the booster stimulus, the following is seen: DNP-BGG evokes a large secondary response in which the antibody avidity is no greater than that existing before the booster, but DNP-OVA evokes a small secondary response in which the anti-DNP avidity is considerably greater than it was before the booster. Paul et al. (8) interpret these data as follows: A single antigen stimulates a number of clones of cells to produce specific antibody, each clone making antibody of a given avidity. "Memory cells" contain the antibody on their surfaces, and those with more avid antibody are more successful in competing for available antigen. When the secondary stimulus is the same as the first (DNP-BGG), the antigen stimulates the same clones of cells stimulated by the original antigen giving a large increase in antibody but no change in average avidity. If the secondary stimulus is DNP-OVA, this antigen contains only a portion of the original antigenic determinant (the DNP part without any BGG contribution), and therefore, it will react preferentially with the few cells containing the surface antibodies with high affinity for DNP. In so doing it will stimulate these cells, thus giving rise to a small anamnestic response but one containing anti-DNP antibodies of high avidity.

Differences in Immunoglobulin Classes

Recent analyses of the structure of antibodies have shown that a given antigen often induces the production of antibodies belonging to several immunoglobulin classes. Furthermore, antibodies of different types and classes may be detected in a certain sequence (21,22). For instance, soluble or particulate proteins often first elicit a rise in 19S antibodies. These antibodies may persist but are then replaced or accompanied by 7S antibodies. In the guinea pig, however, the sequence of antibody appearance depends on the dose of antigen. With 10^{11} particles of ϕX174 Uhr and Finkelstein (23) found that 19S antibody appeared first and then declined as 7S antibody appeared. With 10^9 particles, however, only 19S antibody was detected.

These results are in contrast to those of Nossal et al. (24) using *Salmonella* flagellar antigens in rats. Both intact flagella and polymerized flagellin caused a primary response consisting of 19S antibody, but the soluble low-molecular-weight flagellin caused only a 7S response.

Secondary responses generally consist mainly of 7S antibody. Thus the existence of "memory" for 7S antibody is firmly established. The question of memory for 19S antibody is not easily settled, however. One problem involves the detection of a modest increase in 19S antibodies in the presence of a secondary response containing a large increase in 7S antibodies. Uhr and Finkelstein studied a group of guinea pigs which showed only a 19S response to small doses of ϕX174. Upon rechallenge with antigen, these animals gave only a 19S response which was similar in magnitude to the primary response. Thus no long-lasting 19S memory was demonstrated in the system (22). Similar results were found by Svehag and Mandel (25), who used poliovirus in rabbits.

Long-lasting 19S immunologic memory has been shown in other systems, such as with *Salmonella* flagella in rats (24) and with BSA or HSA in rabbits (26). The problem is quite complex, since many methods of antibody detection are more sensitive to one immunoglobulin species than to another. That is, a given technique may show the appearance of 19S before 7S during the course of immunization merely because that method detects smaller quantities of 19S than of 7S antibodies (27). Thus the results of experiments showing the sequence and magnitude of memory responses of various systems depend upon the type and form (i.e., aggregated or soluble) of antigen, the dose, the route of injection, the species injected, and the methods of antibody measurement.

The facts may be summarized as follows:

1. The usual primary response involves the early detection of 19S followed by 7S antibody. Anamnestic responses usually show positive memory for 7S and little memory for 19S antibody.

2. Some systems show that 19S antibody formation may be induced without detectable 7S antibody and without memory for 19S or 7S antibodies.

3. Some systems show prolonged 19S memory.

POSITIVE MEMORY IN CELLULAR IMMUNITY—THE ACCELERATED ("SECOND-SET") REACTION

Animals receiving skin grafts from allogeneic donors "reject" these grafts within a definite time. This has been called the "first-set" rejection (see Chap. 15). Second grafts from the same (or genetically identical) donors to the same recipients are rejected in accelerated fashion, since they survive for considerably shorter periods than did the original grafts. This has been called the "second-set" phenomenon, and it represents an instance of immunologic memory. This memory is specific, as shown by the following example: An A mouse will reject the first skin graft from a B mouse in 11 days. After rejection, a second graft from a B mouse will survive on the "sensitized" A mouse recipient for only 5 days, but a first graft from a C mouse simultaneously applied will be rejected in 10 days. Thus the memory acquired by the A mouse as a result of having previously rejected B skin is specific for B skin.

The specificity and memory displayed by these grafting experiments are the keystones for the assertion that tissue graft rejection phenomena are immunologic. This memory is long-lasting but has been shown to wane slowly over a period of months (28). It is a property of lymphoid cells, particularly those in the regional nodes draining a rejected graft, since such nodal tissue is most effective in "adoptively" conferring the ability to reject grafts upon normal animals. Serum is not capable of transferring this sensitivity (see Chap. 14). A more clear-cut method of demonstrating the immunologic memory is by the breakdown of tolerance to skin grafts which occurs after adoptive transfer of cells from normal or sensitized donors. Thus, CBA mice tolerant of A skin and retaining an A skin graft will reject the graft after 23 days if implanted with normal CBA nodes, but will reject the skin in 9 to 15 days if implanted with nodes from CBA donors who had been sensitized by previous rejection of an A graft (29). Although quantitative studies of the number of lymph node cells transferred were not made, these experiments are consistent with the notion that immunologic memory includes the acquisition of a greater number of cells specifically reactive for a given antigen. An anamnestic type response has also been shown in experiments where the waning of previously induced cellular immunity has been heightened by a tissue stimulus which is quantitatively insufficient for immunization of a normal animal (30).

An anamnestic response is more difficult to demonstrate in delayed hypersensitivity systems of the tuberculin type. It probably occurs, since the ability to transfer delayed hypersensitivity to tuberculin by means of lymphoid cells from sensitized but not from normal donors suggests that the sensitized donors had a larger pool of specifically reactive cells. In addition, when cells were transferred to inbred guinea pigs 20 days after the donors were immunized to PPD, the recipients had larger skin reactions to PPD than did guinea pigs receiving cells from donors immunized 10 days before transfer (31). In general, however, remarkably little work has been done in terms of quantitative aspects of immunologic memory in the tuberculin type of cellular hypersensitivity. Part of the difficulty lies in the fact that, unless one is very careful, circulating antibody will be produced in the course of inducing and measuring delayed hypersensitivity. This could interfere with the interpretation of further skin tests because of the appearance of Arthus reactions. Salvin and Smith (32) were careful to measure anamnestic responses in guinea pigs in whom delayed hypersensitivity had been induced by such small amounts of diphtheria toxoid or egg albumin that circulating antibody was not detected. In these guinea pigs, reinjection of antigen gave an accelerated Arthus-type reaction. Moreover, the degree of memory (as measured by the shortness of induction period of the Arthus reaction) was greatest if the second dose of antigen was given at the height of the primary delayed hypersensitivity response. Nevertheless, this anamnesis was not properly a secondary delayed hypersensitivity response.

Arnason and Waksman (33) studied the "retest" phenomenon in guinea pigs with delayed hypersensitivity to BSA or tuberculin. These animals had retest reactions when the site of primary sensitization was rechallenged with specific antigen. This reaction evolved faster and faded more quickly than did reactions to the same challenge in previously uninjected sites of the same animals. The authors felt that it depended on preformed local or circulating antibody and that it was probably not a Schwartzman or an Arthus reaction.

NEGATIVE IMMUNOLOGIC MEMORY—TOLERANCE †

There are few areas in modern immunology more puzzling than that of tolerance. Although the phenomenon itself (the failure of an animal to produce a specific immunologic response under conditions in which such

† In this section, the terms *tolerance* and *paralysis* will be used interchangeably. The distinction between *paralysis* by large doses of soluble antigens and *tolerance* to cells has become much less clear in recent years. The two phenomena are undoubtedly very closely related.

a response might ordinarily be expected) is not difficult to recognize, knowledge of its mechanism is vague. This is not surprising, since knowledge of the mechanism underlying tolerance implies knowledge of the (molecular) mechanism underlying antibody formation. The problem has been recently reviewed (34).

Natural Tolerance

Under ordinary conditions, animals do not make antibodies against their own tissue antigens, either soluble or cellular. This phenomenon was stated as a biological principle by Ehrlich, who called it "horror autotoxicus" (fear of poisoning one's self). While it is generally true that an animal does not produce antibodies or immune reactions against its own antigens, it is not true that the animal cannot do so.

Immunization of an animal with his own or isogenic tissues or tissue antigens does not lead to measurable antibody production [except in some cases using large amounts of adjuvant (35)]. If the antigenic stimulus is a tissue graft, such as skin, this graft will be permanently accepted by the animal itself (autograft) or by an isogenic animal (isograft). Another identical graft placed on the recipient will also be tolerated indefinitely: no immunologic memory is demonstrable.

The lack of immunologic response to isogenic antigens contrasts with the responses occurring when the same antigens are introduced into allogenic animals. In this case circulating antibodies are produced and tissue grafts are rejected. In some cases, antigens are species specific rather than strain specific. For instance, human serum albumin (HSA) appears to be antigenically identical in almost all humans and, therefore, isosensitization does not occur, i.e., injection of one person's HSA into another human will not cause the production of anti-HSA. This is not true with human gamma globulin (HGG), since there is a system of genetically determined allotypic HGG antigen, the Gm and Inv system (see Chap. 3). In this case, HGG from one person may immunize another person if the allotypic antigenic determinants differ (36). The degree of immunologic response increases as the phylogenetic disparity between the antigen donor and antibody producer widens. Thus bovine serum albumin is more antigenic for mice than is rat serum albumin.

It becomes obvious that an animal has some means by which, immunologically speaking, it can tell the difference between self and not-self. A substance recognized as self calls forth no immunologic response. A substance recognized as not-self induces an immunologic response. This may be interpreted as an adaptive and protective response to the environment. The response to not-self may be seen as an attempt to preserve individual integrity.

A theory explaining how an animal distinguishes self from not-self was proposed in 1949 by Burnet and Fenner (37). These authors recognized that the ability to make antibody develops slowly during embryonic development and that fetal animals were generally immunologically incompetent. At the same time, these developing animals had the means for disposing of effete "expendable" body cells, presumably with specific surface markers. This mechanism for disposing of "self" antigens when necessary (without making antibody against them) "hardened" during development, so that later on, the introduction of not-self antigens was recognized as such and provoked an immune response. This theory was in accord with the findings of Owen (38), who studied multiovular twin calves of distinct genetic erythrocyte types between which there had been placental anastamoses. These calves were chimeras with regard to erythrocyte serotypes. The two parental serotypes did not segregate, one in one calf and one in the other, as would happen in ordinary fraternal twins. Instead, each calf after birth contained erythrocytes of both serotypes, his "own" and his "brother's." Thus the introduction of a genetically foreign stem line of cells during early embryonic life did not evoke an immune response by the recipient leading to the antibody mediated destruction of the "foreign cells." Instead, the not-self cell line was free to establish itself and replicate as self. The immunologically immature animal was "fooled" into accepting not-self antigens as self. The same antigens given to an immunologically competent recipient would evoke an antibody response in the host and would be destroyed. This theory suggested a number of experiments which greatly increased our knowledge of immune mechanisms.

This hypothesis was later broadened to include the "forbidden clone" theory (39). This theory states that all clones of immunologically competent lymphoid cells which contact self-antigens in embryonic life are destroyed. Any "sequestered" self-antigens which do not have an opportunity to meet lymphoid cells will have corresponding intact lymphoid clones able to make antibodies against the cells. Under ordinary circumstances, the antigens remain sequestered and the lymphoid clones remain unstimulated. Conditions such as trauma or infection might make the antigens accessible to the lymphoid cells and thus lead to the "autoantibodies" directed against these antigens. Such sequestered antigens are thought to include the optic lens, thyroglobulin, and spermatic tissue (see Chap. 14).

Acquired Tolerance to Cells

The hypothesis of Burnet and Fenner predicted that the phenomenon observed naturally in calves by Owen might be demonstrated artificially. That is, the introduction of foreign cells in embryonic life should lead to a state of immunologic tolerance toward those cells. The experiment to prove this hypothesis was successfully carried out by Billingham et al. (40). Normal adult CBA mice rejected A-line skin grafts in 11 days (see Fig. 8-4). CBA embryos were then injected in utero with adult A-line spleen cells. At 8 weeks after birth, the CBA mice accepted A-line skin grafts for greatly prolonged periods of time (over 75 days). Thus the CBA mice were rendered tolerant to A tissue being exposed to it in utero. Further experiments showed (1) that the tolerance was specific since these CBA mice, tolerant of A-line skin grafts, rejected a skin graft from a third strain in a normal first-set manner, and (2) that the tolerated A-line graft retained its antigenic individuality, since it was rapidly rejected if the tolerant CBA mouse was adoptively immunized by being given lymphoid cells from a CBA mouse which had rejected an A graft.

Acquired tolerance is more easily induced if the donors and recipients

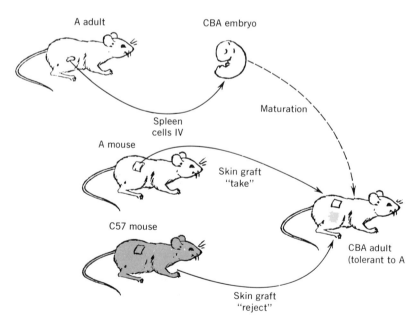

Fig. 8-4 Acquired tolerance to cells as demonstrated by the experiment of Billingham et al. (40).

are closely related at histocompatibility loci. If viable immunocompetent cells are injected, however, a graft-versus-host reaction may occur (see Chap. 15).

Recently, tolerance has been induced by the sophisticated method of obtaining blastocysts from genetically different mice and letting them grow together in tissue culture (41). After a short interval, the embryos are transplanted into pseudopregnant foster mothers. Many of these artificially hybridized embryos come to term, and the resultant animals are true chimeras and will accept skin grafts from either parent strain. These mice have been named *allophenic animals*. Successful allophenic chimeras have been produced using two strains which differed at the strong H-2 histocompatibility locus. A *histocompatibility locus* is a genetic region responsible for the expression of cellular antigens which are important in producing transplant rejections. A "strong" locus is one controlling antigens which provoke vigorous immune cellular responses in transplant situations.

If the ability to fool an animal into accepting foreign cells as self depends upon the immunologic immaturity of that animal, then such phenomena might be induced in animals made immunologically unresponsive in other ways. A tolerant state may be induced in adult animals by giving whole-body irradiation to the recipient before introducing the foreign cells. Upon recovery from x-ray, the recipients are often found to be recolonized by donor cells and therefore to be chimeras containing two genetically distinct populations of cells (42). Such "radiation chimeras" are specifically tolerant of tissue grafts from animals syngenetic with the donor-cell line. This is to be expected, since the existence of the chimeric state itself represents the nonrejection of donor cells.

Acquired Tolerance and Paralysis to Nonliving Antigens

Animals injected with soluble antigens may, under certain circumstances, fail to develop immune responses to these antigens. In a situation analogous to the neonatal induction of tolerance to cellular antigens, newborn rabbits injected with soluble bovine serum albumin (BSA) failed to make circulating antibody when later challenged with BSA (43). Normal rabbits not given BSA at birth responded to the subsequent challenge by making circulating anti-BSA. Further exploration of this phenomenon showed that (1) the phenomenon was specific for the immunizing antigen, (2) for a stated dose of BSA, the earlier in life it was given, the greater the incidence of induction of tolerance, (3) tolerance was a temporary phenomenon and tended to disappear with time, but the duration of tolerance was greater with larger inducing doses of

BSA, and tolerance could be maintained with repeated injections of small doses of antigens, (4) tolerant rabbits did not contain some inhibitor of antibody response, since they supported the vicarious production of anti-BSA by adoptive transfer of cells from rabbits sensitized to BSA, (5) cells from tolerant rabbits did not make anti-BSA when transferred to normal rabbits (43). These data appear similar to those seen when tolerance is produced by living cellular inocula except that with nonliving non-replicating antigens, repeated exposure to antigen is necessary to maintain the tolerant state. Thus a cardinal feature of maintenance of tolerance appears to be the persistence of antigen.

Tolerance to soluble antigens may also be induced in adult animals. At first, this appears to contradict the hypothesis of Burnet and Fenner (37) that tolerance induction depends on the immunologic immaturity of the animals. We must observe, however, that the induction of tolerance to nonliving antigens in mature animals is dependent on the observance of a variety of circumstances which almost make it appear to be a special case. For instance, the induction of "paralysis" in adult mice by pneumococcal polysaccharide may depend upon the relative inability of the mouse to metabolize this antigen, which would thus tend to persist longer in the tissues. The very form of the antigen or manner of introduction may be crucial. For instance, adult mice may be rendered tolerant to BGG if it is given in unaggregated form, but the same antigen given in aggregated form or with Freund's adjuvant or with bacterial endotoxin (non-cross-reacting) causes the production of antibody, not the induction of tolerance (44,45). Again, the route of antigen introduction may be crucial, since guinea pigs fed or injected intravenously with picryl chloride are then unable to develop dermal contact sensitization with this hapten, but contact sensitization with the hapten sensitizes the animal by itself and does not lead to tolerance (46). The dose of antigen has been shown to be critical by Mitchison (47). Mice given various doses of BSA may become tolerant ("paralyzed") after small doses ("low-dose") or after large doses ("high-dose") of antigen. The low-dose paralysis occurs early. The high-dose paralysis occurs later and appears together with some evidence of transient antibody production. D-amino acid polymers in large doses do not evoke detectable antibody in rabbits, but repeated small doses do lead to antibody production specific for the D-configuration. No booster response occurs in this situation, since further doses of D-amino acid polymers lead to the disappearance of circulating antibody (48). Under certain circumstances, tolerance may be produced in adult animals which are already immunized (49). This is important, since it may be pertinent to the establishment of specific unresponsiveness in homotransplantation or autoimmune situations. The induction of tolerance in immunized recipients depends upon the repeated injection of very large doses of antigen, since this is an effort to convert the animal into a state of antigen excess and obviate the production of more antibody by the antigen. As might be expected, irradiation of the recipient hastens the induction of tolerance by antigen (50).

Termination of the Tolerant State

In tolerance induced by living cells, the tolerant state may last indefinitely if the tolerance is induced in neonates and a stable chimeric state is established. As mentioned above, this stable chimerism may be terminated by the adoptive transfer of immunized lymphoid cells. Thus, CBA mice rendered tolerant to A-line cells by the neonatal injection of these cells and bearing an A-line skin graft will reject the graft if they are supplied with CBA lymphoid cells from mice immunized against A cells (40). When tolerance is produced by the injection of nonliving antigens, it may be abrogated by the injection of normal lymphoid cells from compatible animals (51). This is strong evidence that the tolerant state involves a "central failure" of the immunologic apparatus and not some general alteration of the cellular environment of the tolerant animal. The duration of the tolerant state depends upon the persistence of antigen (43). A long series of experiments by Weigle (52) has shown that tolerance to an antigen such as bovine serum albumin can be broken by injection of a cross-reacting antigen such as human serum albumin. Recent evidence (53) has suggested, however, that this may not be a true "termination of tolerance." Termination of tolerance on a cellular level may represent instead the production of antibody in response to the cross-reacting antigen by cells not involved in the immune response to the original antigen.

The persistence of tolerance also depends upon the state of the lymphoid system. In mice made tolerant to BGG, tolerance persists longer in thymectomized mice than in sham-operated controls (54). Whole-body irradiation also hastens the waning of tolerance, but only if the thymus is present (55). These experiments indicate that lymphoid cell turnover is associated with the waning of tolerance and that procedures which retard this (thymectomy) will delay the waning of tolerance, and procedures which accelerate this (whole body irradiation with the thymus present) will accelerate the reappearance of antibody production.

Hypotheses for Immunologic Tolerance

A knowledge of the mechanism by which tolerance or specific immunologic unresponsiveness is induced and maintained is critical for any immunologic theory. In one sense it is the obverse of antibody production or hypersensitiveness, and it is likely therefore that the mystery of tolerance will be solved only when we can answer the riddle of the induction of antibody synthesis at a molecular level.

Several points appear convincing at this time: (1) The maintenance of the tolerant state depends upon the persistence of antigen [although this has been disputed (56)]. (2) The waning of tolerance is connected with lymphoid cell turnover and repopulation. The simplest thought is that constant inhibition of antibody synthesis by various cells depends on a constant supply of antigen. When the antigen level drops below a critical point, cells will be able to respond to antigens again by making antibody. (3) Also, at least in the case of one nonliving antigen (BGG), tolerance takes a finite amount of time to develop. (4) It is now clear that in the tolerant state we are not dealing with cells which are making antibody which is then masked in some way, for instance by the presence of circulating antigen. It is not clear, however, whether the tolerant state involves the presence of cells capable of making a specific antibody but actually inhibited from doing so ("tolerant cells") or whether the tolerant state involves the absence of cells capable of making a specific antibody. In the first case, the maintenance of the tolerant state requires a constant level of antigen to keep the cells tolerant and also to make newly formed lymphoid cells tolerant as they are formed under thymus-directed lymphopoiesis. In the second case, there are no cells capable of making the antibody in question in the tolerant animal, and again antigen is required to assure the constant elimination of newly formed antigen-sensitive cells as they might arise under thymus-directed lymphopoiesis.

The presence of specifically tolerant cells has not been demonstrated. In terms of the "two-cell theory of antibody production" (first cell = antigen processor and perhaps purveyor of information to second cell = antibody producer), tolerance could inhere in either the first or the second cell. In one system in which the distribution of labeled antigen was examined by autoradiography and electron microscopy, however, there was no difference in the uptake and persistence of antigen between normal and tolerant animals (57). Judged by these criteria, the "foreignness" of the antigen seemed the same in tolerant and normal animals. These experiments do not favor the hypothesis that in situations leading to antibody production the antigen is processed by the "first cell," while in tolerance the antigen is not processed by the "first cell" but impinges directly on the "second cell," thereby rendering it tolerant. On the other hand, they do not exclude this hypothesis. Since the nature of the information (if any) normally passed from the first cell to the second cell is not known with certainty, we are in no position to determine whether in the tolerant state this information is lacking, defective, or inadequate in some other way.

Theorists who think that the tolerant state implies the absence of cells able to make specific antibody have been impressed by the ability of "nonspecific" adjuvants to inhibit the development of tolerance. As mentioned above, the concomitant use of adjuvants such as Freund's adjuvant, endotoxin, and even cytotoxic drugs like actinomycin D together with a "tolerogenic" antigen will result in antibody formation rather than tolerance. These adjuvants possess in common the ability to cause lymphoid cell proliferation (sometimes preceded by lymphoid destruction, as in the case of actinomycin D and antimetabolites). Now it is generally recognized that the process of antibody formation appears to include two processes, both the division of lymphoid cells and their maturation from antigen-sensitive precursors into antibody producers (58). Ordinarily, the antigenic stimulus contains both stimuli: the specific stimulus for maturation and the nonspecific stimulus for proliferation. If, however, an antigen contained only the specific stimulus for maturation, it might send the antigen-sensitive precursor immediately along the path to full maturation without division and without the potential for further division. In this case there would be no memory, and the antigen would be "tolerogenic." This has been called *suicidal maturation* or *maturing off the clone*. Under these circumstances, a small amount of antibody would be briefly produced by the precursors as they matured, and it is of interest that Mitchison (47) found that antibody had been formed during the period of induction of high dose tolerance. In such a case, the addition of various unrelated substances, such as adjuvants, could be used to supply the "nonspecific stimulus" which would make a tolerogenic antigen into an immunogenic antigen.

It should be clear from this discussion that although a large amount of data is available concerning immunologic tolerance, we are quite ignorant about the fundamental processes involved. Theories abound, among the most original of which is Smithies's theory of "antibody viruses" (59). According to this model, the antibody response is mediated by self-replicating antibody viruses, each of which contains nucleic acid material with information coding for a specific antibody and which carries a protein coat containing that antibody. Contact with antigen causes proliferation of the viruses and an antibody response. Tolerance occurs when antigen combines with the viruses in a situation in which replication cannot take place and the viruses are eliminated.

THE BASIS OF IMMUNOLOGIC MEMORY

The nature of immunologic memory may lie in the presence or absence of a pool of specifically reactive precursor cells which are ready to respond to antigens. This idea is based on various schemes set forth by Sercarz and

Coons (60) and modified by Nossal (61) describing a sequence of X-Y-Z cells related to antibody production. Makinodan and Albright (62) also proposed a similar scheme and named the cells PC_0, PC_1, and PC_2 cells. A possible model for induction of positive and negative immunologic memory is outlined in Fig. 8-5.

During embryonic life, an animal may acquire immunologic competence by developing a large number of lymphoid cells from progenitor cells. (This process is somehow under the influence of the thymus.) Among these lymphoid cells are groups of a few cells (precursors), each capable of reacting with a limited number of antigens (perhaps only one). These are the immunologically competent, antigen target cells. When an

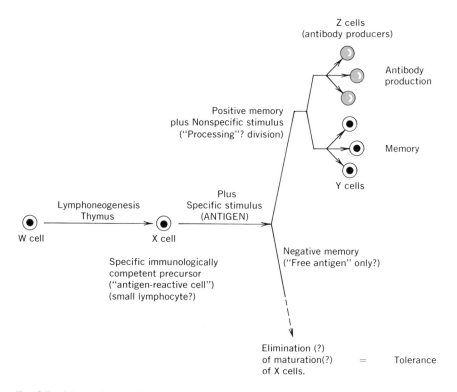

Fig. 8-5 Scheme for positive and negative immunologic memory. In this scheme a specific stimulus (antigen) plus a nonspecific stimulus leads to antibody production and positive memory. The specific stimulus alone leads to elimination or maturation of X cells producing tolerance or negative memory. In the case of maturation of a small clone of cells, small amounts of antibody might be produced while tolerance is being established.

antigen target cell reacts with an appropriate antigen in a situation involving positive memory, it undergoes "maturation" and mitosis. Among the progeny of this cell are different types of cells. Some make immunoglobulins (antibody-forming cells) and some may be involved in delayed hypersensitivity reactions. Others, either derived from antigen target cells or even from antibody-forming cells, have the capacity of reacting again with a new antigenic stimulus and starting the process all over again. These are *memory cells*. Memory cells appear to have a longer life-span than antibody-forming cells, since they persist after antibody production diminishes. They may persist for the lifetime of the animal.

This analysis does not imply that there is anything fundamentally different between the precursor cell, which reacts with the first introduction of antigen, and the "memory" cell, which reacts with a subsequent injection. Such a distinction has been claimed (61) partly on the basis of experiments with antibody production in vitro. While anamnestic responses (presumably the responses of memory cells) are steadily obtainable in vitro, primary responses (presumably the responses of antibody-forming cells) are exceedingly difficult to obtain. However, this may be only a quantitative difference. Under the conditions of this theory, a normal animal has a limited number of antigen target precursor cells able to react with a given antigen. In terms of this theory, the memory systems for each immunoglobulin class would be separate. That is, the cellular events regulating 19S and 7S antibody production would involve different lines of immunocompetent cells, although feedback-type interactions between these different lines of cells and their antibody products undoubtedly occur (see Chap. 5).

Positive Memory

After reaction with antigen in which a "primary" response occurs, the animal is left with an increased number of similar specifically reactive memory cells ready to give a magnified response to a second stimulus of the same antigen. The acquisition of an enlarged pool of these Y cells represents the acquisition of positive immunologic memory.

Negative Memory

"Natural" tolerance to an antigen implies the absence of a pool of specifically reactive precursor cells. Exposure to an antigen does not result in the above cellular transformations. The specifically reactive precursor cells are presumed to have been destroyed (if they were ever present), perhaps in embryonic life.

"Acquired" Immunologic Tolerance

Acquired immunologic tolerance implies either the elimination or inhibition of the pool of specifically reactive precursor cells normally present. In acquired tolerance of the cellular type involving chimerism, the very existence of the chimeric state (B cells surviving in A) indicates that the A host does not have competent precursor cells capable of reacting against B cells. In acquired tolerance to nonliving antigens it is far from clear whether the precursor cells are inhibited or eliminated. Either result could come about by contact with free antigen (specific stimulus only).

WHAT IS THE "MEMORY CELL"?

The above analysis suggests that the question, "what is the memory cell?" may be similar or identical to the question, "what is the specifically reactive immunocompetent cell capable of reacting with antigen in the primary response?" The answer to this question is not known with certainty. There is good evidence that it is a small lymphocyte [reviewed by Gowans and McGregor (63); also see Chap. 6]. A summary of some of this evidence is as follows:

1. Small lymphocytes are known to transform into large pyroninophilic cells during a graft-versus-host reaction. A similar transformation occurs in response to a soluble antigen in areas where small lymphocytes are prominent.

2. Rats depleted of small lymphocytes by chronic drainage of the thoracic duct have impaired primary responses.

3. The depression of immunocompetence to sheep erythrocyte antigen produced by a whole-body irradiation of rats can be restored by small lymphocytes from normal rats but not by small lymphocytes from rats made tolerant to sheep erythrocytes.

4. Small lymphocytes, long thought to be "end cells" incapable of mitosis or indeed of transformation into any other type of cell, have been shown to undergo remarkable changes in vitro. Under the "nonspecific" influence of phytohemagglutinin or the "specific" influence of antigens to which the cell donor has been sensitized, small lymphocyte-like cells from the peripheral blood, thoracic duct, lymph node, or thymus undergo transformation to large "blastlike" cells with concomitant transformation from an essentially resting cell to one synthesizing appreciable amounts of protein, RNA, and DNA (64). This ability to transform into an actively synthesizing cell, together with the recent data showing that small lymphocytes may have a remarkably long life-span in vivo (65,66), indicates that the small lymphocyte has the capabilities of acting as the immunocompetent precursor. One must emphasize, however, that the above evidence is circumstantial, and the direct observation of a small lymphocyte interacting with antigen to transform and to produce specific antibody has yet to be firmly demonstrated.

REFERENCES

1. Wolfe, H. R., Amin, A., Mueller, A. P., and Aronson, F. R.: *Int. Arch. Allergy*, **17**:106, 1960.
2. Makinodan, T., and Peterson, W. J.: *Develop. Biol.*, **14**:112, 1966.
3. Jílek, M., and Šterzl, J.: *Folia Microbiol. (Prague)*, **12**:6, 1967.
4. Sell, S., and Weigle, W. O.: *J. Immunol.*, **83**:257, 1959.
5. Glenny, A. T., and Südmersen, H. J.: *J. Hyg.*, **20**:176, 1921.
6. Gottlieb, S., McLaughlin, F. X., Levine, L., Latham, W. C., and Edsall, G.: *Amer. J. Public Health*, **54**:961, 1964.
7. Dixon, F. J., and Maurer, P. H.: *J. Immunol.*, **74**:418, 1955.
8. Paul, W. E., Siskind, G. W., Benacerraf, B., and Ovary, Z.: *J. Immunol.*, **99**:760, 1967.
9. Fazekas de St. Groth, S., and Webster, R. G.: *J. Exp. Med.*, **124**:331, 1966.
10. Eisen, H. N.: *Cancer Res.*, **26**:2005, 1966.
11. Dixon, F. J., Maurer, P. H., and Deichmiller, M. P.: *J. Immunol.*, **72**:179, 1954.
12. Claman, H. N.: *J. Immunol.*, **91**:29, 1963.
13. Heidelberger, M., MacLeod, C. M., Kaiser, S. J., and Robinson, B.: *J. Exp. Med.*, **83**:303, 1946.
14. Jerne, N. K., Nordin, A. A., and Henry, C. C.: in "Cell-bound Antibodies," B. Amos and H. Koprowski (eds.), Wistar Institute Press, Philadelphia, 1963.
15. Leduc, E. H., Coons, A. H., and Connolly, J. M.: *J. Exp. Med.*, **102**:61, 1955.
16. Nossal, G. J. V.: *Brit. J. Exp. Pathol.*, **40**:118, 1959.
17. Makinodan, T., Kastenbaum, M. A., and Peterson, W. J.: *J. Immunol.*, **88**:31, 1962.
18. Jerne, N. K., and Avegno, P.: *J. Immunol.*, **76**:200, 1956.
19. Eisen, H. N., and Siskind, G. W.: *Biochemistry*, **3**:996, 1964.
20. Steiner, L. A., and Eisen, H. N.: *Bacteriol. Rev.*, **30**:383, 1966.
21. Bauer, D. C., and Stavitsky, A. B.: *Proc. Nat. Acad. Sci. U.S.*, **47**:1667, 1961.
22. Uhr, J. W., and Finkelstein, M. S.: *Progr. Allergy*, **10**:37, 1967.
23. Uhr, J. W., and Finkelstein, M. S.: *J. Exp. Med.*, **117**:457, 1963.

24. Nossal, G. J. V., Ada, G. L., and Austin, C. M.: *Australian J. Exp. Biol. Med. Sci.*, **42**:283, 1964.
25. Svehag, S. E., and Mandel, B.: *J. Exp. Med.*, **119**:21, 1964.
26. Porter, R. J.: *Proc. Soc. Exp. Biol. Med.*, **121**:107, 1966.
27. Altemeier, W. A. III, Robbins, J. B., and Smith, R. T.: *J. Exp. Med.*, **124**:443, 1966.
28. Billingham, R. E., Brent, L., and Medawar, P. B.: *Proc. Roy. Soc. (Biol.)*, **143**:58, 1954.
29. Billingham, R. E., Brent, L., and Medawar, P. B.: *Ann. N.Y. Acad. Sci.*, **59**:409, 1955.
30. Steinmuller, D.: *J. Immunol.*, **85**:398, 1960.
31. Bauer, J. A., and Stone, S. H.: *J. Immunol.*, **86**:177, 1961.
32. Salvin, S. B., and Smith, R. F.: *J. Immunol.*, **84**:449, 1960.
33. Arnason, B. G., and Waksman, B. H.: *Lab. Invest.*, **12**:737, 1963.
34. Leskowitz, S.. *Annu. Rev. Microbiol.*, **21**:157, 1967.
35. Witebsky, E., and Rose, N. R.: *J. Immunol.*, **76**:408, 1956.
36. Fudenberg, H. H., Stiehm, E. R., Franklin, E. C., Meltzer, M., and Frangione, B.: *Cold Spring Harbor Symp. Quant. Biol.*, **29**:463, 1964.
37. Burnet, F. M., and Fenner, F.: "The Production of Antibodies," 2d ed., Macmillan, Melbourne, 1949.
38. Owen, R. D.: *Science*, **102**:400, 1945.
39. Burnet, F. M.: *Brit. Med. J.*, **2**:720, 1959.
40. Billingham, R. E., Brent, L., and Medawar, P. B.: *Nature (London)*, **172**:603, 1953.
41. Mintz, B., and Silvers, W. K.: *Science*, **158**:1484, 1967.
42. Micklem, H. S., and Loutit, J. F.: in "Tissue Grafting and Radiation," Academic Press, Inc., New York, 1966.
43. Smith, R. T.: *Advan. Immunol.*, **1**:67, 1961.
44. Dresser, D. W.: *Immunology*, **5**:378, 1962.
45. Claman, H. N.: *J. Immunol.*, **91**:833, 1963.
46. Chase, M. W.: *Federation Proc.*, **25**:145, 1966.
47. Mitchison, N. A.: *Proc. Roy. Soc. (Biol.)*, **161**:275, 1964.
48. Gill, T. J. III, Kunz, H. W., and Papermaster, D. S.: *J. Biol. Chem.*, **242**:3308, 1967.
49. Dorner, M. M., and Uhr, J. W.: *J. Exp. Med.*, **120**:435, 1964.
50. Claman, H. N., and Bronsky, E. A.: *J. Allergy*, **38**:208, 1966.
51. Dietrich, F. M., and Weigle, W. O.: *J. Immunol.*, **92**:167, 1964.
52. Weigle, W. O.: "Natural and Acquired Immunologic Unresponsiveness," The World Publishing Company, Cleveland, 1967.
53. Paul, W. E., Siskind, G. W., and Benacerraf, B.: *Immunology*, **13**:147, 1967.
54. Claman, H. N., and Talmage, D. W.: *Science*, **141**:1193, 1963.
55. Claman, H. N., and MacDonald, W.: *Nature (London)*, **202**:712, 1964.
56. Nossal, G. J. V.: *Ann. N.Y. Acad. Sci.*, **129**:822, 1966.

57. Ada, G. L., Nossal, G. J. V., and Pye, J.: *Australian J. Exp. Biol. Med. Sci.*, **43**:337, 1965.
58. Talmage, D. W., and Pearlman, D. S.: *J. Theoret. Biol.*, **5**:321, 1963.
59. Smithies, O.: *Science*, **149**:151, 1965.
60. Sercarz, E., and Coons, A. H.: in "Mechanisms of Immunological Tolerance," M. Hasek, A. Lengerova, and M. Vojtiskova (eds.), Academic Press, Inc., New York, 1962.
61. Nossal, G. J. V.: *Australian Ann. Med.*, **14**:321, 1965.
62. Makinodan, T., and Albright, J. F.: *Progr. Allergy*, **10**:1, 1967.
63. Gowans, J. L., and McGregor, D. D.: *Progr. Allergy*, **9**:1, 1965.
64. Bach, F. H., and Hirschhorn, K.: *Sem. Hematol.*, **2**:68, 1965.
65. Nowell, P. C.: *Blood*, **26**:798, 1965.
66. Bloom, A. D., Neriishi, S., and Archer, P. G.: *Lancet*, **II**:10, 1968.

9
Immunoenhancement

Various means employed to increase the level of an immune response can be included under the subject heading of *immunoenhancement*. For example, one can boost the production of antibody by manipulation of the dose, route, and sequence of antigen administration. In addition, there are a wide variety of nonspecific means of increasing the immune response. These vary from physical or chemical alteration of the antigen to alteration of the physiology of the animal to be immunized. Thus, immunoenhancement may be caused by variation of the specific stimulus, the antigen, or it may be caused by altering a variety of nonspecific factors.

Since adjuvants are the agents most commonly employed to produce immunoenhancement, they will be discussed in detail. It also appears useful to consider adjuvant action because a better understanding of this phenomenon may lead to further clarification of some of the steps in antibody synthesis which are still obscure.

ADJUVANTS

Adjuvants include a wide variety of materials that nonspecifically enhance antibody production to unrelated antigens. Some are large molecules and are also antigenic, others are small organic compounds, and still others are physical agents, such as x-radiation. In this chapter no attempt will be made to cover all agents that exert an adjuvant effect on antibody production. A few selected adjuvants will be described and their possible modes of action discussed.

Adjuvants are frequently used by investigators desiring a large amount of specific antibody as a reagent for research. If the antigen is available in small amounts, the use of an adjuvant is especially helpful, since it allows the investigator to reduce the amount of antigen necessary to induce a large quantity of antibody. In addition, some adjuvants alter the type of immune response induced. For example, complete Freund's adjuvant is frequently used to induce delayed hypersensitivity. Adjuvants are often incorporated in vaccines for human use (e.g., diphtheria toxoid and influenza vaccine). Use of adjuvants in these vaccines may reduce the number of injections a person must be given and does reduce the amount of specific antigen that must be obtained, thus allowing immunization of a larger number of people.

On the other hand, adjuvants are of interest in trying to elucidate the mechanism of immunoglobulin synthesis. Definition of the mode of action of any agent that increases the immune response also contributes to the knowledge of the events that are necessary for antibody formation and of the events that limit the amount of antibody produced.

Possible Mechanisms of Adjuvant Action

Although the mechanism of enhancement of antibody production has not been proven for any adjuvant, there are several events in the immune response which have been postulated to be affected by adjuvants. The first events that might be affected are antigen processing and antigen distribution. Less than 5 percent of antigen administered in soluble form appears to be effective in stimulating antibody formation (1). If the percent of antigen administered that actually stimulates antibody production can be increased, the effective antigen dose will be increased without increasing the total amount of antigen administered. The result will be enhanced antibody production.

One method of increasing the amount of soluble antigen injected that is effective in stimulating antibody production is to make that antigen particulate. In general, antibody production is stimulated more readily by particulate than by soluble antigens (2–4). Particulate antigens are probably phagocytosed more readily than are soluble antigens. If processing of antigen by macrophages is a requirement for antibody production, then the increased phagocytosis and/or digestion of a particulate antigen could result in an enhanced immune response by increasing antigenic stimulation. As has been described in Chap. 7, there is evidence that RNA or RNA-antigen complexes extracted from macrophages incubated with antigen stimulate antibody production (5,6). At present there is little or no evidence that adjuvants enhance antibody production by altering the digestion of antigen; however, some agents are known to increase phagocytosis and may enhance the immune response through their effect on phagocytosis (7).

It is well known that the antibody response to a second injection of antigen is usually higher than the response to a first injection of the same antigen (8). This is the classical secondary, or anamnestic, response. Some adjuvants may enhance antibody production by inducing both primary and secondary responses after a single injection of antigen and adjuvant. In most cases, adjuvants of this type render the antigen relatively insoluble. The antigen and adjuvant are mixed together and injected locally so that a "depot" of antigen and adjuvant is formed. The antigen is released slowly from this depot over a period of several days to weeks. In this way the antigenic stimulus is prolonged, and both a primary and secondary response may occur. It is probably also significant that many vehicles capable of causing a depot effect also cause a local inflammation at the injection site. Thus, these adjuvants not only cause slow release of antigen but may also attract cells (i.e., macrophages) important in antibody synthesis to the site of highest antigen concentration.

A second way in which adjuvant may increase the immune response is through an effect on antibody-forming cells. Increased numbers of antibody-forming cells have been observed after administration of antigen and adjuvant (9). Increased mitosis has been demonstrated in the spleens of animals receiving these adjuvants (10). Thus, some adjuvants may enhance antibody production by increasing the rate of proliferation of either the precursors of antibody-forming cells or the antibody-forming cells themselves. In either case the end result would be an increase in the number of cells producing a specific antibody, and therefore, an enhanced immune response would be obtained. On the other hand, an enhanced antibody response would be obtained in the absence of an increase in antibody-forming cells if the adjuvant increased the amount of antibody produced per cell. However, there is no evidence to support this last hypothesis at the present time.

Examples of Adjuvants

Freund's Adjuvant

One of the best-known materials for inducing a heightened and prolonged immune response is Freund's adjuvant. Freund's "incomplete" adjuvant consists of mineral oil and an emulsifying agent. Freund's "complete" adjuvant also contains killed *Mycobacteria*. For immunization, the adjuvant is mixed vigorously with an aqueous solution of the antigen, producing a water-in-oil emulsion with the antigen in the water phase.

Freund (11) developed this adjuvant following the observation of Dienes and Schoenheit (12) that large amounts of antibody and delayed hypersensitivity to protein antigen were induced when protein antigen was injected into a tuberculous animal. Couland (13) found that the immune response to tubercle bacilli was enhanced when the organisms were injected in paraffin oil. However, immunization of animals with proteins suspended in paraffin oil did not result in an enhanced response (14). Freund then incorporated an emulsifying agent in the adjuvant mixture. The resulting water-in-oil emulsion proved to be an excellent adjuvant for inducing high levels of circulating antibody that persisted for a long time. When *Mycobacteria* were added to the adjuvant, not only high levels of circulating antibody but also delayed hypersensitivity to protein antigens were induced (15). Since that time, use of complete Freund's adjuvant has proved to be the method of choice for the induction of delayed hypersensitivity to protein antigens.

Freund et al. (16) extended this work to the study of autoimmunity. They found that homologous and even autologous antigens, when incorporated in complete Freund's adjuvant, induced the production of auto-antibodies. Thus, Freund was one of the first investigators to induce experimental autoimmune aspermatogenesis and allergic encephalomyelitis. These phenomena will be discussed in Chap. 14.

The mechanism of action of Freund's adjuvant is still not completely understood. When antigen is injected in Freund's adjuvant, the antigen is in the aqueous phase of a water-in-oil emulsion. Thus, the antigen is deposited locally in a relatively insoluble form. The small droplets of antigen are slowly released from the emulsion, resulting in antigenic stimulation over a long period of time (17). Thus, the mechanisms described for the depot hypothesis are probably at least part of the cause of the augmented antibody response seen when antigen is injected in Freund's adjuvant.

Many investigators have obtained evidence in support of the depot hypothesis. For example, excision of the injection site a short time after injection of antigen in Freund's adjuvant results in a reduction of the adjuvant effect (18). In addition, antigen in a biologically active form has been found persisting at the injection site for weeks to months after injection (19). It is difficult to assess the importance of this persisting antigen in view of the fact that an augmented response was observed when the injection site was excised at 2 weeks (18). It is true, however, that slow release of antigen is an effective means of inducing antibody, since a prolonged and enhanced antibody response was induced by daily injections of a small amount of protein antigen in aqueous phase (20).

Although it is clear that slow release of antigen over a long period of time is important, it is not the only explanation for the action of Freund's adjuvant. The materials in Freund's adjuvant cause a granuloma or sterile abscess at the injection site (21). The intensity of this reaction varies with the oil used and with the presence or absence of Mycobacteria. Formation of an intense local reaction is one disadvantage of Freund's adjuvant, since it limits the use of this material in humans. On the other hand, granuloma formation may contribute to the adjuvant action, since the granuloma contains a large number of macrophages, cells that may be important in the immune response. Although some investigators have found higher titers of antibody in fluid aspirated from the injection site than in the circulation (22), antibody-forming cells were not found in the local granuloma (23), but were found in the draining lymph nodes.

Another function of the oil vehicle in the adjuvant is to aid in dissemination of the antigen to the lymph nodes. In fact, oil droplets associated with antigen have been observed in the cervical lymph nodes 3 weeks after injection (23). The observed dissemination of antigen and adjuvant might also explain the failure of extirpation of the injection site 2 weeks after injection to abolish the adjuvant effect.

Alterations in antigen processing do not explain all of the characteristics of Freund's adjuvant. For example, an enhanced antibody response has been observed even when antigen is given intravenously and Freund's complete adjuvant subcutaneously (24). Thus, intimate contact between antigen and adjuvant does not appear to be necessary. In addition, induction by Freund's complete adjuvant of a humoral factor which had adjuvant activity has been reported (25). Serum taken from animals 1 to 9 weeks after injection of Freund's complete adjuvant exerted an adjuvant effect when given to other animals with antigen. Perhaps the Mycobacteria present in the complete adjuvant are responsible for these observations. Mycobacteria incorporated in mineral oil stimulate macrophage proliferation at the site of injection, in the lymph nodes, and even in the lungs (26,27). The fraction of Mycobacteria causing the stimulation is Wax D, a peptidoglycolipid (28). One of the major constituents is mycolic acid. Both increased antibody production and enhanced delayed hypersensitivity are induced when Wax D is incorporated in the adjuvant. Thus, fractions derived from *Mycobacteria* cause both a quantitative and qualitative change in the immune response. The means by which this material aids in the induction of delayed hypersensitivity is not understood.

In summary, Freund's adjuvant is a useful material to use for induction of large amounts of antibody persisting for a long period of time. However, because of the rather violent reaction occurring at the injection site, it is used only infrequently in humans. In addition, Freund's complete adjuvant is an excellent agent for the experimental induction of delayed hypersensitivity and autoimmunity.

Particulate Adjuvants

A popular method of enhancing the immune response is to make soluble antigens particulate. Particulate materials are, in general, better antigens than soluble materials (2–4). There are many methods available utilizing a variety of particulate carriers of antigen. One of the most frequently used adjuvants of this type is alum, which was first used by Glenny et al. in 1926 (29). Protein antigens mixed with any of a variety of aluminum compounds form a precipitate that contains antigen adsorbed to the aluminum compound. This mixture is normally injected subcutaneously or intramuscularly. The resulting antibody response is usually higher and more prolonged than that resulting from injection of the soluble antigen.

Many factors have been suggested to play a role in the stimulation of immunization with alum-precipitated antigens. These include slow release of antigen (30), increased phagocytosis of antigen because it has been rendered particulate (31), and an increased cellular response (32).

Persistence of the antigen in granulomatous tissue at the injection site has been demonstrated (33). The antigen present is in a biologically active form, since material extracted from the injection site can induce a secondary response. Antigenic activity was detected even when the extract was obtained 7 weeks after injection. However, the effectiveness of the long-persisting antigenic material in stimulating antibody production is open to some question. Excision of the injection site within a few days after injection of alum-precipitated antigen reduced the immune response, but excision of the site 14 days after injection did not alter antibody formation (34). Thus antigen may be released from the injection site for several days followed by a long period of persistence of localized antigen in which too little antigen to induce an immune response is released.

The cellular studies of White et al. (35) supported these conclusions.

They found small amounts of the adjuvant and antigen present in the macrophages and in lymph node sinuses. In addition, antibody-forming cells were observed for a longer period of time in the lymph nodes of animals given alum-precipitated antigen than in those of animals given soluble antigen. These results suggested that antigenic stimulation persisted longer in the animals treated with alum-precipitated antigen than in those not given adjuvant. Persistence of antigen, however, may occur in areas other than the injection site. After the cellular response in the lymph node subsided at about 5 weeks, antibody-forming cells were observed in the local granulation tissue. Thus the enhanced response is due, at least in part, to a delayed release of antigen resulting in prolonged stimulus to antibody-forming cells in lymph nodes as well as to production of antibody within the local granulation tissue.

Alum is a convenient adjuvant to use in both laboratory animals and humans. The local response to alum-precipitated antigens is not as intense as the local response to Freund's adjuvant. For this reason alum precipitated vaccines are frequently used in humans. Such vaccines are easy to prepare and cause a heightened and prolonged humoral antibody response, usually without the induction of delayed hypersensitivity.

Many other particulate materials have been used as adjuvants. In many cases the antigen is attached either chemically or physically to particles such as bentonite (36), latex (37), or calcium phosphate (38). It has been suggested that these agents increase the antibody response primarily by increasing phagocytosis and processing of antigen (39). In addition, some of these materials, bentonite for example, may stimulate cell proliferation (40). Thus, some of these agents may act not only by increasing the availability of antigen but also by stimulating proliferation of antibody-forming cells.

Aggregation of a protein antigen by physical or chemical means also increases its ability to induce an antibody response. In fact, Dresser (24,41) found that the supernatant of centrifuged BGG induced immunologic tolerance, and the precipitate induced antibody production. However, when the supernatant was injected with an adjuvant, antibody production ensued. He suggested that complete antigens contain both a specific and nonspecific, or adjuvant, stimulus. In his system, centrifugation removed the nonspecific stimulus. Possibly aggregation of antigens increases the amount of this nonspecific stimulus and also increases phagocytosis of antigen.

Although passive antibody may suppress antibody production (42), injection of antigen in antigen-antibody complexes may also enhance antibody production (43,44). The ratio of antigen to antibody is critical in determining the effect on antibody production. For enhancement to occur complexes should be made at the equivalence point or in slight antigen excess. Injection of complexes prepared in antibody excess are likely to lead to suppression of antibody production. Both humoral antibody and delayed hypersensitivity may be induced by antigen-antibody complexes (45). Enhancement may occur through slow release of antigen as the complexes dissociate in vivo or through increased phagocytosis and processing of the aggregated material, so that immunocompetent cells are stimulated more intensely.

In summary, the antibody response may be increased by manipulation of the antigen. Increasing the size of the antigen injected results in many cases in an increased antibody response.

Toxic Adjuvants

There are a variety of adjuvants, most of which have toxic properties, which appear to affect antibody production in a similar way. Included among these are such diverse materials as bacterial endotoxins, x-radiation, nucleotide analogs, colchicine, and oligonucleotides. All of these adjuvants appear to affect some early stage of antibody production and result in an increased number of antibody-forming cells. In contrast to Freund's adjuvant and alum, these agents do not appear to cause a prolonged immune response. Thus, prolonged stimulation by antigen probably is not involved.

The adjuvant action of bacterial endotoxins has been studied for many years. An augmented antibody response to tetanus toxoid had been observed when the individual was given a divalent vaccine containing both the toxoid and killed *Salmonella typhi* (46). The component of the microorganism which exerted the adjuvant effect was the cell wall lipopolysaccharide, endotoxin. Indeed, it was found that endotoxins obtained from a large variety of gram-negative organisms enhanced antibody production in laboratory animals (47). However, endotoxins appeared to enhance antibody production only in animals in which some effects of toxicity could be demonstrated (e.g., elevation of temperature). That is, the adjuvant effect was not seen in animals that were made tolerant to endotoxin or animals that were normally resistant to endotoxin. Thus, the toxicity was associated with the adjuvant action. More recently, adjuvant activity has been demonstrated in chemically detoxified endotoxins (48). The authors, however, suggested that the adjuvant action of these preparations could have been due to small quantities of unmodified endotoxin.

Since endotoxin exerts its adjuvant action only when given near the time of antigen injection, it was suggested that endotoxin acts at some early stage in antibody production (49,50). In addition, endotoxin also partially restores antibody production in rabbits treated with x-radiation or cortisone (49,51). Both of these latter agents are thought to inhibit antibody production by inhibiting some early step in the immune response (52).

The antibody response in animals given antigen and endotoxin is characterized by a short induction period and a higher peak of antibody titer, which occurs earlier than in animals given only antigen. The cellular response correlates well with the serologic findings. Histologically, increased mitotic figures are observed early in the response, and differentiation of the antibody-forming cells is observed earlier in rabbits given endotoxin and antigen than in those given only antigen (10). Two methods of enumerating antibody-forming cells, fluorescent antibody technique and the localized hemolysis in gel technique, have shown that more antibody-forming cells occur earlier in animals given both endotoxin and antigen than in animals given only antigen (53,54). Thus endotoxin appears to enhance the immune response by accelerating and increasing the production of antibody-forming cells.

Endotoxin increases the rate of phagocytosis of colloidal particles 24 hours after injection of rabbits (55). However, the effect of endotoxin on phagocytosis does not appear to be important in the adjuvant action. If increased phagocytosis were the mechanism of action, it would be expected that endotoxin given to rabbits 12 to 24 hours before antigen would result in enhanced antibody production. Endotoxin given at that time was not effective as an adjuvant.

There is a long list of other toxic agents that enhance antibody formation. Examples are x-radiation (56), colchicine (57), 6-mercaptopurine (58), and 5-fluorouracil (50). Many of these agents are also known to inhibit antibody formation (see Chap. 10). However, given in the proper dose and at the proper time with respect to antigen injection, these all enhance antibody formation. They have several characteristics in common with endotoxin. They are all cytotoxic and are all effective in enhancing antibody production if given near the time of antigen injection. Proliferation of cells has been observed after administration of many of these agents, and they shorten the induction period of the immune response. Thus, it is probable that all these agents enhance antibody formation through a similar mechanism.

Increase of antibody production by the toxic agents may be mediated by oligonucleotides. Partially degraded RNA or DNA has been shown to enhance antibody formation when given with antigen (59,60). The effective components are nucleotides of 2 to 10 bases (61). Polyadenylic acid plus polycytidylic acid may also be used (62). These agents enhance the peak titer of the immune response, shorten the induction period, and restore antibody production in x-radiated animals (60). Moreover, an increase in the number of antibody-forming cells has been observed following immunization with oligonucleotides and antigen (62). Several investigators (49,61,63) have suggested that oligonucleotides are the actual adjuvants when toxic agents are used as adjuvants. It was postulated that nucleic acids released from injured cells are partially digested by endogenous nucleases, and the resulting oligonucleotides then would act as the actual adjuvants. In support of this hypothesis, bacterial oligonucleotides have recently been shown to elevate levels of enzymes concerned with the formation of precursors of DNA (64). It is possible that an increased concentration of precursors of DNA allows accelerated DNA synthesis resulting in increased proliferation of antibody-forming cells or their precursors and therefore increased antibody production.

Several materials that enhance antibody production and the characteristics of the augmented immune responses have been described in the preceding pages. Some of these agents appear to affect antigen, others antigen processing, and others antibody-forming cells. Adjuvants are useful for two purposes: (1) as agents to increase the total amount of antibody or the amount of antibody of a certain type that is produced and (2) as aids in the study of the mechanism of immune response.

REFERENCES

1. McConahey, P. J., Cerottini, J. C., and Dixon, F. J.: *J. Exp. Med.*, **127**:1003, 1968.
2. Stelos, P., Taliaferro, L. G., and D'Alesandro, P. A.: *J. Infect. Dis.*, **108**:113, 1961.
3. Nossal, G. J. V., Ada, G. L., and Austin, C. M.: *Australian J. Exp. Biol. Med. Sci.*, **42**:283, 1964.
4. Torrigiani, G., and Roitt, I. M.: *J. Exp. Med.*, **122**:181, 1965.
5. Fishman, M., and Adler, F. L.: *J. Exp. Med.*, **117**:595, 1963.
6. Fishman, M., Hammerstrom, R. A., and Bond, V. P.: *Nature (London)*, **198**:549, 1963.
7. Cutler, J. L.: *J. Immunol.*, **84**:416, 1960.
8. Dixon, F. J.: *J. Allergy*, **25**:487, 1954.
9. Braun, W., and Firshein, W.: *Bacteriol. Rev.*, **31**:83, 1967.
10. Ward, P. A., Johnson, A. G., and Abell, M. R.: *J. Exp. Med.*, **109**:463, 1959.
11. Freund, J.: *J. Allergy*, **28**:18, 1957.
12. Dienes, L., and Schoenheit, E. W.: *Proc. Soc. Exp. Biol. Med.*, **24**:32, 1926.
13. Coulaud, E.: *Rev. Tuberc. (Paris)*, **2**:850, 1934.

14. Freund, J., and Bonanto, M. V.: *J. Immunol.*, **48**:325, 1944.
15. Landsteiner, K., and Chase, M. W.: *J. Exp. Med.*, **73**:431, 1941.
16. Freund, J., Lipton, M. M., and Thompson, G. E.: *J. Exp. Med.*, **97**:711, 1953.
17. Freund, J.: *Annu. Rev. Microbiol.*, **1**:291, 1947.
18. Freund, J.: *Amer. J. Clin. Pathol.*, **21**:645, 1951.
19. Halbert, S. P., Mudd, S., and Smolens, J.: *J. Immunol.*, **53**:291, 1946.
20. Herbert, W. J.: *Nature (London)*, **210**:747, 1966.
21. Rist, N.: *Annu. Inst. Pasteur*, **61**:121, 1938.
22. Freund, J., Schryver, E. M., McGuiness, M. B., and Geitner, M. B.: *Proc. Soc. Exp. Biol. Med.*, **81**:657, 1952.
23. White, R. G., Coons, A. H., and Connolly, J. M.: *J. Exp. Med.*, **102**:83, 1955.
24. Dresser, D. W.: *Nature (London)*, **191**:1169, 1961.
25. Dawe, D. L., Segre, D., and Myers, W. L.: *Science*, **148**:1345, 1965.
26. Pernis, B., Bairati, A., and Milanesi, S.: *Pathol. Microbiol.*, **29**:837, 1966.
27. Moore, R. D., and Schoenberg, M. D.: *Brit. J. Exp. Pathol.*, **45**:488, 1964.
28. Raffel, S.: *J. Infect. Dis.*, **82**:267, 1948.
29. Glenny, A. T., Pope, C. G., Waddington, H., and Wallace, U.: *J. Pathol. Bacteriol.*, **29**:31, 1926.
30. Glenny, A. T., Buttle, G. A. H., and Stevens, M. F.: *J. Pathol. Bacteriol.* **34**:267, 1931.
31. Edsall, G.: *Med. Clinics N. Amer.*, **49**:1729, 1965.
32. Landsteiner, K.: "The Specificity of Serological Reactions," 2d ed., Harvard University Press, Cambridge, 1945.
33. Harrison, W. T.: *Amer. J. Public Health*, **25**:298, 1935.
34. Holt, L. B.: "Developments in Diphtheria Prophylaxis," William Heinemann, Ltd., London, 1950.
35. White, R. G., Coons, A. H., and Connolly, J. M.: *J. Exp. Med.*, **102**:73, 1955.
36. Claman, H. N.: *J. Immunol.*, **91**:833, 1963.
37. Litwin, S. D., and Singer, J. M.: *J. Immunol.*, **95**:1147, 1965.
38. Relyveld, E. H., and Raynaud, M.: in "International Symposium on Adjuvants of Immunity," R. H. Regamey, W. Hennessen, D. Ikić, and J. Ungar (eds.), S. Karger, New York, 1967.
39. Finger, H.: *Arch. Hyg. Bakteriol.*, **149**:732, 1965.
40. Burness, A. T. H., and Moss, J.: *Nature (London)*, **213**:833, 1967.
41. Dresser, D. W.: *Immunology*, **5**:378, 1962.
42. Pearlman, D. S.: *J. Exp. Med.*, **126**:127, 1967.
43. Terres, G., and Wolins, W.: *J. Immunol.*, **86**:361, 1961.
44. Morrison, S. L., and Terres, G.: *J. Immunol.*, **96**:901, 1966.
45. Uhr, J. W., Salvin, S. B., and Pappenheimer, A. M.: *J. Exp. Med.*, **105**:11, 1957.
46. Greenberg, L., and Fleming, D. S.: *Canad. J. Public Health*, **39**:131, 1948.

47. Johnson, A. G., Gaines, S., and Landy, M.: *J. Exp. Med.*, **103**:225, 1956.
48. Johnson, A. G., and Nowotny, A.: *J. Bacteriol.*, **87**:809, 1964.
49. Kind, P., and Johnson, A. G.: *J. Immunol.*, **82**:415, 1959.
50. Merritt, K., and Johnson, A. G.: *J. Immunol.*, **91**:266, 1963.
51. Ward, P. A., and Johnson, A. G.: *J. Immunol.*, **82**:428, 1959.
52. Taliaferro, W. H.: *Ann. N.Y. Acad. Sci.*, **69**:745, 1957.
53. Johnson, A. G.: in "Bacterial Endotoxins," M. Landy and W. Braun (eds.), Quinn, Boden Company, Inc., Rahway, N.J., 1964.
54. Braun, W.: in "Molecular and Cellular Basis of Antibody Formation," Academic Press, Inc., New York, 1965.
55. Benacerraf, B., and Sebestyen, M. M.: *Federation Proc.*, **16**:860, 1957.
56. Taliaferro, W. H., and Taliaferro, L. G.: *Proc. Nat. Acad. Sci. U.S.*, **53**:139, 1965.
57. Jaroslow, B. N., and Taliaferro, W. H.: *J. Infect. Dis.*, **116**:139, 1966.
58. Chanmougan, D., and Schwartz, R. S.: *J. Exp. Med.*, **124**:363, 1966.
59. Merritt, K., and Johnson, A. G.: *J. Immunol.*, **94**:416, 1965.
60. Jaroslow, B. N., and Taliaferro, W. H.: *J. Infect. Dis.*, **98**:75, 1956.
61. Johnson, A. G., in "Ontogeny of Immunity," R. T. Smith, R. A. Good, and P. A. Miescher (eds.), University of Florida Press, Gainesville, 1967.
62. Braun, W., and Nakano, M.: *Science*, **157**:819, 1967.
63. Braun, W., and Nakano, M.: in "International Symposium on Adjuvants of Immunity," R. H. Regamey, W. Hennessen, D. Ikić, and J. Ungar (eds.), S. Karger, New York, 1967.
64. Firshein, W.: *J. Bacteriol.*, **90**:327, 1965.

10
Immunosuppression

Perhaps the most profitable approach to the study of immunosuppression is one in which an attempt is made to relate the various means of abrogating the immune response to interference with some specific step in the normal mechanism. With this in mind, a model must first be established which, although not entirely accurate, will fit in reasonably well with the factual information now available concerning the development of the normal immune system. The sequence of events outlined in Fig. 10-1 will serve this purpose.

The central cell in the immune system is the so-called antigen target precursor cell, which arises from a relatively undifferentiated stem cell. This process, although still not understood, is generally believed to be dependent upon the thymus (see Chap. 4). The precursor cells respond to stimulation with antigen by differentiating into pyroninophilic blast cells, which divide and differentiate further into a population of antibody-producing cells, either directly or indirectly through an intermediate cell. The secondary, or anamnestic, response is believed to be due to stimulation of a pool of memory cells by a second injection of the same antigen, thereby inducing their further proliferation and differentiation into antibody-producing cells.

In the discussion to follow, an attempt will be made to relate the various forms of immunosuppression to the model just described.

LYMPHOID ABLATION

Thymectomy

In 1961 Archer and Pierce (1) found that rabbits that were thymectomized before six days of age had a markedly inhibited ability to make circulating antibodies against bovine serum albumin (BSA). Later, an extensive study of the immune response in neonatally thymectomized rats by Jankovíc et al. (2) showed that these animals also had reduced responses to BSA and, in addition, had a decreased ability to reject skin homografts, were immunologically deficient when tested for delayed hypersensitivity to BSA, the tuberculin skin test, and susceptibility to induced allergic encephalomyelitis. Miller (3) and other investigators

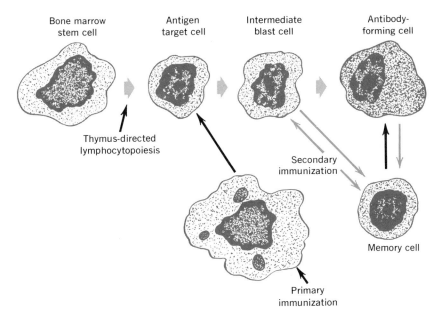

Bone marrow stem cell   Antigen target cell   Intermediate blast cell   Antibody-forming cell

Thymus-directed lymphocytopoiesis

Secondary immunization

Memory cell

Primary immunization

Fig. 10-1 Schematic diagram representing a possible pathway for the maturation of cells of the immune system.

[see Miller et al. (4)] examined the effects of neonatal thymectomy on the immune response in mice and found that these animals produced little or no circulating antibody to a number of antigens, were incapable of rejecting skin homografts, and showed decreased resistance to virus-induced tumors. Humphrey et al. (5) observed, however, that although antibody responses to sheep erythrocytes and to *Salmonella typhi* H and O antigens tended to be much lower in thymectomized than in intact mice, some of the thymectomized animals responded as well as the controls. This heterogeneity of response was also true if the antigen was pneumococcus type III polysaccharide or hemocyanin. In interpreting their results, these authors suggested that the thymus is the source of potentially competent stem cells and that some "random seeding" of other tissues had occurred before the animals were thymectomized.

An immunosuppressive effect of thymectomy on the adult animal was not as easily demonstrated. Several groups of investigators [see Miller et al. (4)] removed the thymus from adult rabbits, mice, and guinea pigs and reported little or no depression in the circulating antibody responses to a number of antigens. A normal homograft response was also observed in mice which were thymectomized as adults.

A significant advance was made when it was discovered that adult mice, when thymectomized after sublethal doses of total body x-radiation, behaved like neonatally thymectomized animals in that regeneration of their immune competence was postponed or inhibited (6). These animals recovered at a normal rate if they were grafted with thymus tissue from nonirradiated donors. More recently, several investigators (7,8) have reported that if adult mice are thymectomized, after approximately 3 months the animals become lymphopenic and immunologically incompetent, much like neonatally thymectomized mice.

It would appear that persistence of the normal immune mechanism in the adult mouse is dependent upon the continued presence of a thymus, which serves either as a source of stem cells or as a mediator of their differentiation into antigen-sensitive precursor cells. It may even do both. It follows that thymectomy either depletes the reserve of stem cells or interferes with their differentiation.

Bursectomy

The bursa of Fabricius is a lymphoid structure found in birds which arises during embryonic development as an outpocketing of the cloacal entoderm (9,9a) (Fig. 10-2). It has been the object of considerable interest in recent years, since it is an important component in the immune mechanism of birds and it seems to be at least partially analogous to the thymus in mammals.

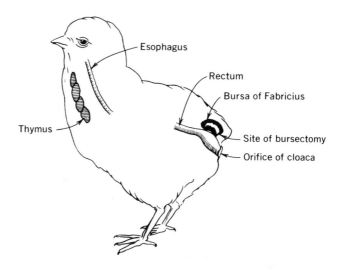

Fig. 10-2 The bursa of Fabricius is a lymphoid structure which develops embryologically as an outpocketing of the cloacal entoderm. The chicken thymus develops from the third and fourth pharyngeal pouches and is composed of 14 separate lobes, 7 of which are distributed along each side of the bird's neck. From Kemenes and Pethes (9a) with permission.

The effect of bursectomy on antibody production has been studied in several laboratories [reviewed by Warner and Szenberg (10)]. Glick et al. (11) reported that removal of the bursa at 12 days of age reduced the production of agglutinins to *Salmonella typhimurium* in chickens when the birds were challenged at 8 to 20 weeks, and Chang et al. (12) showed that bursectomy at 2 or 5 weeks of age reduced the antibody response to sheep erythrocytes when the birds were challenged at 12 weeks. Bursectomy at 10 weeks, however, had little effect on chickens challenged at 20 weeks with these same antigens. Wolfe et al. (13) bursectomized chickens at 1 to 5 weeks and challenged them with bovine serum albumin (BSA) at 6 weeks of age. As illustrated in Fig. 10-3, the birds which were bursectomized at 1 week made no detectable precipitating antibodies; the other groups gave increasing responses, with those animals bursectomized at 5 weeks being indistinguishable from the controls. The appearance in chickens of natural agglutinins to rabbit erythrocytes was also observed to be depressed if the birds were bursectomized, and the degree of depression was again related to the time of bursectomy. In contrast to the above, it has been reported that bursectomy has no effect on homograft survival time, or delayed hypersensitivity reactions in chickens (10).

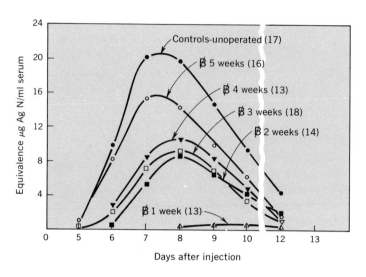

Fig. 10-3 Antibody responses of chickens injected at 6 weeks of age with 40 mg BSA/kg body weight. The antibody titers are expressed as μg of antigen nitrogen combining at equivalence with 1 ml of serum. Numbers in parentheses indicate the number of animals per group. $ = surgically bursectomized birds. From Wolfe et al., unpublished data.

The lymphocyte populations in the spleen as well as the differential white counts in the blood appear normal in bursectomized chickens. There is, however, a striking depletion of plasma cells (14). Also, when surgically bursectomized and subjected to sublethal doses of total body x-ray at 1 day of age, chickens have been found to lack round "bursa-dependent" follicles in their spleens at 6 weeks (15). Cooper et al. (16) have also reported that "IgM-like" and "IgG-like" immunoglobulins were extremely low or absent in these birds. It has been suggested that plasma cell development in the chicken is dependent upon the presence of a bursa. The finding that bursectomy had no effect on homograft immunity or delayed hypersensitivity reactions has led to the hypothesis (17) that there are two relatively independent immune systems in the chicken, one dependent on the bursa and the other dependent on the thymus (18) (see Fig. 10-4). Cooper et al. (16) have suggested that the tonsils, Peyer's patches, or other gut-associated lymphoid tissue may be the mammalian equivalent of the avian bursa (see Chap. 4).

Splenectomy

There is an abundance of data (19) indicating that, following an intravenous or intraperitoneal injection of antigen, most of the circulating antibody produced during the immune response is synthesized in the spleen. It is, therefore, not surprising that removal of the spleen follow-ing antigenic stimulation results in a decreased production of antibody.

The importance of the spleen in antibody production is best demon-strated by injecting small amounts of antigen intravenously. Wolfe et al. (20) showed that the immunosuppressive effect of splenectomy in

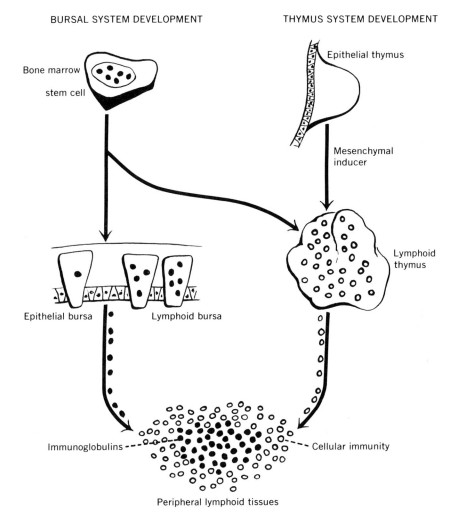

BURSAL SYSTEM DEVELOPMENT   THYMUS SYSTEM DEVELOPMENT

Fig. 10-4 Diagram illustrating the development of the two immune systems in the chicken. The thymus is believed to control cellular immunity, while the production of plasma cells and the synthesis of circulating antibodies are believed to be functions of the bursa of Fabricius. From Good (18) with permission.

chickens was greatest when only a small amount of antigen was used. The effect was masked with larger doses of antigen, indicating that extrasplenic sites were then being stimulated to make antibody.

The relation of the route of antigen injection to the degree of immune suppression produced by splenectomy has been explored in several laboratories (21–24). Rowley (21) showed that almost no antibody was produced in splenectomized rats following small intravenous injections of heated sheep red cell stromata. However, if the antigen was given intraportally, intraperitoneally, or intradermally, the animals made normal amounts of antibody. These results were confirmed by Wissler et al. (22). Draper and Sussdorf (23) compared the immune response to sheep cells in intact and splenectomized rabbits. Hemolysin titers were lower in splenectomized animals following the injection of antigen into the liver or femoral bone marrow, higher after injection into the appendix, kidney fat, or subcutaneous tissue of the lumbar region, and the same as intact controls after injection into the peritoneal cavity, thigh muscle, mesenteric lymph nodes, spleen, or rear footpads. These results indicate that nonsplenic sites are important contributors to antibody production provided they receive sufficient amounts of antigen. Rosenquist and Wolfe (24) compared intravenous and subcutaneous injections of bovine serum albumin in splenectomized chickens and observed a delay of the precipitin response in both groups when compared with intact controls. The delay was even longer in the splenectomized birds that were injected subcutaneously than in those that were injected intravenously. The authors suggested that the additional delay in the former group may reflect the longer time required for a given amount of subcutaneously injected antigen to reach and stimulate nonsplenic lymphoid tissue.

The age at which splenectomy is performed appears to have some relationship to the severity of the effect produced. Rosenquist and Wolfe (24) reported that in fowls splenectomized at 4, 9, or 17 weeks, only the last group showed a depressed response. The effect of splenectomy on the younger birds was only manifested by a delay in the response. It appears that in the younger animals nonsplenic tissue is more able to compensate for the removal of this organ (24a). Unfortunately, a similar study has not been carried out with mammals.

Taliaferro and Taliaferro (25–27) thoroughly investigated the effect of varying the time of splenectomy in relationship to antigen injection on hemolysin production in rabbits and reported that removal of the spleen within 4 days following immunization significantly reduced the production of antibody. Splenectomy after 6 days was ineffective, indicating that most of the antibody synthesis in the spleen occurs during the initial exponential rise of the immune response. Inhibition of antibody production also resulted when the spleen was removed within 28 days before immunization; splenectomy 98 days prior to immunization had no effect, further indicating that with sufficient time compensation for the loss of the spleen does occur.

Recent work (28) indicates that splenectomy may selectively inhibit the production of 19S antibody in both the primary and secondary responses. Although intact rats made no detectable primary response to intravenously injected soluble bovine gamma globulin (BGG), similar animals, when injected with BGG plus endotoxin, responded with an early 19S response and a later 7S response. In contrast, splenectomized rats had no early 19S response, but had an enhanced late 7S response when injected with BGG either alone or together with endotoxin.

Secondary stimulation of intact rats with BGG resulted in an accelerated response and the production of both 19S and 7S antibodies. Secondarily stimulated splenectomized animals were only able to make a delayed, predominantly 7S, response. Pierce (28) postulated that the 19S primary response antibody produced in the spleen "sensitized" the intact animals for a subsequent secondary response when restimulated with the same antigen.

Thoracic Duct Drainage

A reduction in the weight of the lymph nodes, a depletion of small lymphocytes from the cortex of the nodes, and a marked lymphopenia has been produced in rats (29) by cannulating the thoracic duct and draining lymph from the fistula for several days. It was shown that first-set skin homografts persisted significantly longer in rats treated in this manner, with the degree of prolongation dependent upon the degree of genetic difference between donor and host. Lymphocyte-depleted rats also showed a severely depressed response to injections of either sheep erythrocytes or tetanus toxoid. The sheep cells were injected intravenously, and the toxoid was administered as two injections given 3 weeks apart, the first intraperitoneally and the second intravenously. If depletion of lymphocytes by thoracic duct cannulation was carried out before the second of the two injections of tetanus toxoid, the secondary response was not affected.

The unresponsive state produced by thoracic duct drainage is apparently not due to stress, and can be corrected by intravenous injections of suspensions consisting almost entirely of small lymphocytes (29). It appears that the mechanism of action of this treatment is similar to that of splenectomy, in that it results in a generalized depletion of antigen target precursor cells.

Antilymphocyte Serum

The selective destruction of lymphoid cells by immunologic mechanisms is not a new approach to immunosuppression. Since the phenomenon was first observed in vitro by Metchnikoff in 1899 (30), a large number of workers have used it in studies directed at learning more about the normal functioning of the immune mechanism. Waksman et al. (31) reported that guinea pigs, when treated with antilymphocyte serum (ALS) produced in rats, showed reduced numbers of circulating lymphocytes and a depression of the delayed hypersensitivity reaction. Later, Woodruff and Anderson (32) found that rabbit anti-rat lymphocyte serum prolonged skin homograft survival time in rats and also observed that the immunosuppressive effects of ALS and thoracic duct drainage were additive. Monaco et al. (33) showed that treatment with ALS produced a profound reduction in peripheral lymphocytes and depletion of lymphoid organs in mice. These animals were immunologically deficient both in their ability to make humoral antibodies against sheep erythrocytes and rabbit gamma globulin and in their ability to reject skin homografts.

From the above discussion it would appear that ALS acts in a manner similar to thoracic duct drainage and splenectomy, i.e., by depletion of antigen-sensitive precursor cells. Recent work (34), however, especially in the field of human organ transplantation, has revealed that the effectiveness of ALS, produced in horses by immunization with human spleen cells in suppressing the rejection of renal homografts is not always accompanied by lymphopenia. Levey and Medawar (35,36) studied the problem and suggested that ALS may act by attaching to the surface of lymphocytes, causing an immunologic paralysis or "blindfolding" of these cells to other antigenic stimuli. This hypothesis was later rejected when it was found that the immunosuppressive effect persisted in the progeny of the originally treated cells. Levey and Medawar (36) next suggested that ALS might be acting as a stimulant to lymphoid cells, much like phytohemagglutinin, committing them to hyperplastic activity, thereby preempting their participation in normal immune reactions. An alternative hypothesis, proposed by the same authors, is that ALS might act by attaching itself to the cells of the homograft, exerting a protective function at the site of the graft itself.

It is still not certain that the immunosuppressive properties of ALS depend upon its specificity for lymphocytes, since it is possible to produce antiserum against epidermal cells and L cells, which have similar properties. Recently Turk and Willoughby (37) have reported the curious finding that although antiserum to thymus cells suppressed skin hypersensitivity reactions in rabbits and caused disappearance of cortical lymph nodes, a similar antiserum produced against lymph node cells depressed skin hypersensitivity without producing any detectable lymphoid depletion. They concluded that the first antiserum affected both the central stem cell and peripheral precursor cell components of the immune mechanism, while the lymph node antiserum had only a peripheral effect. ALS has also been shown to erase the immunologic memory of presensitized animals. Positive skin tests to tuberculin, mumps, and trichophyton were abolished within 3 to 4 days by ALS treatment (34). The significance of these findings is still uncertain.

INHIBITION OF ANTIGEN UPTAKE

RES Blockade

As reviewed by Jaffe (38) a large body of experimental evidence, replete with much controversy, implicated the phagocytic cells of the reticuloendothelial system (RES) as the main antibody former. This suggestion was based on the fact that blockade of these cells by loading them with carbon particles or other insoluble materials depressed or abolished antibody production.

The role of the RES macrophages in antibody production is now believed to be that of an antigen processor, especially in the case of particulate antigens (39). The so-called RES blockade method of suppressing the immune response may be due to an overloading or physical blocking of the cells which are necessary for the processing of antigen or, perhaps even more likely, to a depletion of serum opsonins. Recent work with perfused liver systems has shown that the blocking of Kupffer cells by bacteria or carbon particles can be overcome by introducing normal serum into the perfusate [see the review by Rowley (40)].

Passive Antibody

Smith (41) first recognized that if excess amounts of specific antibody are mixed with antigen before injecting it into an animal, it is possible to get a significant depression of the immune response. The same is true if the antibody is injected after the antigen, e.g., passively administered diphtheria antitoxin inhibited primary and secondary responses in guinea pigs when given as late as 5 days after immunization with toxoid adjuvant.

Not all antibody is equally effective in inhibiting the production of circulating antibody. Although 7S antibody produced against ϕX bacteriophage (42) was effective in inhibiting both the 19S and 7S primary responses to this antigen, 19S antibody was only effective in inhibiting 19S production. (Fab)$_2$ fragments have also been shown to be effective inhibitors of antibody production (43). Animals inhibited by passive antibody show an absence of the usual splenic cellular response to antigen.

It is now generally believed (42,44) that inhibition of antibody production by passive antibody is mediated through its interaction with the antigen, thereby preventing the latter from becoming accessible to reactive cells. This conclusion is based on the specificity of the effect with the degree of suppression related to the avidity of the passive antibody and the similarity of the effects of excess antibody or reduced antigen dosage on antibody production.

An alternative explanation has been proposed by Rowley and Fitch (43). They reported that in vivo or in vitro exposure of normal spleen cells to humoral antibody against sheep erythrocytes made them less responsive to a subsequent challenge by this antigen following transfer to irradiated hosts. They postulated that there are sites on or in the antigen-sensitive precursor cells which are sterically similar or identical to sites on the antigen and that the antibody exerts its inhibitory effect by combining with them. This hypothesis is attractive because it also provides a homeostatic mechanism for the control of antibody formation in the normal immune response as well as a model for explaining immunologic tolerance (see Chap. 8).

Competition of Antigens

Animals which are injected with a mixture of several antigens will often produce antibody against all the components of the mixture. In fact, the total amount of antibody produced may greatly exceed that which is produced in response to the injection of one of the components alone. Nevertheless, Abramoff and Wolfe (45) have described situations in which the immunogenicity of one antigen appears to be impaired by the previous, simultaneous, or subsequent injection of one or more other antigens (Fig. 10-5). Such interference with the immune response to one antigen is termed *competition of antigens* [See reviews by Adler (46,47)], and may manifest itself in varying degrees, ranging from complete suppression to a mere delay in the attainment of the maximum level of antibody observed in control animals. Among the variables which must be considered in any study of this phenomenon are the genetic constitution and physiological status of the test animals, the route and method of immunization, the absolute amounts and relative proportions of the antigens injected, past immunization history, and the kind of antigen selected.

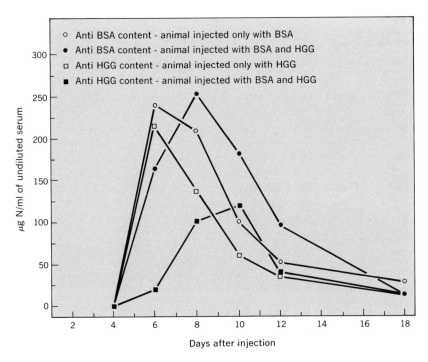

Fig. 10-5 Antibody production in chickens injected with 20 mg of BSA, HGG, or a combination of these antigens per kg body weight. Antibody titers are expressed as μg of antibody nitrogen per ml of undiluted serum. From Abramoff and Wolfe (45) with permission.

The mechanism by which introduction of one antigen interferes with the production of antibody against a second antigen remains obscure. Most discussions of competition of antigens have attempted to explain the phenomenon either in terms of a competition for a limited number of pluripotential stem cells or in terms of some "humoral" mechanism. The latter usually involves competition for some precursor necessary for protein synthesis, e.g., amino acids.

An interesting study in support of a humoral feedback inhibition explanation for competition of antigens has recently been reported by Radovich and Talmage (48). Spleen cells from nonimmunized donor mice and from donor mice injected with horse erythrocytes 2 days before transfer were mixed with sheep erythrocytes and injected intravenously into irradiated recipients. The inhibition of the response to sheep red cells was greater in mice receiving 50 million spleen cells from donors preinjected with horse erythrocytes than in those receiving 10 million cells from the same donors. Under these conditions it might be expected that competition would increase for a limited number of precursor cells if fewer such cells were injected. On the other hand, competition for a humoral factor would increase with injection of more cells. They also found that competition was maximal in this system when 4 days separated the two injections of antigen. They suggest that a humoral factor may be produced as a result of the response to the first antigen, and is acting as an inhibitor preventing a response to the second antigen.

EFFECT OF X-RAYS

In 1908 Benjamin and Sluka (49) were the first to systematically study the effect of ionizing radiation on antibody formation. They found that rabbits, when exposed to total-body x-rays before immunization, eliminated antigen more slowly and had lower levels of precipitating antibody than rabbits irradiated 4 days after immunization. These findings have since been substantiated and extended in other species with several antigen-antibody systems (50). Kohn (51) reported a depression of the primary response in rats when 300 r was given at various times during the week before and 5 days after a single injection of sheep erythrocytes. An x-ray dose of 175 r given 3 days before the antigen resulted in a greater depression of the hemolysin response than 600 r given 2 days after antigen stimulation. Fitch et al. (52) studied the ability of the rat to form hemolysins when a single intravenous injection of sheep erythrocytes or typhoid vaccine was given a few days before or 1 and 6 days after 500 r. Dixon et al. (53), using I^{131}-labeled bovine gamma globulin, and Taliaferro et al. (50), using sheep erythrocytes, systematically studied the time of antigenic stimulation in relation to x-radiation in rabbits. All of these investigators reported an early radiosensitive phase of the immune response and a later relatively radioresistant phase (Table 10-1).

It is now generally accepted that the primary effects of ionizing radiation on biologic systems are produced by the interaction of radiation energy with atoms and molecules of living cells. Part of this energy is absorbed, and as a result, molecular structures are disrupted, and highly reactive free radicals and peroxides are produced. The latter compounds may themselves react with other cell constituents, e.g., nucleic acids, causing further damage. The end result, depending upon the dose of radiation administered, may range in severity from the temporary derangement of some normal cellular function to the death of the organism.

Intense total body irradiation causes shrinkage of lymphoid organs such as the spleen, thymus, and lymph nodes. There is a depletion of lymphocytes from these organs as well as from the peripheral blood and lymph. In the bone marrow, a severe hypoplasia of the blood-forming

TABLE 10-1
Various Radiation-Antigen Time Relationships

Experimental group	No. of animals	PERCENT INJECTED ANTIGEN IN TOTAL BLOOD VOLUME					FRACTION OF RABBITS SHOWING IMMUNE ANTIGEN DISAPPEARANCE RATE				Maximum antibody concentration†	
		4 Day	7 Day	9 Day	11 Day	13 Day	4-7 Day	7-9 Day	9-11 Day	11-13 Day		
Controls	16	13.9	0.1	0			16/16				16.4	10
400 r 6 hr after antigen	9	12.7	0.5	0			9/9				14.2	7
400 r simultaneously with antigen	18	11.5	1.8	0.2	0		12/18	17/18	18/18		12.7	5
400 r 5 hr before antigen	9	12.5	2.9	0.4	0.1	0	4/9	8/9	9/9	9/9	7.7	4
400 r 12 hr before antigen	9	11.8	4.4	1.7	0.6	0.1	0/9	3/9	6/9	2/7	2	2
400 r 48 hr before antigen	8	13.8	4.7	2.6	1.5	0.8	0/8	0/8	0/8		0	
800 r 3 days after antigen	29	—	4.8	0.7	0.1	0	0/29	27/29	29/29		16.1	21‡
800 r 1 hr after antigen	8	—	5.5	2.2	0.7	0.2	0/8	2/8	6/8	8/8	6.4	6§

† μg of antigen nitrogen precipitated by 1 ml antiserum at P80 with standard deviation.
‡ Antibody results on 10 rabbits.
§ Antibody results on 5 rabbits.
SOURCE: From Dixon et al. (53) with permission.

tissue is evident. Plasma cells, polymorphonuclear leukocytes, and macrophages appear to be the least sensitive to x-rays. However, there is some evidence that transport of antigen by macrophages of the perifollicular sinus of the spleen may be inhibited by irradiation (54), probably by damage to some follicular component.

In conjunction with the extensive destruction of lymphoid cells, there is in those cells a loss of reproductive integrity which may survive immediate death. It is believed that synthesis of DNA per se is not very sensitive to irradiation (55), but that replication of DNA in the cell is inhibited or delayed by interference with other processes in the cell cycle. The synthesis of RNA appears to be inhibited by irradiation in certain cases. A relationship between this inhibition and damage inflicted on the DNA macromolecule has been suggested.

In any case, the effects of irradiation on immune processes are probably not due to a direct interference with those metabolic processes or activities which are already being carried out by the affected cells. As indicated above, a very general response of cells to low doses of radiation is the loss of reproductive integrity, and the studies concerning the cellular aspects of the radiosensitive and radioresistant phases of antibody production all suggest that mitosis is an early and necessary step in the immune response. Taliaferro and Talmage (56) measured the rate of S^{35} amino acid incorporation into antibody at different times following immunization. Their data indicate that little, if any, antibody is synthesized during the latent period, suggesting that this period is one during which the responding cells are preparing for synthesis of antibody, probably by dividing and synthesizing mRNA. The importance of cell division during the latent period has since been directly demonstrated by the use of FUDR (5-fluorouracil deoxyriboside), which specifically blocks the synthesis of DNA. This compound was found to have its greatest suppressive effect when given to mice within 48 hours of the antigen (57).

It was formerly thought by most investigators that the secondary, or anamnestic, immune response is relatively radioresistant when compared with the primary response. A definitive attempt to clarify this question was carried out by Makinodan et al. (58). They compared the primary and secondary anti-sheep RBC responses of normal and irradiated mouse spleen cells following transfer to irradiated hosts (Fig. 10-6). They concluded that (1) the slopes of the regression lines for primary and secondary responses remained unaltered after radiation treatment; and (2) the magnitude of decrease in both responses after a given dose of x-ray treatment was about the same.

Claman (59) irradiated rabbits after the primary or secondary injection of bovine gamma globulin and noted that irradiation produced a fall

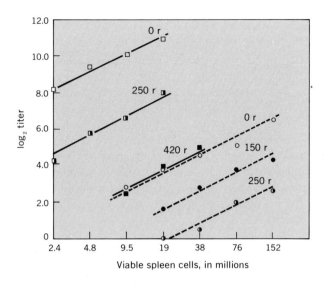

Fig. 10-6 Effect of x-radiation on 6-day primary and secondary anti-sheep erythrocyte responses of cultured mouse spleen cells. The abscissa indicates the number of spleen cells transferred to irradiated hosts, and the ordinate shows the $\log_2$ titer. - - - primary response ——— secondary response. From Makinodan et al. (58) with permission.

in titer of the primary but not the secondary response. Irradiation also inhibited the response of primarily immunized animals to a subsequent injection of the same antigen. Claman suggested that irradiation following the primary injection of antigen inhibited the maturation of antigen-sensitive precursor cells to form antibody-producing cells. The resulting decline in titer represented the naturally occurring gradual loss of antibody-producing cells. The ineffectiveness of x-rays in depressing the secondary response in these experiments suggested that the transformation of precursor cells to producers had already been completed by this time. La Via (60) also showed that antibody titers of rats immunized with a single dose of *S. typhi* and irradiated during the plateau phase of antibody production were unaffected, perhaps by the same mechanism postulated by Claman (59) for the secondary response of the rabbit.

There are several ways in which the immune mechanism of organisms exposed to ionizing radiation may be protected. The most obvious means of achieving this end is to shield a portion of the lymphoid tissue. Jacobson and Robson (61) have shown that shielding of the spleen or appendix of rabbits gives 70 percent protection of both primary and secondary hemolysin responses to sheep erythrocytes. Essentially normal titers can be obtained following immunization of animals splenectomized 1 day after irradiation, providing the antigen is injected intraperitoneally. Taliaferro et al. (50), using careful quantitative methods, confirmed in principle the findings of Jacobson and Robson but found much less protection.

Several nonspecific substances, e.g., kaolin, carbon suspensions, various bacterial proteins, and lipopolysaccharides, have also been reported to confer some measure of protection to the immune mechanism if they are administered before moderate doses of radiation. Stender et al. (62) have produced a high degree of protection of the response in rats to heat-killed *Brucella* antigen by injecting carbon suspensions or proteins from *E. coli* subcutaneously into the thigh several days before 200 to 350 r. In these experiments the antigen was administered by the same route 2 days after irradiation.

Cytological and histological investigations and autoradiographic studies using tritiated thymidine revealed that the nonspecific agents caused an activation of the lymphoreticular tissues and a proliferation of immunologically competent cells. These cells could be induced by antigen and were capable of developing into plasma cells and producing antibody. After large doses of x-ray, the proliferation of antibody-forming cells was delayed, presumably because of physical damage to the mitotic process.

There are several chemical compounds which, when given at the appropriate time, protect living organisms from the lethal effects of ionizing radiation. At the present time five different groups of such substances are distinguished: (1) sulfur-containing compounds (cysteine, cysteamine); (2) pharmacologically active substances (cyanide, serotonin, tryptamine); (3) metabolites (glucose, pyruvic acid); (4) compounds with specific protective characteristics (thiourea); (5) vitamins and hormones. A few of these have been studied in connection with irradiation and antibody formation.

Makinodan et al. (63) injected mice with sheep erythrocytes 1 day following 950 r total-body irradiation. These mice were also given syngeneic marrow immediately after irradiation. The immune response of these animals was protected somewhat if they were injected with MEG (2-mercaptoethylguanidine hydrobromide) 10 minutes before irradiation. Simic et al. (64) conducted similar studies with rats and were able to demonstrate a similar protective effect of MEA (β-mercaptoethylamine) or AET (β-aminoethylisothiouroniumchloride hydrochloride) on the hemolysin response to sheep red cells if the drugs were administered 5 minutes before irradiation. The latter authors suggested that MEA and AET protect some biochemical mechanism essential for the proliferation and differentiation of the antibody-forming cells after stimulation with antigen. This mechanism may be associated with the metabolism of nucleic acids in the irradiated spleen.

There are also several materials which, if injected together with antigen, have been reported to restore the antibody-forming capacity of irradiated animals. Much work in this area has been done by Taliaferro et al. (50).

Colchicine, which appears to be the most active of all the restorative agents, will, if injected at the same time as antigen, increase the mean peak hemolysin titer nine- to tenfold in irradiated (400 r) and in unirradiated rabbits. It exerts no detectable restorative activity, however, if doses of x-ray higher than 600 r are used, presumably because there would be too few surviving cells to produce measurable amounts of antibody (65). Colchicine is believed to have restorative activity because of its in vivo cytotoxic activity, which can kill cells and release their nucleic acid degradation products. A similar mechanism has been invoked to explain the heightened immune response sometimes observed when animals are irradiated or treated with FUDR (57) shortly before immunization.

Several other materials have been tested for their restorative activity, as measured by peak titer (Table 10-2). Yeast, HeLa cells, and rabbit and mouse spleen cells, all of which contain a rich pool of nucleic acid precursors, showed various degrees of activity. Nucleic acid digests, which

TABLE 10-2

Restoration of Peak Hemolysin Titer from X-ray Induced Depression by a Variety of Materials Administered at the Same Time as Antigen to Rabbits Irradiated on the Previous Day [†]

86% or more restoration	*Partial restoration: 41 to 64%*	*None*
Tissue preparations		
Yeast extract (2000)	Mouse spleen (0.3)	Rabbit kidney (0.4–1.5)
HeLa cells (0.2–0.8)	Rabbit spleen (0.4–1.6)	Rabbit muscle (0.9–2.1)
Nucleic acids, digests,	DNA incubated with	Polymerized DNA (100)
and derivatives	DNase (100 + 10)	Polymerized RNA (100)
	RNA incubated with	DNase (10)
	RNase (100 + 10)	Adenine (10)
	RNase (10)	Adenosine (10)
	Kinetin (4, 10, 12)	Adenylic acid (10)
		Crude guanosine (57)
		Mixtures of nucleosides (100), nucleotides (100), and nucleotide diphosphates (20)
Other materials		
Colchicine (3.6)	3-indoleacetic acid (10)	Croton oil (3 ml of a 1:30 dilution per kg)

[†] Numbers in parentheses equal the milligram amounts given per rabbit; numbers in brackets equal approximate wet weight in grams.
SOURCE: From Taliaferro et al. (50) with permission.

contained polynucleotides of various sizes, were also active. Other cellular preparations of lower nucleic acid content, e.g., rabbit kidney and muscle, were inactive [reviewed in (50)].

Since Jacobson and Robson (61) first demonstrated that a significant percentage of the immune capacity of an irradiated animal may be protected by encasing the spleen in a lead shield, there have been many attempts to both minimize the lethal effects of radiation and to restore the immune capabilities of the animal by injecting hematopoietic cells. Excellent reviews of this subject have been written by Koller et al. (66), Gengozian (67), and Micklem and Loutit (68).

Harris et al. (69) were probably the first to demonstrate that transferred lymph node cells could be stimulated with specific antigen and elicit their immune response in an irradiated host. They reported that blood leukocytes and peritoneal exudate cells were less active than lymph node cells and they were unable to demonstrate any antibody production by transferred thymus cells. La Via et al. (70) were successful in partially restoring the hemolysin response in irradiated rats with homologous spleen cells.

Makinodan and his associates conducted an extensive series of experiments dealing with the recovery of the immune mechanism in irradiated mice with or without injections of isologous hematopoietic tissue [see review by Gengozian (67)]. After irradiated mice were injected with syngeneic bone marrow, they were found to recover the ability to respond normally to injections of sheep erythrocytes by approximately 1 month after irradiation. Similarly, mice took twice as long to recover a normal responsiveness to rat erythrocytes. These results suggested that irradiation must have impaired some early phase of the immune response, probably the "antigen recognition" mechanism, which was not directly replaced by the transfused bone marrow.

More recently, the role of the macrophage in antibody production has been explored in a similar system by Gallily and Feldman (71). When peritoneal exudate cells were incubated in vitro with *Shigella* and injected into sublethally irradiated (550 r) mice, the animals produced circulating antibody. Neither mice subjected to the same dose of radiation before injection with antigen alone nor mice exposed to 910 r before injection with sensitized macrophages were able to respond. It was concluded that the macrophages from normal donor animals, following incubation with antigen, elicited the production of antibody by the lymphoid cells of the irradiated recipients. It follows that two populations of cells of differing radiation sensitivities are involved in the immune response to this and probably other antigens.

From the preceding it can easily be seen that the efficacy of transplanted hematopoietic tissue, while useful as a means of alleviating radiation-induced injuries, also provides researchers with an invaluable immunologic tool. The use of lethally irradiated animals, usually mice, as hosts for transplants of isologous lymphoid tissue, has provided a unique method which permits study, in a more quantitative manner, of the immunologic activity of the different types of cells.

IMMUNOSUPPRESSIVE DRUGS

The immunosuppressive drugs which are of interest in immunosuppression may, for convenience, be grouped into six general classes: (1) the alkylating agents; (2) the antimetabolites; (3) the antibiotics; (4) the steroids; (5) the folic acid antagonists; (6) the plant alkaloids. There are other compounds with immunosuppressive properties which do not fit into this classification, e.g., the salicylates, the ataractic drugs, and the methyl hydrazines. Since these are of lesser importance, they will not be discussed here. Their description and possible significance in immunosuppressive therapy have been described in a review by Gabrielsen and Good (72).

Alkylating Agents

These include such compounds as the nitrogen mustards, bisulfan, triethylene melamine, and cyclophosphamide. These chemicals interact directly with protein and DNA molecules, causing their denaturation. It is believed that they affect constituents of the cell nucleus most severely (73) (see Fig. 10-7). They are also powerful lympholytic agents. Their action is similar in some respects to that of x-rays, and for this reason they were once called *radiomimetic drugs*. However, none of these agents mimics more than a fraction of the effects of x-radiation.

The alkylating agents, like x-rays, are most effective in blocking the inductive phase of antibody production. Hektoen and Corper (74) showed that mustard gas, when administered to dogs or rabbits several days after antigen stimulation, had no immunosuppressive effect on their immune response. The same agent, however, when given before or together with antigen, caused a marked depression of antibody production. This depression was temporary, lasting only 2 to 3 weeks. Similar results have been obtained with other alkylating agents.

More recently, studies with cyclophosphamide (75–78) have indicated that this derivative of nitrogen mustard is effective in suppressing the immune response of rabbits, guinea pigs, and mice to a number of anti-

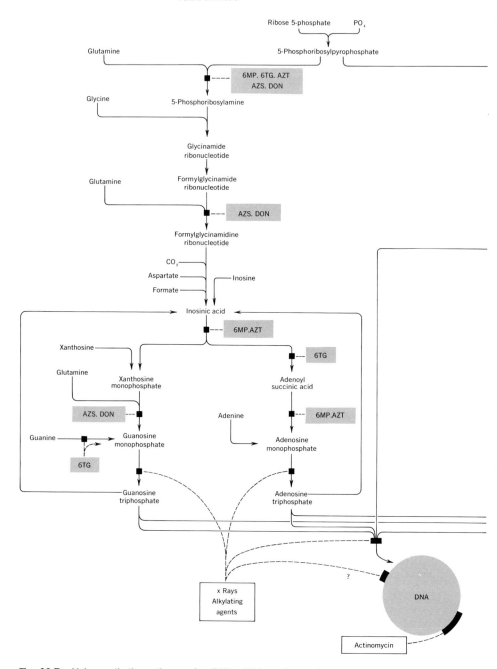

Fig. 10-7 Main synthetic pathways for DNA, RNA, and protein synthesis, indicating points of action of immunosuppressive drugs. From Berenbaum (73) with permission.

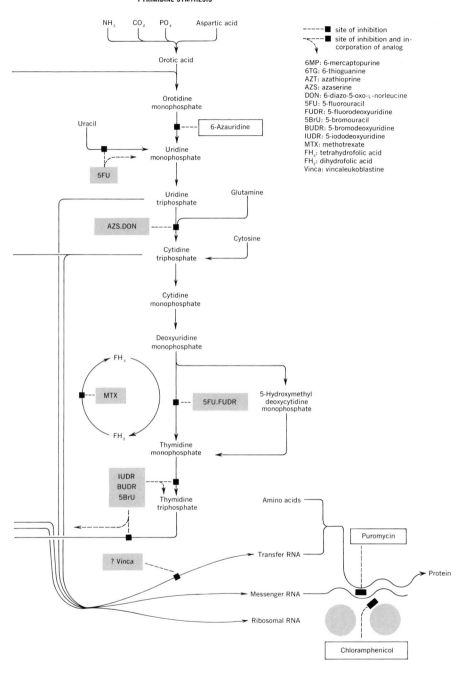

PYRIMIDINE SYMTHESIS

```
NH₃    CO₂    PO₄    Aspartic acid
```

Orotic acid

Orotidine
monophosphate

Uracil   6-Azauridine

5FU

Uridine
monophosphate

Uridine   Glutamine
triphosphate

AZS.DON

Cytidine   Cytosine
triphosphate

Cytidine
monophosphate

Deoxyuridine
monophosphate

FH₄

MTX   5FU.FUDR   5-Hydroxymethyl
                         deoxycytidine
                         monophosphate

FH₂

Thymidine
monophosphate

IUDR
BUDR   Thymidine
5BrU   triphosphate

                         Amino acids

                                        Puromycin

? Vinca

            Transfer RNA

                                        Protein

            Messenger RNA

            Ribosomal RNA

                         Chloramphenicol
```

------■  site of inhibition
------■  site of inhibition and in-
         corporation of analog

6MP: 6-mercaptopurine
6TG: 6-thioguanine
AZT: azathioprine
AZS: azaserine
DON: 6-diazo-5-oxo-L-norleucine
5FU: 5-fluorouracil
FUDR: 5-fluorodeoxyuridine
5BrU: 5-bromouracil
BUDR: 5-bromodeoxyuridine
IUDR: 5-iododeoxyuridine
MTX: methotrexate
FH₄: tetrahydrofolic acid
FH₂: dihydrofolic acid
Vinca: vincaleukoblastine
```

gens. However, unlike other alkylating agents, this drug is effective not only during the latent period, but will suppress antibody production when administered several days after the injection of antigen.

Alkylating agents have also been used effectively to suppress delayed hypersensitivity reactions in rabbits (79). This suppression was not due to leukopenia because the skin reaction remained negative even after the leukocyte counts had returned to normal (80).

Antimetabolites

These include the purine antagonists such as 6-mercaptopurine (6-MP) and its derivatives as well as the halogenated pyrimidines.

The purine antagonists (6-MP, azathioprine, thioguanine, 8-azathioguanine) act principally by blocking the interconversion of nucleosides, particularly the formation of adenylic acid from inosinic acid (see Fig. 10-7). In addition, azathioprine may bind sulfhydryl groups. The end result of treatment with purine inhibitors is interference with nucleic acid and protein synthesis.

6-MP has a greater effect on delayed hypersensitivity reactions than on humoral antibody production. Appropriate 4-day treatment of rabbits with 6-MP effectively blocked their delayed hypersensitivity reaction to BGG, but the animals made normal amounts of humoral antibodies (81). The production of delayed hypersensitivity is, therefore, probably not a necessary prelude to antibody synthesis.

6-MP is apparently only effective in inhibiting the production of circulating antibodies in rabbits if it is administered at the same time as antigen or shortly thereafter. Once antibody appears in the serum, the drug is relatively ineffective. Treatment of rabbits with 6-MP before injection of antigen also fails to inhibit antibody production. The drug appears to act on a later phase of induction than the alkylating agents. The production of antibody-forming cells is prevented by 6-MP treatment, and Schwartz (82) postulates that these are the target cells for this drug. He also found that the relationship between the dosage of 6-MP and the degree of suppression of the primary response was linear, suggesting that the action of the drug was due, not to inhibition of mitosis, but to suppression of a first-order biochemical process essential to the induction of antibody production.

The pyrimidine analogs include such drugs as 5-fluorodeoxyuridine (FUDR), 5-bromodeoxyuridine (BUDR), and 5-fluorouracil (5-FU). These compounds are either incorporated into DNA (see Fig. 10-7), producing molecules that cannot support mitosis, or they compete with the normal substrates for enzymatic sites. In either case, cell division is prevented. The pyrimidine analogs are chiefly important as carcinostatic and virostatic compounds and have generally been too toxic to use in suppressing immunity in experimental animals.

By employing tissue culture techniques Dutton (83,84) and O'Brien and Coons (85) were able to examine the effect of BUDR on the secondary response of spleen cells in vitro. They found that cells already producing antibody when the culture was started continued to do so, while recruitment, via cell division, to the antibody-forming population was blocked by BUDR. They also showed that the antibody produced in their cultures depended upon cell division during the second, third, and probably fourth day after antigen stimulation.

In one of the few in vivo experiments with pyrimidine analogs, Merritt and Johnson (57) observed that a daily injection of 1 mg FUDR for 12 days inhibited the primary response of mice to BGG. On the other hand, when a single dose of 8 mg was given, either 1 hour before or 4 days after antigen, a distinct adjuvant effect was observed. This enhancement has still not been explained, but is probably related to the similar phenomenon which results when x-ray is administered in low doses shortly before the injection of antigen.

The amino acid analog β-3-thienylalanine has also been studied in vivo and has been shown to have an effect very similar to that of 6-MP (86). In fact it is most effective when given with antigen and shortly after. It is relatively inefficient if administered at a later time. It acts by blocking RNA synthesis and subsequent RNA-dependent synthesis of antibody (87).

Antibiotics

These include a large group of substances which are produced by various species of *Streptomyces*. The most commonly known ones are puromycin, mitomycin C, the actinomycins, chloramphenicol, and azaserine. These have all been studied with respect to their ability to inhibit the immune response.

Puromycin is structurally similar to the amino acid-bearing end of sRNA. For this reason it is believed to compete with sRNA for sites on the ribosome, thereby inhibiting the transfer of amino acids. Thus it is a specific inhibitor of protein synthesis. Studies of the effect of puromycin on antibody synthesis in vivo have been limited because toxic doses must be administered before any measurable effect can be seen. Smiley et al. (88) and Ambrose and Coons (89) found, however, that low doses of puromycin were effective in inhibiting antibody production in tissue culture usually without killing the cells.

Mitomycin C acts by depolymerizing DNA, thereby inhibiting its replication. It is also an alkylating agent, inhibiting RNA and protein synthesis if used in high enough concentrations in vivo. It has been used with some success in an effort to suppress the rejection of kidney allografts in dogs by Otte and Grosjean (90). Bloom et al. (91) used mitomycin C to inhibit the capacity of cells from picryl chloride–sensitized guinea pigs to transfer reactivity to normal recipients. More recently, Sakauchi and Dewitt (92) have shown that mitomycin C inhibits antibody production in rats to injections of allogeneic lymphocytes if the drug is given at the time of antigen stimulation. It does not inhibit antibody production when given at the height of the immune response. These results indicate that the immunosuppressive effect is not due to direct inhibition of protein synthesis.

The mechanism of action of the actinomycins has been inferred from the work on actinomycin D by Goldberg and Reich (93). This drug inhibits DNA-dependent RNA synthesis by binding the guanidine residues of DNA. It has proven very effective in inhibiting antibody production in vitro, provided the incubation period is long enough. Fishman et al. (94) have reported that actinomycin D selectively inhibits 19S antibody production. However, Uhr (95) has demonstrated that the secondary response may also be inhibited by actinomycin D. David (96) demonstrated the effect of actinomycin D on delayed hypersensitivity reactions. Peritoneal exudate cells from sensitized guinea pigs are inhibited from in vitro migration by specific antigen. Low doses of actinomycin D prevent this inhibition, and the cells migrate. High doses of the drug kill the cells.

Study of the immunosuppressive activity of the actinomycins in vivo has been limited by their high toxicity. Jerne et al. (97) have reported that a single dose of actinomycin D, given to mice 1 day after an immunizing injection of sheep erythrocytes, strikingly suppressed the production of circulating antibody, as measured by the localized hemolysis in gel technique. Hanna and Wust (98,99) studied the effect of actinomycin D on the production of hemagglutinins to sheep erythrocytes in mice. They reported that 12 μg of the drug, an LD_{30} dose, given at any time between 12 hours before and 8 hours after the injection of antigen, delayed the appearance of circulating antibody for approximately 2 days. The eventual rate of appearance of circulating antibodies and the maximum titer were similar to that observed in those animals receiving sheep red cells alone. Correlated with the delay in response was the destruction of most of the large lymphocytic cells of the lymphatic nodules. The authors suggested that cells committed to respond to the injected antigen were more susceptible to destruction by actinomycin D than were the unstimulated cells.

Chloramphenicol is similar to puromycin in that it inhibits the transfer of amino acids to ribosomes. It appears to be a specific inhibitor of protein synthesis. Ambrose and Coons (89) found that relatively low doses of chloramphenicol sharply inhibited the in vitro secondary response to BSA and diphtheria toxoid. When chloramphenicol was present for the first 6 days of culture, there was a 90 percent reduction in the response; when the drug was added after the first 6 days, the response was 40 percent of normal. Weisberger et al. (100), by using high doses of chloramphenicol (0.5 to 0.6 g/kg/day) for 10 to 12 days, were able to suppress the primary response of rabbits to BGG.

Azaserine is a glutamine analog in bacterial systems, but probably functions as an alkylating agent in mammalian cells. It is not very effective as an immunosuppressive agent when used alone, but has been demonstrated to act synergistically with 6-MP in inhibiting tumor growth. Combinations of Azaserine and azathioprine are effective in prolonging kidney survival in dogs (101), and this combination has also been used in human renal transplants (102).

Steroids

Adrenal steroids may inhibit immune responses in any or all of several different ways. Their ability to inhibit proliferative responses is well known (103). In addition, they are powerful lympholytic agents (104), especially destructive to thymus cells. The stabilizing effect of steroids on lysosomal membranes (105) may be inhibitory to the afferent limb of the immune response, i.e., the uptake and processing of antigen. The efferent limb of the response may be suppressed by the reported anticomplementary action of steroids (106), and local manifestations of delayed hypersensitivity reactions may be prevented by the anti-inflammatory activity of these compounds (107).

The effect of treatment with steroids on the production of circulating antibodies has been studied by many investigators [see Gabrielsen and Good (72)]. Perhaps the most extensive investigation in this area was carried out by Fagraeus and Berglund (108), who showed that cortisone treatment can depress the antibody response to S. typhi H in both rabbits and rats as well as the response to sheep erythrocytes in rats. With low doses of cortisone (4 mg/100 g body weight), suppression was achieved only if the drug was administered before the injection of antigen. Cortisone was effective in suppressing antibody production only if given in higher doses for prolonged periods of time. These workers also found that the inhibition of hemolysin production by cortisone in rats could be reversed by injections of allogeneic or xenogeneic thymus or spleen cells.

The effectiveness of adrenal steroids in prolonging the survival of skin or kidney allografts has been repeatedly demonstrated in both experimental animals and humans [see Gabrielsen and Good (72)]. As early as 1951 Billingham et al. (109) showed that treatment with cortisone prolonged skin allograft survival in rabbits by a factor of 3 or 4. More recent work has been concerned with problems of human organ transplantation. Moderate prolongation of kidney allograft survival in prednisolone-treated dogs has been reported by Zukoski et al. (110). Marchioro et al. (111), also working with dogs, successfully used prednisolone to overcome rejection crises in azathioprine-treated kidney recipients. This latter finding has proved especially useful in human organ transplant programs.

Folic Acid Antagonists

These include such compounds as Aminopterin (4-aminopteroylaspartic acid) and methotrexate (4-amino-N^{10}-pteroylaspartic acid). These are powerful immunosuppressive agents which act by inhibiting the activity of dihydrofolic reductase, an enzyme which is required for the conversion of folic acid to folinic acid. Folinic acid is essential for the metabolism of one-carbon fragments, particularly transmethylation. This latter process is of particular importance in the synthesis of purines, pyrimidines, and some amino acids. It is very important in nucleic acid and protein synthesis.

The effect of methotrexate on the development of delayed hypersensitivity and humoral antibody production has been investigated by Friedman et al. (112). They were able to suppress completely both types of immune responses to diphtheria toxoid and ovalbumin in incomplete adjuvant. Larger doses of methotrexate were required to produce a suppression when the antigens were administered in complete adjuvant. Friedman and Buckler (113) later found that when lymph node cells from tuberculin-inoculated guinea pigs, in which tuberculin hypersensitivity had been blocked by methotrexate, were transferred to normal recipients, the recipients became tuberculin-sensitive in 2 weeks. In contrast, when lymph node cells from tuberculin-sensitive donors were transferred to methotrexate-treated recipients, tuberculin sensitivity did not develop unless the drug treatment was stopped. They concluded that methotrexate suppresses the multiplication of sensitized cells rather than the acquisition of tuberculin sensitization. Turk and Stone (80) have reported data which are consistent with this idea. By histologic studies they showed that whereas methotrexate inhibited the development of delayed hypersensitivity in guinea pigs, it failed, unlike 6-MP, to inhibit the appearance of blast cells in the local lymph nodes.

Plant Alkaloids

There are two kinds of plant alkaloids which have been used as immuno-suppressants. Colchicine, with its spindle-blocking properties, has been known for some time and has been widely used experimentally as an inhibitor of mitosis in metaphase. Prior to the discovery of its immuno-suppressive properties, its major clinical use has been in the treatment of gout. The *Vinca* drugs (vinblastine and vincristine), which have been discovered more recently, are also spindle inhibitors and inhibit mitosis in metaphase. However, it has generally been found that their immuno-suppressive properties are not as great as those of colchicine.

Plant alkaloids are very toxic. Colchicine, in particular, is extremely lympholytic, even destroying nondividing cells. It has also been reported to interfere with phagocytosis (114). Colchicine-treated leukocytes can engulf bacteria, but the degranulation, vacuolization, and changes in acid phosphatase activity which usually accompany phagocytosis are inhibited. The immunosuppressive properties of colchicine and possibly the *Vinca* alkaloids are probably due to a combination of general toxicity and an interference with the uptake and processing of antigen.

In addition to the several reports of immunosuppression of antibody production by treatment with colchicine [see Gabrielsen and Good (72)], there have been reports of immune enhancement in colchicine-treated rabbits (50). The mechanism for this phenomenon is believed to be similar to that which sometimes occurs following x-radiation or treatment with pyrimidine analogs.

REFERENCES

1. Archer, O., and Pierce, J. C.: *Federation Proc.*, **20**:26, 1961.
2. Janković, B. D., Waksman, B. H., and Arnason, B. G.: *J. Exp. Med.*, **116**:159, 1962.
3. Miller, J. F. A. P.: *Lancet*, **II**:748, 1961.
4. Miller, J. F. A. P., Marshall, A. H. E., and White, R. G.: *Advan. Immunol.*, **2**:111, 1962.
5. Humphrey, J. H., Parrott, D. M. V., and East, J.: *Immunology*, **7**:419, 1964.
6. Globerson, A., Fiore-Donati, L., and Feldman, M.: *Exp. Cell Res.*, **28**:455, 1962.
7. Miller, J. F. A. P.: *Nature (London)*, **208**:1337, 1965.
8. Metcalf, D.: *Nature (London)*, **208**:1336, 1965.
9. Burnet, M.: *Sci. Amer.*, **207**:50, 1962.
9a. Kemenes, F., and Pethes, G.: *Z. Immunitäts Allergieforsch.*, **125**:446, 1963.

10. Warner, N. L., and Szenberg, A.: *Annu. Rev. Microbiol.*, **18**:253, 1964.
11. Glick, B., Chang, T. S., and Jaap, R. G.: *Poultry Sci.*, **35**:224, 1956.
12. Chang, T. S., Rhiens, M. S., and Winter, A. R.: *Poultry Sci.*, **36**:735, 1957.
13. Wolfe, H. R., Carroll, M. A., and Cote, W. P.: *Federation Proc.*, **21**:22, 1962.
14. Isaković, K., and Janković, B. D.: *Int. Arch. Allergy*, **24**:296, 1964.
15. Cooper, M. D., Peterson, R. D. A., and Good, R. A.: *Nature (London)*, **205**:143, 1965.
16. Cooper, M. D., Peterson, R. D. A., and Good, R. A.: in "Phylogeny of Immunity," R. T. Smith, P. Miescher, and R. A. Good (eds.), University of Florida Press, Gainesville, 1966.
17. Warner, N., and Szenberg, A.: in "The Thymus in Immunobiology," R. A. Good and A. E. Gabrielson (eds.), Harper & Row, New York, 1964.
18. Good, R. A.: *Hosp. Pract.*, **2**:38, 1967.
19. McMaster, P. D.: in "The Cell," vol. 5, J. Brachet, and A. E. Mirsky (eds.), Academic Press, New York, 1961.
20. Wolfe, H. R., Norton, S., Springer, E., Goodman, M., and Herrick, C. A.: *J. Immunol.*, **64**:179, 1950.
21. Rowley, D. A.: *J. Immunol.*, **64**:289, 1950.
22. Wissler, R. W., Robson, M. J., Fitch, F. W., Nelson, W., and Jacobson, L. O.: *J. Immunol.*, **70**:379, 1953.
23. Draper, L. R., and Süssdorf, D. H.: *J. Infect. Dis.*, **100**:147, 1957.
24. Rosenquist, G. L., and Wolfe, H. R.: *Immunology*, **5**:211, 1962.
24a. Keily, Sr. D., and Abramoff, P.: *J. Immunol.*, **102**:1058, 1969.
25. Taliaferro, W. H., and Taliaferro, L. G.: *J. Infect. Dis.*, **87**:37, 1950.
26. Taliaferro, W. H., and Taliaferro, L. G.: *J. Infect. Dis.*, **89**:143, 1951.
27. Taliaferro, W. H., and Taliaferro, L. G.: *J. Infect. Dis.*, **90**:205, 1952.
28. Pierce, C. W.: *Lab. Invest.*, **16**:782, 1967.
29. Gowans, J. L., and McGregor, D. D.: *Progr. Allergy*, **9**:1, 1965.
30. Metchnikoff, E.: *Ann. Inst. Pasteur*, **13**:737, 1899.
31. Waksman, B. H., Arbouys, S., and Arnason, B. G.: *J. Exp. Med.*, **114**:997, 1961.
32. Woodruff, M. F. A., and Anderson, N. A.: *Nature (London)*, **200**:702, 1963.
33. Monaco, A. P., Wood, M. L., Gray, J. G., and Russell, P. S.: *J. Immunol.*, **96**:229, 1966.
34. Starzl, T. E., Porter, K. A., Iwasaki, Y., Marchioro, T. L., and Kashiwagi, N.: in "Antilymphocyte Serum," Ciba Foundation Study Group No. 29, Little, Brown and Company, Boston, 1967.
35. Levey, R. H., and Medawar, P. B.: *Ann. N.Y. Acad. Sci.*, **129**:164, 1966.
36. Levey, R. H., and Medawar, P. B.: *Proc. Nat. Acad. Sci. U.S.*, **56**:1130, 1966.
37. Turk, J. L., and Willoughby, D. A.: *Lancet*, I:249, 1967.
38. Jaffé, R. H.: *Physiol. Rev.*, **11**:277, 1931.

39. Fishman, M.: *J. Exp. Med.*, **114**:837, 1961.
40. Rowley, D. A.: *Advan. Immunol.*, **2**:241, 1962.
41. Smith, T.: *J. Exp. Med.*, **11**:241, 1909.
42. Uhr, J. W., and Finkelstein, M. S.: *Progr. Allergy*, **10**:37, 1967.
43. Rowley, D. A., and Fitch, F. W.: in "Regulation of the Antibody Response," B. Cinader (ed.), Charles C Thomas, Springfield, Ill., 1968.
44. Uhr, J. W., and Möller, G.: *Advan. Immunol.*, **8**:81, 1968.
45. Abramoff, P., and Wolfe, H. R.: *J. Immunol.*, **77**:94, 1956.
46. Adler, F. L.: in "Mechanisms of Hypersensitivity," J. H. Shaffer, G. A. Lo Grippo, and M. W. Chase (eds.), Little, Brown and Company, Boston, 1959.
47. Adler, F. L.: *Progr. Allergy*, **8**:41, 1964.
48. Radovich, J., and Talmage, D. W.: *Science*, **158**:512, 1967.
49. Benjamin, E., and Sluka, E.: *Wien. Klin. Wochschr.*, **21**:311, 1908.
50. Taliaferro, W. H., Taliaferro, L. G., and Jaroslow, B. N.: "Radiation and Immune Mechanisms," Academic Press, Inc., New York, 1964.
51. Kohn, H. I.: *J. Immunol.*, **66**:525, 1951.
52. Fitch, F. W., Wissler, R. W., LaVia, M. F., and Barker, P: *J. Immunol.*, **76**:151, 1956.
53. Dixon, F. J., Talmage, D. W., and Maurer, P. H.: *J. Immunol.*, **68**:693, 1952.
54. Hunter, R. L., and Wissler, R. W.: *J. Reticuloendothel. Soc.*, **4**:444, 1967.
55. Nygaard, O. F.: in "Ionizing Radiation and Immune Processes," C. A. Leone (ed.), Gordon and Breach, New York, 1962.
56. Taliaferro, W. H., and Talmage, D. W., J. Infect. Dis., **97**:88, 1955.
57. Merritt, K., and Johnson, A. G.: *J. Immunol.*, **91**:266, 1963.
58. Makinodan, T., Kastenbaum, M. A., and Peterson, W. J.: *J. Immunol.*, **88**:31, 1962.
59. Claman, H. N.: *J. Immunol.*, **91**:29, 1963.
60. LaVia, M. F.: Unpublished observations.
61. Jacobson, L. O., and Robson, M. J.: *J. Lab. Clin. Med.*, **39**:169, 1952.
62. Stender, H. S., Strauch, D., and Winter, H.: in "Ionizing Radiation and Immune Processes," C. A. Leone (ed.), Gordon and Breach, New York, 1962.
63. Makinodan, T., Shekarchi, I. C., and Congdon, C. C.: *J. Immunol.*, **79**:281, 1957.
64. Simic, M. M., Sljivic, V. S., Petrovic, M. Z., and Cirkovic, D. M.: "Antibody Formation in Irradiated Rats," *Bull. Boris Kidric Inst. Nucl. Sci.*, **16**(Suppl. 1):1–151.
65. Taliaferro, W. H., and Jaroslow, B. N.: *J. Infect. Dis.*, **107**:341, 1960.
66. Koller, P. C., Davies, A. J. S., and Doak, M. A.: *Advan. Cancer Res.*, **6**:181, 1961.
67. Gengozian, N.: in "Ionizing Radiation and Immune Processes," C. A. Leone (ed.), Gordon and Breach, New York, 1962.

68. Micklem, H. S., and Loutit, J. F.: "Tissue Grafting and Radiation," Academic Press, Inc., New York, 1966.
69. Harris, T. N., Harris, S., and Farber, M. B.: *Proc. Soc. Exp. Biol. Med.*, **86**:549, 1954.
70. LaVia, M. F., Robson, M., and Wissler, R. W.: *Proc. Soc. Exp. Biol. Med.*, **96**:667, 1957.
71. Gallily, R., and Feldman, M.: *Immunology*, **12**:197, 1967.
72. Gabrielsen, A. E., and Good, R. A.: *Advan. Immunol.*, **6**:91, 1967.
73. Berenbaum, M. C.: *Brit. Med. Bull.*, **21**:140, 1965.
74. Hektoen, L., and Corper, H. J.: *J. Infect. Dis.*, **28**:279, 1921.
75. Santos, G. W., and Owens, A. H., Jr.: *Blood*, **20**:111, 1962.
76. Santos, G. W., and Owens, A. H., Jr.: *Bull. Johns Hopkins Hosp.*, **114**:384, 1964.
77. Potel, J.: in "Cyclophosphamide," G. H. Fairley and J. M Simister (eds), Williams & Wilkins, Baltimore, 1965.
78. Finger, H.: *Experientia*, **21**:163, 1965.
79. Cohen, S. G., and Mokychic, W. E.: *J. Infect. Dis.*, **94**:39, 1954.
80. Turk, J. L., and Stone, S. H.: in "Cell-bound Antibodies," B. Amos and H. Koprowski (eds.), Wistar Institute Press, Philadelphia, 1963.
81. Borel, Y., and Schwartz, R.: *J. Immunol.*, **92**:754, 1964.
82. Schwartz, R. S.: *Progr. Allergy*, **9**:246, 1965.
83. Dutton, R. W., Dutton, A. H., and Vaughan, J. H.: *Biochem. J.*, **75**:230, 1960.
84. Dutton, R. W., and Pearce, J. D.: *Immunology*, **5**:414, 1962.
85. O'Brien, T. F., and Coons, A. H.: *J. Exp. Med.*, **117**:1063, 1963.
86. LaVia, M. F.: *Proc. Soc. Exp. Biol. Med.*, **114**:133, 1963.
87. Hotham-Iglewski, B., and LaVia, M. F.: *Proc. Soc. Exp. Biol. Med.*, **131**:895, 1969.
88. Smiley, J. D., Heard, J. G., and Ziff, M.: *J. Exp. Med.*, **119**:881, 1964.
89. Ambrose, C. T., and Coons, A. H.: *J. Exp. Med.*, **117**:1075, 1963.
90. Otte, H., and Grosjean, O.: *Compt. Rend. Soc. Biol.*, **158**:909, 1964.
91. Bloom, B. R., Hamilton, L. D., and Chase, M. W.: *Nature (London)*, **201**:689, 1964.
92. Sakauchi, G., and Dewitt, C. W.: *Transplantation*, **5**:248, 1967.
93. Goldberg, I. H., and Reich, E.: *Federation Proc.*, **23**:958, 1964.
94. Fishman, M., van Rood, J. J., and Adler, F. L.: in "Molecular and Cellular Basis of Antibody Formation," J. Sterzl (ed.), Academic Press, Inc., New York, 1965.
95. Uhr, J. W.: *Science*, **142**:1476, 1963.
96. David, J. R.: *J. Exp. Med.*, **122**:1125, 1965.
97. Jerne, N. K., Nordin, A. A., and Henry, C.: in "Cell-bound Antibodies," B. Amos and H. Kaprowski (eds.), Wistar Institute Press, Philadelphia, 1963.
98. Wust, C. J., and Hanna, M. G., Jr.: *Proc. Soc. Exp. Biol. Med.*, **118**:1027, 1965.
99. Hanna, M. G., and Wust, C. J.: *Lab. Invest.*, **14**:272, 1965.

100. Weisberger, A. S., Daniel, T. M., and Hoffman, A.: *J. Exp. Med.*, **120**:183, 1964.
101. Alexandre, G. P. J., Murray, J. E., Dammin, G. J., and Nolan, B.: *Transplantation*, **1**:432, 1963.
102. Murray, J. E., Merrill, J. P., Harrison, J. H., Wilson, R. E., and Dammin, G. J.: *New Engl. J. Med.*, **268**:1315, 1963.
103. Baker, B. L.: in "Pituitary Adrenal Function," R. C. Christman (ed.), AAAS, Washington, D.C., 1951.
104. Dougherty, T. F.: *Physiol. Rev.*, **32**:379, 1952.
105. de Duve, C.: in "Injury Inflammation and Immunity," L. Thomas, J. W. Uhr, and L. Grant (eds.), Williams & Wilkins, Baltimore, 1964.
106. Gewurz, H., Wernick, P. R., Quie, P. G., and Good, R. A.: *Nature (London)*, **208**:755 1965.
107. Dougherty, T. F., and Schneebeli, G. L.: *Proc. Soc. Exp. Biol. Med.*, **75**:854, 1950.
108. Fagraeus, A., and Berglund, K.: *J. Immunol.*, **87**:49, 1961.
109. Billingham, R. E., Krohn, P. L., and Medawar, P. B.: *Brit. Med. J.*, **1**:1157, 1951.
110. Zukoski, C. F., Callaway, J. M., and Rhea, W. G., Jr.: *Transplantation*, **3**:380, 1965.
111. Marchioro, T. L., Axtell, H. K., LaVia, M. F., Waddel, W. R., and Starzl, T. E.: *Surgery*, **55**:412, 1964.
112. Friedman, R. M., Buckler, C. E., and Baron, S.: *J. Exp. Med.*, **114**:173, 1961.
113. Friedman, R. M., and Buckler, C. E.: *Federation Proc.*, **22**:501, 1963.
114. Malawista, S. E., and Bodel, P.: *J. Clin. Invest.*, **45**:1044, 1966.

11
Theories of Antibody Formation

One of the earliest attempts to explain the immune response in detail was that by Ehrlich (1) in 1900. Ehrlich postulated that antibodies were preformed side chains attached to cells. Some of these side chains, which he thought to be important in the transport of nutrients, might by chance have a structure complementary to some antigen. When an antigen reacted with such a side chain, it interfered with its function. As a response, the cell synthesized large quantities of the identical side chain, some of which was released into the bloodstream as circulating antibody. This concept is amazingly similar to recent concepts of antibody formation. It emphasized the chemical nature of the antigen-antibody interaction and suggested that specificity could be the result of a chance complementary fit.

The weakness in Ehrlich's proposal was the idea that each side chain must have a specific natural function to explain its presence. When the full range of antibody specificity was understood, this idea seemed impossible, and the whole proposal was discarded.

304

In 1930 Breinl and Haurowitz (2), followed by Alexander (3) and Mudd (4), advanced a theory which pictured the antigen as entering a globulin-producing cell and acting as a template. Thus the problem of the specific formation of antibody to thousands of different antigens could be explained. In 1940 Pauling (5) presented a more detailed model based on the variable folding of a polypeptide chain. Karush (6) further expanded this idea by suggesting variable pairing of the cysteine residues as the stabilizing mechanism.

The direct template theories emphasized the reversible nature of the antigen-antibody reaction and provided the stimulus to investigate the chemical structure of the antibody molecule. Championed largely by biochemists, these theories were also tested and disproven by the biochemists. The antibody molecule was found to be composed of a number of peptides and its specificity due to variable pairing of heterogeneous peptides.

In 1941, Burnet and Fenner (7) published their classic monograph on antibody production. They felt that immunology had veered from the mainstream of biology. Since antibody is a protein synthesized by a biologic organism, they believed it to be important to consider how other adaptive proteins are synthesized. Burnet and Fenner based their theory on concepts current at that time concerning adaptive enzymes in bacteria. They postulated that when antigens enter an antibody-forming cell, changes are produced in replicable enzymes responsible for the synthesis of an antibody molecule. This theory introduced the concept of a replicable antibody-synthesizing unit which is inheritable on a cellular level. Thus the theory explained the anamnestic response, the efficiency of antibody synthesis, and the logarithmic rise of antibody levels in the serum following antigenic stimulation. It focused the interest of immunology on the antibody-forming cell and the characteristics of the immune response. Later, these authors proposed that recognition of one's own antigens develops during embryonic life by means of a "self-marker." With progress in the knowledge of induced protein synthesis in bacteria, Burnet modified the theory to implicate the desoxyribonucleic acids (DNA) as the inheritable units responsible for specific antibody synthesis. A similar theory, postulating specific mutations of DNA induced by antigen was advanced simultaneously by Schweet and Owen (8). More recently, Goldstein (9) has described a theory involving modification of the ribonucleic acids (RNA) by antigen. However, it is difficult to explain the molecular mechanism by which an antigen produces a specific mutation in either DNA or RNA. This difficulty probably opened the way once again to the natural selection theories.

In 1955, Jerne (10) first used the term *natural selection* in connection with a systematic theory of antibody production. Jerne postulated that about 1 million different γ-globulin molecules are formed in embryonic life, perhaps by the thymus. Once formed, these molecules can be used by antibody-forming cells as models for the synthesis of identical molecules. Thus, in a sense, the γ-globulin molecule is considered a replicable unit. Those molecules with reactivities to self antigens are removed during fetal life before the appearance of antibody-forming cells. Antigen injected after birth combines selectively with certain γ-globulins possessing complementary configurations (antibodies) and increases the entry of these γ-globulins into antibody-forming cells. As a consequence, the antibody globulin is used preferentially as a model for the synthesis of new protein.

Jerne's theory introduced new concepts of immunologic specificity and tolerance. It explained the presence of preformed "antibodies" to synthetic haptens by eliminating Ehrlich's concept of a specific function for each preexisting antibody and substituting a concept of the randomized production of a wide variety of γ-globulins with overlapping reactivities. Jerne's theory was the first to provide a molecular explanation of immunologic tolerance, i.e., the distinction between self and not-self. Previous explanations had at some point all required homocentric expression such as "self-recognition." In place of self-recognition Jerne substituted recognition of not-self and attributed the lack of antibodies to self to the absence of γ-globulin molecules with which to react.

The main objection to Jerne's theory is experimental evidence that immunologic memory resides in the cells, not in the serum. This objection can be resolved by substituting cell potential for γ-globulin in the randomizing process. In 1957, cell selection theories were advanced almost simultaneously by Talmage (11) and by Burnet (12). Subsequently, these concepts were described in more detail by Burnet in *The Clonal Selection Theory of Acquired Immunity* (13), which introduced the concept of the *forbidden clone* to explain autoimmunity. Cells with the capacity for the formation of antibody against a normal body protein were "forbidden" and eliminated during embryonic life. The assumptions of cell selection were stated explicitly by Lederberg (14), and the implications of selective theories to immunologic specificity were discussed in detail by Talmage (15).

At the present time the single overall theory of antibody formation no longer seems useful. Because of advances in knowledge, particularly at the molecular level, the theories of antibody formation can more profitably be broken down into four major questions:

1. The genetic basis of immunoglobulin diversity
2. Cellular or subcellular selection

3. The role of the macrophage and bone marrow cell

4. The mechanism of tolerance

The first question is obviously the most basic, and its answer will probably determine the answer to the second question and may also affect the solution to the last two.

THE DIVERSITY OF IMMUNOGLOBULIN CHAINS, A GENETIC PUZZLE

The structural basis of antibody diversity has been demonstrated to be in the sequence of amino acids in both the light and heavy chains that make up all immunoglobulins (see Chap. 3). Most studies have involved human or mouse light chains (κ or λ) which can be obtained in nearly pure form from patients or mice with multiple myeloma. A comparison of any two human κ chains (or two mouse κ or two human λ chains) has revealed a striking pattern of diversity (Fig. 11-1). Beginning at the

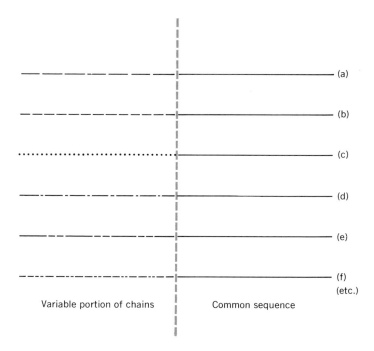

Variable portion of chains | Common sequence

(a)

(b)

(c)

(d)

(e)

(f)
(etc.)

Fig. 11-1 A diagrammatic representation of the variability in one class of light chains. The amino terminus is to the left. From Dreyer and Bennett (28) with permission.

amino terminal end, an average of 40 to 50 of the first 107 to 112 amino acid residues are different in the two chains (Tables 11-1 and 11-2; Fig. 11-2) (16). The two molecules are identical for the remaining carboxyl terminal half of the chain. There is a sharp and easily identifiable boundary between the common and variable portions of these light chains. The available evidence indicates that both normal light and heavy chains have the same pattern of diversity.

An analysis of the genetics of the two parts of the immunoglobulin chains leads to the paradoxical conclusions that the identical common portions derive from a single cistron (c-gene) and that the variable portions come from different cistrons (v-genes).

The evidence that the identical common portions derive from a single c-gene relates to the genetics of the Inv allotype, a variation which has been demonstrated to be due to a single amino acid interchange in the common portion of human κ chains. The mendelian pattern of inheritance of the Inv allotypes (17) and the improbability of identical mutations occurring in two different c-genes are both strong evidences that there is only a single cistron per chromosome set for the common portion of

TABLE 11-1

Comparison of Variable and Common Segments of Two Mouse and One Human (AG) κ Chains

Variable segment (111 residues)	M41/M70	M70/Ag	M41/Ag
Total mutations	49	47	37
One-step	28	32	31
Two-step	17	11	6
Deletions	4	4	0
Common segment			
Total mutations	0	43	43
One-step	—	29	29
Two-step	—	14	14

SOURCE: Data from Gray et al. (18) with permission.

TABLE 11-2

Comparison of Variable Segments of Three Human Chains (112 Residues)

Mutations	Bo/Ha	Bo/SH	Ha/SH
One-step	29	31	31
Two-step	9	14	17
Deletions	0	4	4
Total	38	49	52

SOURCE: Data from Putnam et al. (16) with permission.

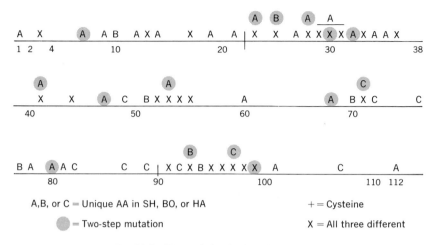

Variation in Three Human λ Chains

Fig. 11-2   The variation in three human λ chains. Numbers represent amino acid residues beginning with the amino terminus. A, B,
and C indicate positions with unique amino acids in one of the chains,
SH, Bo, or Ha, respectively. X indicates different amino acids in all
three chains. A circle represents a two-step mutation. The two
cysteines are indicated by vertical crosslines. The deletion in SH
at positions 29 to 31 is indicated by a horizonal line. From Putnam
et al. (16) with permission.

human κ chains. It should also be noted that the common portion of the
human κ chain differs from the mouse common portion at 43 residues
(18) (Table 11-1). This is strong evidence that a normal rate of mutation
occurred in the evolution of the species and that there is no unusual
structural demand which maintains two identical c-genes.

The evidence that the variable portions derive from multiple v-genes
is less compelling, and two recently advanced hypotheses assume a single
cistron for the entire light chain.

The Somatic Mutational Hypothesis of Brenner and Milstein

This hypothesis (19) postulates the existence of a special "cleavage"
enzyme to recognize and break one of the two DNA chains at the point
separating common from variable portions (Fig. 11-3). Two other enzymes are known to exist which will break down the DNA chain in one
direction (into the variable portion) and then repair it. A high frequency
of breakdown and repair will have the effect of producing a hot spot of
somatic mutation.

Against this hypothesis is the failure to find any mutational gradient
along the variable portion. The Brenner-Milstein hypothesis predicts that

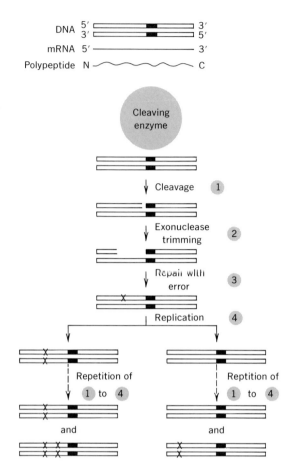

DNA 5′ ━━━━ ■ ━━━━ 3′
    3′ ━━━━ ■ ━━━━ 5′
mRNA 5′ ───────── 3′
Polypeptide N ～～～～ C

Cleaving
enzyme

↓ Cleavage (1)

↓ Exonuclease (2)
    trimming

↓ Repair with (3)
    error

| Replication (4)

↓ Repetition of   ↓ Repetition of
  (1) to (4)   (1) to (4)

and   and

Fig. 11-3   The somatic mutation model.   From Brenner and Milstein
(19) with permission.

the highest rate of mutation would occur near the point separating common from variable portion.   However, the mutations seem rather evenly
or randomly distributed along the variable portion (Figs. 11-2, 11-4,
and 11-5).

The Code Alteration Hypothesis

This hypothesis by Potter et al. (20) and, more recently, Campbell (21)
postulates special or "permissive" codons and a variety of special transfer
RNA molecules for the variable portions of light chains.   Different
immunoglobulin-producing cells would have different sets of transfer RNA
molecules and would thus translate the same messenger RNA in different
ways.   Compelling evidence against this hypothesis is found in the exis-

Variation in Two Mouse and One Human (Ag) κ Chains

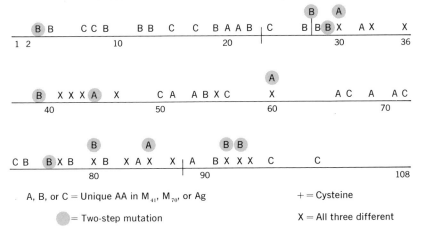

A, B, or C = Unique AA in M₄₁, M₇₀, or Ag   + = Cysteine

⬤ = Two-step mutation   X = All three different

Fig. 11-4 Variation in two mouse and one human (Ag) κ chains. A, B, and C indicate positions with unique amino acids in M₄₁, M₇₀, or Ag, respectively. An insertion of four amino acids in M₇₁ is indicated between positions 27 and 28. Data taken from Gray et al. (18) and Putnam et al. (16) with permission.

Comparison of κ(Ag) and λ(SH) Chains

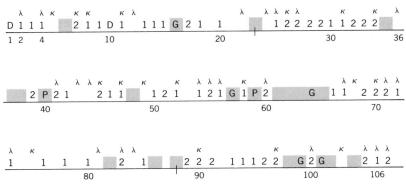

Fig. 11-5 Comparison of κ and λ chains. The numbers indicate one-step and two-step mutations between Ag and SH chains. Boxes enclose 23 positions constant in all λ and κ chains for which information is available. G and P inside the boxes indicate glycine and proline residues. D indicates a deletion in the λ chain. Insertions in the λ chain near position 30 (3 residues) and near position 95 (2 residues) are not indicated. κ and λ indicate that at these positions all known κ or λ chains are constant. Data taken from (16), (18), (22), (30), and (35–41) with permission.

tence of at least two different chain lengths among the variable portions of different human and mouse κ chains (16,17).

There are also strong arguments against the existence of permissive codons, since such codons would have a restrictive effect on the kinds of mutations occurring in all other regions of the DNA. A further argument against the code-alteration hypothesis is that the pattern of amino acid interchanges between different variable segments of the same species (Tables 11-1 and 11-2) is very similar to that between the common segments of mouse and man. There is a striking predominance of one-step mutations and a high correlation between the number of two-step muta- tions and the total number of mutations. This would be expected only if the two-step mutations were the result of two single-step mutations with the same codon. Also, the number of different permissive codons required to explain the amino acid variations in only three λ chains is 60 (Table 11-2) (16). This certainly exceeds the number of codons which could be relegated to a permissive status.

Multiple V-gene Hypothesis

In a recent summary of work on the amino acid sequence of mouse and human κ chains, Smithies (22) showed that an amino acid variant in one position is frequently associated with a different specific variant in other positions (Tables 11-3 and 11-4; Fig. 11-6). This lack of randomness in amino acid variation is difficult to explain by any single v-gene hypothesis.

TABLE 11-3
Subgroups of Eight Human and Two Mouse κ Chains

Chain	\multicolumn{7}{c}{Position}	Other variations
	1	3	4	10	13	15	17	
Ag	ASP	GLN	MET	SER	ALA	VAL	ASP	
Roy	ASP	GLN	MET	SER	ALA	VAL	ASP	
BJ	ASP	GLN	MET	SER	ALA	VAL	ASP	2
Ker	ASP	GLN	MET	SER	ALA	VAL	ASP	
HBJ10	ASP	GLN	MET	SER	ALA	VAL	ASP	
HS4	GLU	VAL	LEU	THR	LEU	PRO	GLU	9
HBJ5	GLU	VAL	LEU	THR	LEU	PRO	GLU	9
HBJ3	ASP	VAL	LEU	SER	VAL	PRO	GLU	9,12,14
M-41	ASP	GLN	MET	SER	ALA	LEU	GLU	
M-70	ASP	VAL	LEU	SER	VAL	LEU	GLN	9,12,14

SOURCE: Data from Gray et al. (18), Smithies (22), Hilschmann and Craig (35), Milstein (36), and Titani et al. (41), with permission.

TABLE 11-4
Subgroups of Ten Human λ Chains

	Position				Other variations
Protein	3	10	13	17	
Ha	VAL	VAL	THR	ARG	
HBJ7	VAL	ALA	THR	GLY	
HBJ11	VAL	ALA	THR	ARG	
BJ98	VAL	VAL	ALA	ALA	12,14,20,21
Bo	ALA	ALA	SER	SER	
HBJ2	ALA	ALA	SER	SER	
HBJ15	ALA	VAL	SER	THR	8 (Ala) 18 (Ile)
HBJ8	ALA	VAL	SER	SER	5,8 (Ala) 18 (Ile)
SH	GLU	VAL	ALA	THR	1,7,9,12,14,19,21

SOURCE: Data from Putnam et al. (16), Gray et al. (18), Smithies (22), and Hood et al. (37), with permission.

The association of certain sets of mutations is found in the myeloma light chains (both λ and κ) from different individuals and even species. For example, among κ chains with aspartic acid in the first position, there is a high frequency (nine out of twelve) of methionine in the fourth. But three out of four κ chains with glutamic in the first position have leucine at position 4, and none has methionine. The total number of such associations already demonstrated is quite large, and the probability is very small that they represent chance coincidence. The fact that the association of certain mutations occurs in the light chains from different individuals and even species indicates that different v-genes for the variable region were already established in the gene pool of the common ancestor of these individuals and species.

Among the multiple gene theories, two postulate a different cistron for each different variable fragment.

Splicing of Peptides

In 1965, Cioli and Baglioni (23) found, in the urine of some patients with myeloma, a peptide fragment corresponding to the variable portion of the myeloma light chain. This has suggested a model in which the common and variable portions derive from different messenger RNA molecules and the peptides are pieced by a specific enzyme (24). Attempts to test this hypothesis by pulse-labeling with radioactive amino acids have so far been inconclusive (25,26). As shown by Dintzis (27) with hemoglobin, the pulse-labeling of a growing peptide chain will result in a single gradient of specific activities along the completed chains with the highest specific

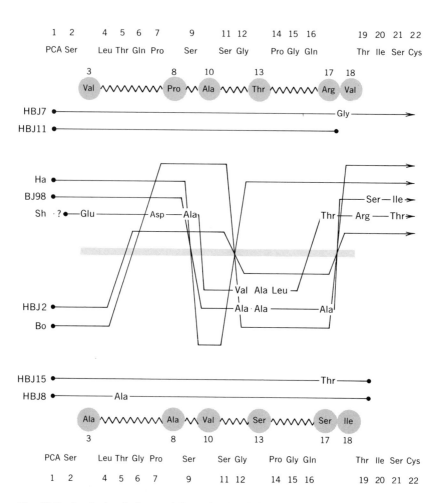

Fig. 11-6 A chart of the variations in λ chains illustrating Smithies' model of recombination. From Smithies (22) with permission.

activity at the COOH end. Experiments with light chains in myeloma cells have shown that the common portion (COOH end) has a higher specific activity than the variable portion but have not ruled out the possibility of a break in the gradient at the point of division between the two portions. Differences in specific activity can be explained by differences in pool size of the two postulated peptides.

An argument against this hypothesis derives from the fact that κ and λ common portions use different sets of variable pieces. If, during evolution, the κ gene separated from the λ gene after the process of peptide-piecing had been developed, a single piecing enzyme would be expected to connect κ common portions with λ variables and vice versa. On the other

314

hand, if the separation of κ and λ genes occurred first, the piecing of the two chains at the identical place is surprising.

Splicing of Cistrons—Hypothesis of Dreyer and Bennett

This hypothesis is similar to the previous one, except that splicing is performed at the DNA level instead of at the peptide (28) (Fig. 11-7). The common cistron is postulated to have some mechanism of inserting itself into the DNA adjoining any one of many variable cistrons. In this respect the common cistron is similar to a bacterial lysogenic phage or episome. The development of two distinct but parallel systems in the κ and λ chains

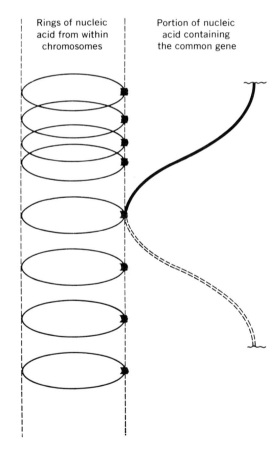

Rings of nucleic
acid from within
chromosomes

Portion of nucleic
acid containing
the common gene

Fig. 11-7 Dreyer and Bennett model of gene splicing. From Dreyer and Bennett (28) with permission.

has the same difficulties as peptide piecing. However, the fact that the κ and λ common genes are unlinked, i.e., on different chromosomes, may provide an explanation of why they use a different set of variable genes.

Recombination Hypotheses

As pointed out by Edelman and Gally (29) (Fig. 11-8) and then by Cohen and Milstein (30) and by Smithies (22) (Fig. 11-9), the number of v-genes need not be as great as the number of variable peptides. A large increase in number of different v-genes might be achieved by somatic recombination between a limited number of different v-genes in the germ line. Edelman and Gally suggested 20 to 50 tandem duplicated genes. Smithies suggested one "master" gene for the entire light chain and an inverted "scrambler" half-gene for the variable portion. Smithies preferred the smaller number of genes because the single inverted duplication would be more stable. On the other hand, the finding of five different amino acids at position 17 in λ chains and also at position 9 in κ chains suggests a larger number of v-genes. Smithies explained this variation as due to heterogeneity of the master and scrambler alleles in the human population (genetic polymorphism). But light chains from the inbred mouse strain (BALB/c) are at least as heterogeneous as human light chains (31), and three mouse κ chains from this strain have three different amino acids as position 4 (24). Thus it is easier to explain the marked variation at certain positions shown in Tables 11-3 and 11-4 by postulating multiple v-genes than by genetic polymorphism and an unusually high rate of recombination in some cells.

In a recent analysis of the first 20 amino acids in 63 human light chains, Hood and Talmage (31a) concluded that the evolution of this part of the light chain involved two separate steps: (1) the development of more than seven subclass genes through gene duplication and prolonged mutational drift and (2) extensive rapid duplication of some of

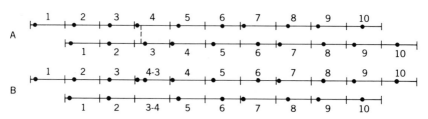

Fig. 11-8 Edelman and Gally's model of recombination. From Edelman and Gally (29) with permission.

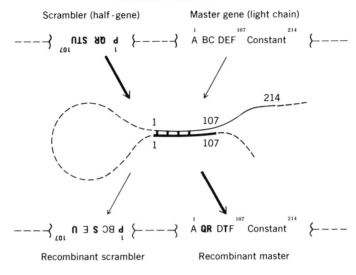

Fig. 11-9 Smithies' model of recombination. From Smithies (22) with permission.

the mature subclass genes followed by random mutation of the duplicated variants. The relationship of the variants in seven subclasses is depicted in Fig. 11-10.

The first step, i.e., the evolution of the subclass genes, was clearly a germ-line evolution, since these different subclasses were found in different individuals and even species. The second step might have been either a germ-line or a somatic process.

At the present time the weight of evidence appears to be shifting back toward a germ-line process. The distinction between the two types of mutations has become less sharp as more data has accumulated. Subclasses of the subclasses are now apparent. Although the existence of large numbers of v-genes (perhaps 1000 or more) might seem to create an unstable genetic situation, the existence of a large amount of reduplication of DNA in higher animals has been established by hybridization techniques.

Although somatic recombination hypotheses explain well the two-step evolution of light chain variants, the specific nature of the changes are against recombination. The random mutations within each subclass are nearly all explicable as the substitution of a single nucleotide. In many cases, including the few instances where it is necessary to postulate that two nucleotides are substituted, the nucleotides inserted are not those from one of the other subclass genes.

Thus, many uncertainties remain in attempts to explain the variability

317

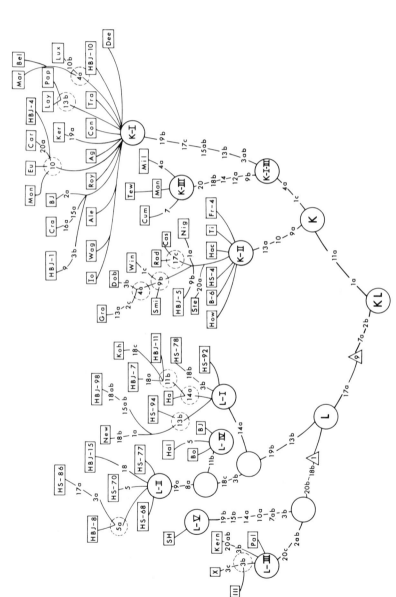

Fig. 11-10 A "phylogenetic" tree constructed from the amino terminal 20 residues of 41 kappa and 22 lambda proteins by the method of Fitch and Margoliash, which reduces the number of mutations to a minimum. The 63 proteins are indicated by closed rectangles. Deletions are indicated by triangles and mutations by numbers. The letters a, b, and c indicate which nucleotide is changed according to the genetic code. Closed circles indicate major classes and subclasses. Dotted circles indicate subdivisions of the subclasses or highly improbable identical mutations occurring in two different individuals. From Hood and Talmage (31a) with permission.

of immunoglobulin chains. There would appear to be more v-genes than c-genes in both κ and λ classes, but no inkling of how in any one cell the c-gene becomes joined to one of the v-genes. Superimposed on this, there is considerable uncertainty regarding the number of v-genes in the germ line, and whether additional diversity is inserted by some somatic process.

CELLULAR OR SUBCELLULAR SELECTION

The evidence from amino acid sequence analysis reviewed above gives strong support to the concept that immunoglobulin diversity has a genetic basis. Present concepts of DNA transcription and RNA translation would require that the genetic diversity is intrinsic, i.e., not the result of the specific action of antigen. This conclusion is based on the fact that information in DNA and RNA is in the form of a one-dimensional code which must be translated by a complex machine in order to be relevant to a three-dimensional structure such as an antigen. For this reason it is infinitely more simple to postulate a preexisting genetic diversity than a preexisting translating machinery for every possible kind of antigen.

If genetic diversity antedates the entry of antigen into the organism, then the role of antigen must be the selection of diverse gene products. If this is so, then the next question here is whether this selection occurs at the cellular or subcellular level. Stated another way, this is a question of the potential of individual cells to respond to antigen. If the potential of a cell is large, then selection must occur at a subcellular level. If the potential of a cell is restricted before exposure to antigen, then the antigen must select between cells of diverse predetermined potential.

Advantages of Cell Selection

There are a number of obvious advantages to the concept that the antigen selects among prediversified cells. The cell is a well-defined entity with the capacity for independent replication, and cell differentiation is a well-established, albeit poorly understood, phenomenon. At the subcellular level, mitochondria, chloroplasts, and centrioles are the only organelles with a proven capacity for independent replication (32–34).

All but one of the genetic models discussed in the previous section require that genetic diversity be accomplished through cellular diversity. The single possible exception is the peptide-splicing model. If there is a different gene for each variable fragment and if mRNAs for all variable fragments are made in every plasma cell, then it is conceivable that the antigen determines which variable fragment is spliced to the common fragment. This would be selection at a subcellular level. However, there are two difficulties with this position. It does not provide an explanation of immunologic memory, and it does not explain the chief finding in favor of peptide splicing, namely the presence of a homogeneous variable fragment in the urine of some patients with multiple myeloma.

Subcellular Selection and the Multipotential or Polyresponsive Cell

Subcellular selection requires the postulation of a polyresponsive cell, that is, a cell with the capacity to respond to any antigen by making the corresponding antibody. Despite the present difficulties of this postulate, it is a popular concept, mainly because of the traditional idea that cell differentiation advances by selective restriction of cell potentials rather than by the acquisition of new potentials. However, the traditional concept of gradual restriction of cell potential refers to the ultimate potential of the cell's descendants rather than to the immediate ability of the individual cell to respond to environmental stimuli. For example, different descendants of the fertilized ovum will ultimately make all the proteins made in the whole body, but the immediate responsiveness of this cell is severely restricted. It cannot afford to waste its energy making antibody, hemoglobin, insulin, or albumin. The ability to make these proteins will arise one by one in different descendants.

The relation of the polyresponsive cell to the question of cell selection is illustrated in Fig. 11-11. There is general agreement on the existence of a precursor cell which has not yet attained the capacity to respond to any antigen. There is good evidence that this cell is present in the bone marrow and develops immunocompetence in the thymus or under the influence of thymic hormone (see Chap. 4).

At the other end of the process of differentiation there is considerable evidence that the ability of individual cells to make different kinds of antibody is severely restricted (42–44). Recent experiments indicate that one cell may be able to make only one kind of antibody at a time, even among the many kinds of antibody reacting with the same antigen. It now seems probable that earlier conclusions that one cell could make two antibodies were erroneous as the result of technical artifacts.

The important question illustrated in Fig. 11-11 is whether the precursor cell advances directly from zero competence to the competence to make a single antibody, or whether it must first achieve the competence to make all possible antibodies and then in the presence of antigen turn around and restrict this potential to that of a single antibody.

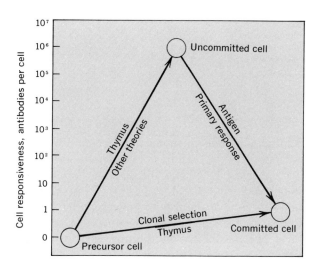

Fig. 11-11 A diagrammatic representation of the relation of cell selection to the multipotential cell. See text.

Attempts have been made to answer this question by determining whether the same stem cell could respond to more than one antigen. Following exposure to antigen, responding cells begin to divide and as a result become more easily killed by radioactively labeled thymidine or its analogs. It has been possible in two different experiments (45,46) to kill the cells responding to one antigen without affecting those capable of responding to another. This fact, plus the small number of cells (1 out of 100,000 spleen cells) (47–49) responding to a complex red cell antigen, suggests that different cells respond to different antigens. On the other hand, evidence that a large fraction of the cell population can make the same antibody may be considered as favoring polyresponsiveness (50).

Arguments for and against the Multipotential Cell

It is always difficult to prove a negative, and the above described failures to find a polyresponsive cell can be explained as due to the use of antigens common to the environment. It has been suggested that in the true primary response, the antigen reacts with a polyresponsive cell (51). Thus, qualitative differences between the primary and secondary response have been interpreted as evidence for a polyresponsive cell (51,52). For example, in the intact animal the secondary response has been found to be much more resistant to irradiation than the primary response (53).

However, there are other explanations for these and other qualitative differences between the two responses, e.g., feedback effects of circulating antibody. When an attempt has been made to equalize nonspecific en-

321

vironmental effects by transferring the cells to an irradiated recipient, the supposed qualitative differences disappeared (54,55) (Fig. 11-12).

Antigenic Competition

Another immune phenomenon frequently considered as evidence for a polyresponsive cell is antigenic competition. For a number of days following the injection of one antigen, the host has a depressed response to a second antigen (56) (Fig. 11-13). This can be explained as the preemption of a limited number of polyresponsive cells. It could also be due to feedback effects of humoral factors. An attempt to distinguish between these two possibilities by diluting out the two responses has given clear evidence for the latter hypothesis (57).

Splenic Nodule Transfer

A few claims have been made that polyresponsiveness of antibody-forming cells has been demonstrated by inducing antibody formation to several antigens in x-radiated animals injected with the cells of a single or a few

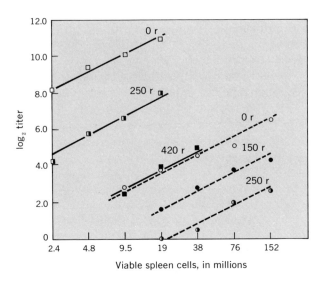

Fig. 11-12 Effect of x-ray dose on 6 day primary and secondary responses of spleen cells (9-44 samples per point). - - - -, primary antibody response; _____, secondary antibody response. From Makinodan et al. (54) with permission.

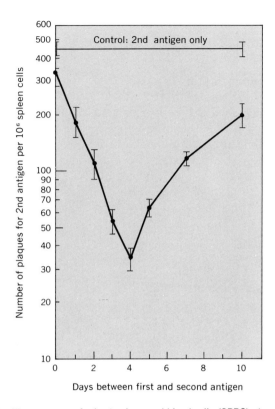

Fig. 11-13 The response of mice to sheep red blood cells (SRBC) at various time intervals after injection of horse red blood cells (HRBC). Vertical bars indicate standard error.

splenic nodules (58,59). This conclusion is based on the non sequitur that because the nodules appear to arise from the action of a single stem cell [probably erythroid (60)], they contain only the progeny of that cell. In fact, it is well known that lymphocytes circulate rapidly throughout the body. A suggestion that the lymphocytes in the splenic nodules get there by infiltration is found in the published micrographs of such nodules (59). The nodules appear to contain approximately the same concentration of lymphocytes as the internodular spaces.

More recent experiments (60) have shown that the lymphoid progeny of a relatively few bone marrow cells contain cells capable of responding to several different antigens. This indicates that the ultimate potential of the bone marrow stem cell is large, like that of the fertilized ovum, but does not provide evidence that a single immunocompetent cell can respond to more than one antigen.

19S to 7S Conversion

During a primary response, it is not uncommon that the earliest antibody is 19S, or IgM. Later there appears 7S, or IgG, antibody. It has been suggested that cells making 19S antibody convert to making 7S antibody (61). The major evidence for this conversion is based on the fact that 19S antibody is more sensitive to reducing agents such as mercaptoethanol. Nossal and Mäkelä (61) found that during the period of overlap between 19S and 7S production, some cells made antibody of intermediate sensitivity to mercaptoethanol. This evidence is not entirely firm, because 7S antibody may sometimes be partially sensitive to reducing agents.

The unequivocal demonstration that single cells convert from 19S to 7S antibody of the same specificity would be strong evidence for a polyresponsive cell. This is true because the 7S and 19S antibodies must utilize different heavy chains. If cells have a predetermined potential to make a limited number of chains, it is very improbable that the same cell would happen to have the potential to make two different heavy chains specific for the same antigen.

In summary, the frequently postulated multipotential or polyresponsive cell has been elusive. Evidence once thought to be strongly favoring its existence has been shown to be based on incorrect assumptions or technical artifacts. On the other hand, it is impossible to categorically rule out the existence of such a cell. Eventually, a decision may be made on the basis of genetic evidence, since the mechanism of gene diversity may necessarily restrict the responsiveness of individual cells.

ROLE OF MACROPHAGE AND BONE MARROW CELLS

In the simplest form of the *cell selection theory* an individual cell of predetermined restricted potential reacts directly with an antigen and is stimulated to make antibody. In general, immunologists who have favored cell selection have doubted that other cells played a significant role in the reaction besides providing a favorable environment for nutrients, gas, pH, etc. This is because a cell with a predetermined restricted potential to make only one kind of antibody would not seem to need the assistance of other cells.

Immunologists who have favored subcellular selection and the multipotential cell also tended to postulate important interactions between cells. One of the oldest and most persisting ideas is that a macrophage first digests an antigen and then transfers to the lymphocyte a more antigenic form. This kind of interaction is much easier to imagine if neither cell has a restricted potential.

However, lymphocytes are extremely mobile cells, and it would not be correct to conclude that the concept of cellular interaction is incompatible with that of cell selection. There is some suggestion of this possibility in the way lymphocytes recirculate rapidly through the follicles of lymph nodes and spleen. Even the most rapid mixing of cells, however, would not produce a significant chance of interaction between two cells of restricted potential. Therefore, in the cell selection theories, one can postulate only certain kinds of cell-to-cell interactions. If one cell has a restricted potential, only a small number of such cells can be present in the animal, and the other cell in the interaction must play a nonspecific role in the sense that a large number of cells must be able to fill this role.

If the antibody-forming cells have a restricted potential, the most likely function in which they would be restricted is the synthesis of specific messenger RNA. As discussed in the first section of this chapter, there are now good reasons for postulating this restriction at the cellular level. Other cells might play a cooperative role in one of two ways: (1) in synthesizing the inducer of messenger RNA synthesis, and (2) in translating the message. The first role is the postulated action of the macrophage referred to above. The second action would seem unnecessary because all cells contain some ribosomes. However, if the limiting factor in antibody production is the number of cells capable of making specific messenger, a large increase in efficiency could be accomplished by restricting the RNA synthesis of the specific cell to messenger synthesis and arranging for other cells to make the ribosomes and translate the message into protein. This would require the transfer of messenger RNA from the specific cell to a nonspecific cell as postulated by Fishman (62) and by Cohen and Parks (63).

No direct evidence exists that digestion by a macrophage is an essential part of antigenic stimulation. Indirect evidence consists in the demonstration (1) that antigen is localized in macrophages; (2) that cytoplasmic bridges are formed between macrophages and other cells (64); (3) that a highly antigenic form of antigen can be found in liver cells (65); (4) that an antigen-RNA complex extracted from macrophages can induce antibody formation by lymphocytes in vitro (62); and (5) that spleen cells can be divided into two populations, both of which are required for antibody formation in vitro (66).

None of these observations is compelling evidence that the macrophage plays a physiological role in antibody formation. The fact that an RNA extract is capable of inducing antibody formation in lymphocytes or that the antibody so produced is of the macrophage allotype is irrelevant. Neither observation is convincing proof that this process takes place to a significant degree in vivo (see Chap. 5 for further discussion).

On the other hand, considerable evidence exists that digestion of antigen by the macrophage has no role in antibody formation.

1. The larger the antigen the more antigenic it usually is. This would not suggest that antigens need to be broken down to be antigenic.

2. The antigenic determinants to which an antibody response is made are surface groups even though enzymatic digestion or denaturation is capable of uncovering new groups (67).

3. A major part of the antibody response is made to complex surface determinants which are lost when the antigen is broken down even slightly (68).

4. It has been possible to induce antibody to synthetic peptides made of D-amino acids (69), for which the animal possesses no known degradative enzymes. It is true that L-amino acids are more antigenic, but this is not surprising in view of the fact that both the species' and individual's experience is largely with the L-forms.

5. A small amount of antibody which, given passively, is barely sufficient to coat the surface groups of a particulate antigen is capable of completely suppressing the antibody response (70).

6. Using a radioactively labeled antigen of high specific activity, Mitchell and Abbot (71) have been able to show that some of the antigen is localized on the surface of specialized cells in the lymph follicles. This antigen is not phagocytosed and persists much longer than the phagocytosed antigen of the macrophage, which is rather rapidly digested (72).

7. Extracellular antigen is probably the important antigen for inducing an antibody response because passive antibody can produce a suppressive effect on the response even if given several days after the antigen (73).

All of these observations indicate that intracellular digestion of antigen is not an essential feature of the antibody response. However, they do not argue against the possibility that undigested antigen is fixed to the surface of certain specialized cells, such as the dendritic processes of reticular cells in lymphoid follicles, and that such fixation greatly augments the interaction of antigen with lymphocytes.

The possibility of transfer of messenger RNA from a lymphocyte to another cell seems farfetched. A strong suggestion that this may nevertheless be so is derived from the recent observation of Mitchell and Miller (74) that in the enhanced antibody response produced by injection of thymus and bone marrow cells into an irradiated recipient [first described by Claman et al. (75)], it is the bone marrow cell which actually makes the antibody. Since bone marrow enhances the response of spleen cells from immune animals (76) as well as thymus cells, its role would appear to be nonspecific and it must, according to this reasoning, have received its messenger from another cell. For a more recent review of this question see 72a.

MECHANISM OF ACQUIRED IMMUNOLOGIC TOLERANCE

One of the most important immunologic problems from both the practical and theoretical points of view is the mechanism of acquired immunologic tolerance. Two Nobel prizes have been given for postulating (77) and then demonstrating (78) its existence, but almost nothing is known about the mechanism of its production. A great deal has been written about possible cellular models, but most of it is not very enlightening.

The difficulty with determining the mechanism of immunologic tolerance is that this determination must surely depend on a solution to the unanswered questions discussed above, as well as a few others. For example, it has not been established whether maturation to the antibody-forming cell is reversible, although the term *suicidal maturation* has been used rather freely.

The following facts would appear to be reasonably well established:

1. Tolerance is at least as specific as positive immunologic memory.

2. Tolerance may be produced in adults, albeit with more difficulty or with fewer antigens than early in life (79, 80).

3. Persistence of tolerance requires the persistence of antigen (81).

4. Thymectomy prolongs the time required for tolerance to disappear (82).

5. Tolerance may be partial in a qualitative (83) as well as a quantitative sense.

6. Factors favoring tolerance are those which do not favor immunity: soluble antigens, low molecular weight, intravenous injections, high and low concentrations of antigen, persistence of antigen, antigens not easily broken down.

7. Development of tolerance requires exposure to antigen for several days (79,84) to several weeks (85).

From these facts the most important conclusion would seem to be that the antigen produces tolerance by prolonged action on extrathymic cells. The role of the thymus appears to be that of instituting and restoring responsiveness to the extrathymic population of cells.

If one prefers to think in terms of a multipotential cell, then the specificity and duration of tolerance requires that the action of antigen on the multipotential cell be slow to develop, specific in effect, and persist through several divisions in such a way that the cell and its progeny will be able to respond to every antigen except the tolerogenic antigen. The action of some thymic hormone must be postulated to speed up the restoration of responsiveness.

In the case of specifically responsive cells of restricted potential, this process need not be so specific at the subcellular level. Any process which eventually ends in cell death will produce the effect of specific tolerance if applied only to responsive cells. The phenomena of partial tolerance and the slow development and slow disappearance of tolerance are somewhat more easy to explain with this model. The fact that loss of responsiveness takes at least 4 days (86) makes it unlikely that tolerance is achieved by allergic death of responsive cells. Rather, an active process such as cell maturation is suggested (87).

Aside from these vague generalizations, it is hard to see what can be gained from more detailed models of cell differentiation and compartmentalization. It is apparent that any model which postulates two partially antagonistic actions of antigen can explain all of the known facts. For example, let us assume that the two actions of antigen on the specific cell are the induction of messenger RNA and ribosome synthesis (RNA and DNA synthesis would work equally well). The induction of ribosome synthesis is postulated to require special conditions, e.g., complement fixation (88), macrophage modified antigen, membrane fixed antigen (89), or some other. In the absence of ribosomes the cell irreversibly matures without division and dies because it cannot make essential enzymes. This leads to tolerance. With ribosomes the cell replicates and more memory cells develop.

It is obvious that with a little time and inclination, one can synthesize dozens of such models, all of which are equally able to explain the various features of immunologic tolerance, including the high and low zones of antigen concentration (85). Acquired tolerance remains one of the most important and puzzling phenomena in immunology today.

REFERENCES

1. Ehrlich, P.: Proc. Roy. Soc. (Biol.), **66**:424, 1900.
2. Breinl, F., and Haurowitz, F.:Z. Physiol. Chem., **192**:45, 1930.
3. Alexander, J.: Protoplasma, **14**:296, 1932.
4. Mudd, S.: J. Immunol., **23**:423, 1932.

5. Pauling, L.: *J. Amer. Chem. Soc.*, **62**:2643, 1940.
6. Karush, F.: *Trans. N.Y. Acad. Sci.*, **20**:581, 1958.
7. Burnet, F. M., and Fenner, F.: "The Production of Antibodies," Macmillan, Melbourne, 1941.
8. Schweet, R. S., and Owen, R. D.: *J. Cell. Comp. Physiol.*, **50**(suppl. 1): 199, 1957.
9. Goldstein, D. J.: *Ann. Allergy*, **18**:1081, 1960.
10. Jerne, N. K.: *Proc. Nat. Acad. Sci. U.S.*, **41**:849, 1955.
11. Talmage, D. W.: *Annu. Rev. Med.*, **8**:239, 1957.
12. Burnet, F. M.: *Australian J. Sci.*, **20**:67, 1957.
13. Burnet, F. M.: "The Clonal Selection Theory of Acquired Immunity," Vanderbilt University Press, Nashville, Tenn., 1959.
14. Lederberg, J.: *Science*, **129**:1649, 1959.
15. Talmage, D. W.: *Science*, **129**:1643, 1959.
16. Putnam, F. W., Shinoda, T., Titani, K., and Wikler, M.: *Science*, **157**: 1050, 1967.
17. Steinberg, A. G.: *Progr. Med. Genet.*, **2**:1, 1962.
18. Gray, W. R., Dreyer, W. J., and Hood, L.: *Science*, **155**:465, 1967.
19. Brenner, S., and Milstein, C.: *Nature (London)*, **211**:242, 1966.
20. Potter, M., Appella, E., and Geisser, S.: *J. Mol. Biol.*, **14**:361, 1965.
21. Campbell, J.: *J. Theor. Biol.*, **16**:321, 1967.
22. Smithies, O.: *Science*, **157**:267, 1967.
23. Cioli, D., and Baglioni, C.: *J. Mol. Biol.*, **15**:385, 1966.
24. Hood, L. E., Gray, W. R., and Dreyer, W. J.: *Proc. Nat. Acad. Sci. U.S.*, **55**:826, 1966.
25. Lennox, E. S., Knopf, P. M., Munro, A. J., and Parkhouse, R.M.E.: *Cold Spring Harbor Symp. Quant. Biol.*, **32**:249, 1967.
26. Fleischman, J. B.: *Biochemistry*, **6**:1311, 1967.
27. Dintzis, H. M.: *Proc. Nat. Acad. Sci. U.S.*, **47**:247, 1961.
28. Dreyer, W. J., and Bennett, J. C.: *Proc. Nat. Acad. Sci. U.S.*, **54**:864, 1965.
29. Edelman, G. M., and Gally, J. A.: *Proc. Nat. Acad. Sci. U.S.*, **57**:353, 1967.
30. Cohen, S., and Milstein, C.: *Nature (London)*, **214**:449, 1967.
31. Potter, M., Dreyer, W. J., Kuff, E. L., and McIntire, K. R.: *J. Mol. Biol.*, **8**:814, 1964.
31a. Hood, L. E., and Talmage, D. W.: *Science*, In press.
32. Luck, D. J. L.: *J. Cell. Biol.*, **16**:483, 1963.
33. Kirk, J. T. O., and Tilney-Bassett, R. A. E.: in "The Plastids," W. H. Freeman and Company, San Francisco, 1967.
34. Sorokin, S. P.: *J. Cell Sci.*, **3**:207, 1968.
35. Hilschmann, N., and Craig, L. C.: *Proc. Nat. Acad. Sci. U.S.*, **53**:1403, 1965.
36. Milstein, C.: *Nature (London)*, **209**:370, 1966.
37. Hood, L., Gray, W. R., and Dreyer, W. J.: *J. Mol. Biol.*, **22**:179, 1966.
38. Milstein, C.: *Proc. Roy. Soc. (Biol.)*, **166**:138, 1966.

330
Biology of the
Immune Response

39. Baglioni, C.: *Biochem. Biopyhs. Res. Commun.*, **26**:82, 1967.
40. Wikler, M., Titani, K., Shinoda, T., and Putnam, F. W.: *J. Biol. Chem.*, 242:1668, 1967.
41. Titani, K., Whitley, E., Jr., and Putnam, F. W.: *Science*, **152**:1513, 1966.
42. Green, I., Vassalli, P., Nussenzweig, V., and Benacerraf, B.: *J. Exp. Med.*, **125**:511, 1967.
43. Green, I., Vassalli, P., and Benacerraf, B.: *J. Exp. Med.*, **125**:527, 1967.
44. Mäkelä, O.: *Cold Spring Harbor Symp. Quant. Biol.*, **32**:423, 1967.
45. O'Brien, T. F., and Coons, A. H.: *J. Exp. Med.*, **117**:1063, 1963.
46. Dutton, R. W., and Mishell, R. I.: *J. Exp. Med.*, **126**:443, 1967.
47. Playfair, J. H. L., Papermaster, B. W., and Cole, L. J.: *Science*, **149**:998, 1965.
48. Kennedy, J. C., Till, J. E., Siminovitch, L., and McCulloch, E. A.: *J. Immunol.*, **96**:973, 1966.
49. Claman, H. N., Chaperon, E. A., and Triplett, R. F.: *Proc. Soc. Exp. Biol. Med.*, **122**:1167, 1966.
50. Bussard, A. E., and Lurie, M.: *J. Exp. Med.*, **125**:873, 1967.
51. Kim, Y. B., Bradley, S. G., and Watson, D. W.: *J. Immunol.*, **97**:189, 1966.
52. Perkins, E. H., and Makinodan, T.: *J. Immunol.*, **92**:192, 1964.
53. Dixon, F. J., Talmage, D. W., and Maurer, P. H.: *J. Immunol.*, **68**:693, 1952.
54. Makinodan, T., Kastenbaum, M. A., and Peterson, W. J.: *J. Immunol.*, **88**:31, 1962.
55. Cohen, E. P., Crosby, L. K., and Talmage, D. W.: *J. Immunol.*, **92**:223, 1964.
56. Adler, F. L.: *Progr. Allergy*, **8**:41, 1964.
57. Radovich, J., and Talmage, D. W.: *Science*, **158**:512, 1967.
58. Trentin, J. J., and Fahlberg, W. J.: in "Conceptual Advances in Immunology and Oncology," Harper & Row, New York, 1963.
59. Mekori, T., Chieco-Bianci, L., and Feldman, M.: *Nature (London)*, **206**:367, 1965.
60. Trentin, J., Wolf, N., Cheng, V., Fahlberg, W., Weiss, D., and Bonhag, R.: *J. Immunol.*, **98**:1326, 1967.
61. Nossal, G. J. V., and Mäkelä, O.: *J. Immunol.*, **88**:604, 1962.
62. Fishman, M.: *J. Exp. Med.*, **114**:837, 1961.
63. Cohen, E. P., and Parks, J. J.: *Science*, **144**:1012, 1964.
64. Schoenberg, M. D., Mumaw, V. R., Moore, R. D., and Weisberger, A. S.: *Science*, **143**:964, 1964.
65. Garvey, J. S., and Campbell, D. H.: *J. Exp. Med.*, **105**:361, 1957.
66. Mosier, D. E.: *Science*, **158**:1573, 1967.
67. MacPherson, C. F. C., and Heidelberger, M.: *Proc. Soc. Exp. Biol. Med.*, **43**:646, 1940.
68. Henney, C. S., and Ishizaka, K.: *Proc. Soc. Exp. Biol. Med.*, **125**:335, 1967.
69. Stupp, Y., and Sela, M.: *Biochim. Biophys. Acta*, **140**:349, 1967.

70. Talmage, D. W., Freter, G. G., and Thomson, A.: *J. Infect. Dis.*, **99**:246, 1956.
71. Mitchell, J., and Abbot, A.: *Nature (London)*, **208**:500, 1965.
72. McDevitt, H. O., Askonas, B. A., Humphrey, J. H., Schechter, I., and Sela, M.: *Immunology*, **11**:337, 1966.
72a. Talmage, D. W., Radovich, J., and Hemingsen, H.: *J. Allerg.*, **43**:323, 1969.
73. Dixon, F. J., Jacot-Guillarmod, H., and McConahey, P. J.: *J. Exp. Med.*, **125**:1119, 1967.
74. Mitchell, G. F., and Miller, J. F. A. P.: *Proc. Nat. Acad. Sci. U.S.*, **59**: 296, 1968.
75. Claman, H. N., Chaperon, E. A., and Triplett, R. F.: *J. Immunol.*, **97**: 828, 1966.
76. Radovich, J., Hemingsen, H., and Talmage, D. W.: *J. Immunol.*, **100**: 756, 1968.
77. Burnet, F. M., and Fenner, F.: "The Production of Antibodies," 2d ed. Macmillan, Melbourne, 1949.
78. Billingham, R. E., Brent, L., and Medawar, P. B.: *Phil. Trans. Roy. Soc. London, Ser. B*, **239**:357, 1956.
79. Dresser, D. W.: *Immunology*, **5**:161, 378, 1962.
80. Rubin, B. A.: *Nature (London)*, **184**:205, 1959.
81. Smith, R. T.: *Advan. Immunol.*, **1**:67, 1961.
82. Claman, H. N., and Talmage, D. W.: *Science*, **141**:1193, 1963.
83. Crowle, A. J., and Hu, C. C.: *Clin. Exp. Immunol.*, **1**:323, 1966.
84. Claman, H. N.: *J. Immunol.*, **91**:833, 1963.
85. Mitchison, N. A.: *Proc. Roy. Soc. (Biol.)*, **161**:275, 1964.
86. Golub, E. S., and Weigle, W. O.: *J. Immunol.*, **99**:624, 1967.
87. Talmage, D. W., and Pearlman, D. S.: *J. Theor. Biol.*, **5**:321, 1963.
88. Pearlman, D. S., Sauers, J. B., and Talmage, D. W.: *J. Immunol.*, **91**:748, 1963.
89. Nossal, G. J. V.: *Ann. N.Y. Acad. Sci.*, **129**:822, 1966.

12
Antigen-Antibody Reactions

This chapter is a survey of some methods currently available to detect and measure humoral antibody.[†] Before reviewing these procedures in detail, it is helpful to first make certain generalizations about immunoglobulins as a class of serum proteins. In spite of the fact that the body of knowledge concerning humoral antibody has become complex over the past 2 decades, certain simplicities have also emerged. As a result, it is currently possible to make four generalizations about antibody:

1. Under normal circumstances, antibodies are produced only in response to antigenic stimulation. This property functionally separates antibodies from other binding proteins in the serum, such as haptoglobin and transferrin. It is worth noting that antigenic stimulation can come from subtle exposure, such as from bacteria in the intestinal tract stimulating the production of isoagglutinins (1,2) and from oral ingestion of milk and other food proteins (3).

[†] ACKNOWLEDGMENTS: It is a pleasure to acknowledge the advice and helpful criticism of Drs. W. B. Dandliker and M. J. Polley. Portions of the investigations reported in this chapter were supported by grants AI-07968, AI-06894, and AI-2E-214 of the National Institutes of Health.

2. All antibodies are globulins that are made up of heavy and light polypeptide chains. At present there are five classes of human immunoglobulins, called IgG, IgA, IgM, IgD, and IgE (see Chap. 3). The IgG immunoglobulins have been further divided into four subgroups, and IgA and IgM, into two subgroups. Despite major differences between the various peptide heavy chains in all these groups, all known antibody molecules have either kappa- or lambda-type light chains.

3. Antibodies are heterogeneous, even when produced following exposure to the purest of antigens (4). They are heterogeneous not only as regards to structure, as alluded to above, but also with respect to the strength of the bond they can form with their corresponding antigen sites and with respect to their function in vivo and in vitro. This is true for pure antigens but even more so for complex antigens because of the increased number of antigenic sites.

4. All antibodies have the capacity to bind with their respective antigens. This binding refers to the Fab portion of the γ-globulin molecule, which contains the antigen-combining site, and not to the Fc portion, which recently has been shown to bind nonspecifically to "protein A" derived from the cell wall of *Staphylococcus aureus* (5). For reasons to be made clear below, statements such as, "all antibodies precipitate with antigen, fix complement in the presence of antigen, or have the capacity to agglutinate antigen-coated erythrocytes" are absent from these broad generalizations.

Many useful but basically different techniques are currently being employed to detect and measure the interaction between antigen and antibody. The observed manifestations utilized in the different tests to detect antibodies depend not only on the quantity of antibody but also on factors such as the quality of antibody and the presence or absence of cofactors such as the complement system. In vivo tests are further influenced by factors contributed by the host. It is not surprising, therefore, that results obtained from different methods are difficult to compare and are frequently interpreted in various ways. In order to evaluate these complicated and, at times, contradictory results, it is helpful to consider all antigen-antibody tests in three general categories: primary, secondary, and tertiary.

The primary interaction between antigen and antibody is the first step in a series of biochemical processes which may or may not finally result in an overt secondary or tertiary reaction as defined below. This binding of antigen to antibody is represented by the following equation:

$$Ag + Ab \underset{kd}{\overset{ka}{\rightleftharpoons}} Ag \cdot Ab$$

In this formulation, Ag represents one of usually multiple antigenic sites on a given antigen molecule, Ab represents one of two or more antigen binding sites on a given antibody molecule, and Ag·Ab represents the combined state after these two molecules interact with one another. Like every other chemical reaction, there is an association and dissociation constant, and the summated effects of the two yield an equilibrium constant (6,7). It is important to note that the total concentration of antibody in a sample is the sum of the free- and bound-antibody sites and that the concentration of free-antibody sites under any given circumstance is governed by the law of mass action according to the following equation:

$$\frac{(Ag)(Ab)}{(Ag \cdot Ab)} = K$$

In these terms, so-called nonavid antibody populations are those which have relatively high K values, and the so-called avid antibody populations are those with relatively low K values. From the practical standpoint, the properties of antigen bound to avid antibody populations are more sensitive to changes in antigen concentrations than are those obtained with nonavid antibody populations. With antisera which contain mostly avid antibody populations, the amount of antigen bound to antibody in the zone of antigen excess closely reflects the total antigen-binding capacity of the serum. Thus, a change in the concentration of antigen added to avid antibody results in a marked change in the proportion of antigen added which is bound by the antibody. In contrast, changes in the concentration of antigen added to antisera containing mostly nonavid antibody populations result in relatively large increases or decreases in the amount of antigen bound to antibody and little change in the proportion of the antigen bound. It should be noted, however, that both the amount and proportion of antigen bound by either avid or nonavid antibody populations are relatively sensitive to changes in antibody concentration under these conditions. For these reasons, if data approximating the total antigen binding capacity of a given antiserum are desired, this can be best studied by increasing the concentration of antibody as well as antigen and conducting the experiment in extreme antigen excess (6,8,9).

A list of primary binding tests is presented in Tables 12-1 and 12-2 and will be referred to more fully later in this chapter.

Secondary tests may be regarded as manifestations that may or may not occur following (n) number of primary interactions. Table 12-3 shows a few commonly used secondary tests. The importance of separating secondary from primary tests is indicated, for example, by the observation that some populations of antibodies have the capacity to form precipitates in the presence of antigen, and other populations of antibodies do

TABLE 12-1

Quantitative Tests That Depend Entirely on the Primary
Interaction between Antigen and Antibody

A. Tests dependent upon separation of bound from free antigen by precipitation
   of antigen-antibody complexes using:
   1. 50% ammonium sulfate
   2. Anti-immunoglobulin
B. Tests dependent upon fluorometric methods:
   1. Fluorescence quenching
   2. Fluorescence enhancement
   3. Fluorescence polarization
C. Tests dependent upon the difference in molecular size of bound- and free-
   antigen molecules:
   1. Equilibrium dialysis
   2. Ultracentrifugation
   3. Gel filtration
D. Tests dependent on the adsorption of antigen to inert surfaces:
   1. Paper chromatography
   2. Silica, talcum powder, Fuller's earth
   3. Dextran-coated charcoal
E. Tests dependent on the differential electrophoretic mobility of bound and free
   antigen:
   1. Disk polyacrylamide gel electrophoresis
   2. Paper or acetate electrophoresis
F. Tests dependent on the adsorption of specific antibody to polymeric surfaces:
   1. Polypropylene, polystyrene
   2. Coupling of antibody to Sephadex
G. Isotope-labeled eluates

TABLE 12-2

Qualitative Tests That Depend Entirely on the Primary
Interaction between Antigen and Antibody

A. Tests dependent on the binding of antigen to insoluble antigen-antibody
   precipitates:
   1. Indirect radioimmunoelectrophoresis
   2. Radioimmunodiffusion
   3. Direct radioimmunodiffusion and radioimmunoelectrophoresis
   4. Immunofluorescence
B. Test dependent on the differential electrophoretic mobility of bound and
   free antigen:
   1. Radio-gel-electrophoresis
   2. Free boundary electrophoresis

TABLE 12-3
Some Secondary Manifestations Which May or May Not
Occur Following (*n*) Number of Primary Interactions

1. Precipitation
   In solution
   In gel
2. Direct agglutination
3. Agglutination of erythrocytes or other particles
   coated with antigen
4. Complement fixation
5. Hemolysis

not (6). This is true whether the reaction is carried out in solution, by way of the quantitative precipitin or the P-80 test (10), or whether the precipitin reaction is carried out in a gel or agar medium. Similarly, agglutination tests, whether direct or indirect, measure the capacity of antisera to agglutinate antigen-coated particles. Some IgM antibody populations are 50 to 500 times more efficient in performing this capacity than are some 7S IgG antibody populations (11). Thus, agglutination tests do not tell how much antibody is present, but tell the antigen agglutinating capacity of antisera, just as precipitation tests measure precipitating capacity rather than total antibody content. Similarly, complement fixation tests measure the capacity of certain antigen-antibody reactions to utilize some of the eleven components of complement, but, again, it is known that other antibody populations, such as reagins and IgA antibody, do not have capacity to fix complement (12). Finally, hemolysis sometimes is an important secondary capacity to measure, but hemolysis is completely dependent upon the complement system, and some antibody populations are more efficient in causing hemolysis than others (13). As a group, the secondary tests are useful tools under certain circumstances, but when employed to study antibody populations of unknown and/or heterogeneous composition, they must be regarded as capacity tests rather than tests which necessarily reflect total antibody content. Not only will secondary manifestations frequently fail to reflect the total antibody content of an unknown antiserum, but of equal importance, a negative secondary manifestation test does not indicate the absence of antibodies. Secondary tests will be referred to later in this chapter, when they will be compared with primary tests performed on identical sera.

Tertiary tests are also manifestations of primary antigen-antibody interactions, but because they occur in vivo, they are even more complex than secondary manifestations. Some secondary tests performed in vitro, such as immune hemolysis and immune adherence, become tertiary mani-

TABLE 12-4
Some Tertiary Manifestations of Antigen-Antibody
Interaction

---

1. P-K test for reagin
2. Passive cutaneous anaphylaxis
3. Arthus reaction
4. Antibody-induced glomerulitis
5. Clearance of antigen from circulation by antibody
6. Tissue injury and possible symptoms
7. Protection

---

festations of antigen-antibody interaction when they occur in vivo. Some examples of these interesting relationships between secondary and tertiary tests will be considered in detail in the section of this chapter that concerns the complement system. Tertiary tests are not only subject to variables which control primary and secondary tests, but they have some of their own variables, a few examples of which are the antibody receptor and the chemoreceptor sites present in the host, the levels of complement in the host, the presence or absence of leukocytes, and the number of mast cells. These tertiary tests, which are even further removed from the primary interaction than are the secondary tests, are similar to secondary tests in that they are "capacity tests" which do not quantitate antibody content. Similar to secondary tests, negative tertiary tests do not indicate the absence of antibodies. A list of some tertiary manifestations of antigen-antibody interactions is presented in Table 12-4. It is stressed that protection and/or tissue injury resulting from antigen-antibody interactions in vivo are tertiary manifestations and will be discussed below especially as they are related to the complement system.

PRIMARY BINDING TESTS

As mentioned above, the binding of antigen to antibody is the initial step in a series of processes that may or may not result in a secondary or tertiary reaction. These tests reflect how much antigen a given serum can bind and are not dependent on many of the variables that control secondary and tertiary tests. As a result, primary binding tests may be positive when other tests are negative. Prior to a discussion of the individual tests listed in Table 12-1, it is of interest to point out certain characteristics that quantitative primary binding tests have in common.

1. Each test requires either a purified antigen or antibody preparation.

2. Each test utilizes a sensitive method to quantitate either antigen or antibody, usually with the help of isotopic or fluorescent labels.

3. Each method allows the investigator to separate the soluble antigen-antibody complexes from the antigen or antibody free in solution.

Quantitative Tests That Depend Entirely on the Primary Interaction

Tests Dependent Upon Separation of Bound from Free Antigen by Precipitation of Antigen-Antibody Complexes.

Ammonium sulfate method to measure antigen-binding capacity. The ammonium sulfate test is a primary test suitable for certain non-dialyzable antigens. It measures the capacity of antisera to combine with soluble macromolecular antigens and detects both precipitating and non-precipitating antibodies. The antigen originally employed for this procedure was bovine serum albumin (BSA), and the test was based on the principle that I^{131}-labeled bovine serum albumin (I^{131}-BSA) is soluble in 50 percent saturated ammonium sulfate (SAS/2), whereas soluble I^{131}-BSA-antigen-antibody complexes are insoluble under the same conditions (6). When a constant amount of I^{131}-BSA is added to serial dilutions of anti-BSA, a point is reached when antigen excess is achieved, spontaneous precipitation of I^{131}-BSA-antibody aggregates cannot occur, and equilibrium in solution is established. After the addition of ammonium sulfate, the I^{131}-BSA bound to antibody is precipitated. The use of ammonium sulfate does not appreciably alter the proportions of I^{131}-BSA which are bound to antibody or in solution prior to the addition of SAS/2, because SAS/2 markedly inhibits the formation and dissociation of I^{131}-BSA-antibody complexes (6).

In practice, constant amounts of labeled antigen are added to serial dilutions of the test antiserum. The percent of precipitated antigen following SAS/2 is determined at the various serum dilutions, and the dilution of antiserum which would precipitate 33 percent of the antigen added is calculated and referred to as the ABC-33 end point. The radioactivity in the SAS/2 precipitate is an indication of antigen binding capacity rather than the amount of antigen or antibody spontaneously precipitated, and results are expressed as μg I^{131}-BSA nitrogen (N) bound to antibody per ml of undiluted serum. The 33 percent precipitation end point was arbitrarily selected, because spontaneous precipitation does not occur at this degree of antigen excess, but enough of the I^{131}-labeled antigen is in the precipitate to permit accurate counting procedures. The procedure and calculations involved have been described in detail (6,14).

This test has been applied to compare antigen binding capacity with antigen precipitating capacity in rabbit and human sera (15), to discriminate between trace amounts of homologous and heterologous cross-reacting antigenic groups (16,17), to study association and dissociation rates of antigen-antibody interactions (7,18,19), to detect antibody in species where precipitating antibody is difficult to detect (20–22), to detect circulating antigen-antibody complexes in vivo (23,24), and to determine the maximum binding capacity of a given antiserum (8,9).

An important limitation of this test is that the labeled antigen must be soluble in 40 to 50 percent SAS and that the fractionation procedure must have no appreciable effect upon the equilibrium established between free and antibody-bound antigen prior to the addition of ammonium sulfate.

Although originally developed for use in the BSA-anti-BSA system, this method has been used with varying degrees of success with other antigens. Some of these are ten additional mammalian albumins (25,26), egg albumin (27), alpha lactalbumin (28), type-specific streptococcal M protein (29), crude (30) and purified antigen derived from ragweed pollen (31), somatic antigen from gram-negative bacteria (32), a protein fraction of rabbit spinal cord with capacity to elicit experimental allergic encephalomyelitis (33), DNA (34), two preparations of *Salmonella enteritidis* endotoxin (35), and the separated Fab and Fc components of human IgG (36).

In a number of other procedures free antigen has been similarly separated from bound antigen by precipitation with solvents such as sodium sulfite (37), sodium sulfate (38), or a solution of 50 percent alcohol in 5 percent saline (39). It is not known whether the proportion of antigen bound to antibody to that free in solution is appreciably altered by addition of these solvents, and published details are inadequate to completely evaluate these systems.

Anti-immunoglobulins to precipitate antigen-antibody complexes. This method is frequently referred to as the coprecipitation technique (40,41) or the double-antibody system (42). Soluble I^{131}-antigen-antibody complexes are precipitated by heterologous anti-IgG just as in the ammonium sulfate test they are precipitated by SAS/2. To illustrate its sensitivity, this procedure was compared with the ammonium sulfate test using a rabbit anti-BSA antiserum, and the results are illustrated in Fig. 12-1. Constant amounts of I^{131}-BSA were added to two sets of dilutions of an antiserum. The antigen-antibody complexes were precipitated in the one set by SAS/2 and in the other by a sheep anti-rabbit IgG antiserum. The percent of radioactive antigen precipitated was calculated and found to be almost identical using either method (43). Figure 12-1 also indicates that the dilution of antiserum which would have precipi-

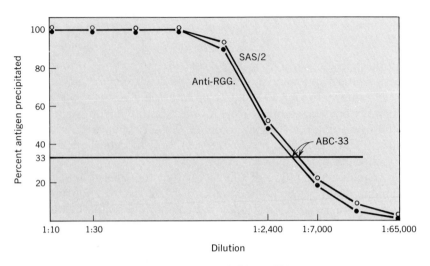

Fig. 12-1 Percent of I¹³¹-BSA antigen precipitated in a rabbit serum after the addition of SAS and/or anti-rabbit gamma globulin. The ABC-33 end point, or the dilution of antiserum that would precipitate 33 percent of the antigen added, is approximately 1:5000 using either method. From Minden et al. (86) with permission.

tated 33 percent of the antigen is 1:5000. This is the ABC-33 end point that is usually selected in the ammonium sulfate test described above.

A limitation of the anti-immunoglobulin procedure is that it requires large amounts of concentrated antibody to precipitate the antigen-antibody complexes. Moreover, cross-reactions between the anti-IgG and the I¹³¹-labeled test antigen prohibit the use of certain antigens. This procedure has been successfully used to measure antibodies to such antigens as insulin (41), horse serum albumin (44), BSA (43), human growth hormone (42), and an extract of human tubercle bacilli (45).

Tests Dependent Upon Fluorometric Methods

The availability of new instruments, such as the spectrofluorophotometer, has helped establish fluorescence as a new and highly useful dimension for the measurement of antibody. Fluorometry has a high degree of sensitivity, far greater than that of absorption spectrophotometry. At the present time, three techniques have been examined in sufficient detail to be considered as practical procedures for the measurement of selected antigen-antibody reactions.

Fluorescence quenching. Nearly all proteins emit fluorescent energy in the ultraviolet spectral region, and this energy yield is diminished when certain molecules attach to the proteins. Although the potentially fluorescent amino acid residues in proteins are phenylalanine, tyrosine, and trypto-

340

phan, even when proteins contain all three amino acids, the fluorescent spectrum is essentially that of tryptophan. The emission band of tryptophan residues is 350 μ, and an important requirement is that the absorption spectrum of the attached hapten overlap the emission band of the protein. The result is that the antigen-antibody interaction is quantitatively measurable with the quenching of the antibody fluorescence as the indicator. This largely limits the method to ligands such as DNP which absorb in the 300 to 360 μ region.

Similar to equilibrium dialysis, this is a quantitative procedure. A particular advantage is the ease and rapidity of measurements as compared with equilibrium dialysis. It requires minute amounts of antibody, with as little as 40 μg of purified antibody being sufficient. The ratio of bound over free antigen is easily determined, permitting the kinetics of a hapten-antibody system to be readily measured over wide ranges of conditions such as pH, temperature, and ionic strength, not approachable by other methods.

A principal limitation, as noted above, is that the antigen cannot be of a heterogeneous nature and must satisfy special spectral conditions. Since antibody constitutes only a small fraction of a serum's total protein emission, the procedure cannot be used with whole serum and is best used with purified immunospecific antibody. This procedure has yielded valuable information on the affinities of antibodies during the immune response (46) and offers future promise. Uncertainties remain, however, concerning interpolation of the results obtained, and the validity of results are usually verified by comparison with data obtained using equilibrium dialysis (47,48).

Fluorescence enhancement. Fluorescence enhancement is based on the principle that some molecules are nonfluorescent in aqueous solution but are highly fluorescent when bound to certain proteins. When a suitable fluorescent antigen is added in increasing amounts to antibody or antibody components and an antigen-antibody reaction takes place, fluorescence increases in a manner that can be quantitated by measurements in a spectrofluorophotometer at 435 μ (49). The basis for the assumption of fluorescence on binding to protein is not fully understood. The procedure has been applied to only a few haptens, such as naphthalene sulfonic acid (50). However, it is a relatively simple, sensitive, and quantitative test and does not require purified antibody. As in equilibrium dialysis, it allows for the calculation of bound- over free-antigen ratios, permitting study of the kinetic qualities of the antigen-antibody interaction.

An important limitation is that the antigen in question must satisfy spectral conditions that will result in increased fluorescence when bound to antibody.

Fluorescence polarization. In this test, measurements of polarization of fluorescence have been applied to the detection of antigen-antibody interactions. The interaction occurs between one kind of molecule which bears a fluorescent label and another which may or may not be fluorescent. The concept and mechanism of this technique have been fully described (51,52), but in essence it is the influence of molecular size and shape on fluorescence polarization which makes it useful in the study of antigen-antibody interactions. When a hapten or protein antigen becomes bound to an antibody molecule, a reduction in the rate of Brownian motion occurs that results in a corresponding increase in fluorescence polarization. The polarization of antigen has been shown to increase quantitatively with antibody concentration and is measured in a fluorescence polarimeter (53).

In practice, the antigen is labeled with a fluorescent molecule which absorbs and emits in the regions of the spectrum where other groups of protein do not interfere. A prerequisite is that the molecular size of the component to be detected should not be too small in comparison with the detecting agent.

The test is adaptable for basic studies of both the kinetics and equilibrium of the antigen-antibody reaction. It has been employed using ovalbumin (51), bovine serum albumin (54), and penicillin (55) as antigens. It is rapid, simple, and highly sensitive, with as little as 0.4 $\mu g/ml$ of antibody globulin having been detected with this method (55). Analysis of the data yields the association constant, site concentration, heterogeneity constant, reaction order, and rate constant of the reaction.

An important limitation is that when the test is performed on whole serum, there is excessive background fluorescence. Accordingly, results are better if globulin or purified antibody is used.

Tests Dependent upon the Difference in Molecular Size of Bound- and Free-Antigen Molecules

Equilibrium dialysis. Historically, equilibrium dialysis is the first primary binding test and is used to study the interaction between antibody and haptens (56). The size of the hapten molecule must be small enough to freely pass a semipermeable membrane. In practice, cellophane dialysis bags containing constant amounts of antibody preparation are dialyzed for 18 to 24 hours in a series of baths of buffered solutions containing graded concentrations of hapten. The concentration of antigen is then measured both inside and outside the dialysis bag. The concentration of hapten is usually determined by measurements of its color, its absorptive properties, by fluorescence, or by means of an isotope label. If there is no bound antigen, the concentration of hapten is the same on both sides of the membrane. If hapten molecules are bound to antibody, the hapten-antibody complex is too large to pass the semipermeable membrane, and the concentration of hapten is greater within the dialysis bag. The concentration of hapten bound to antibody is determined by subtracting the concentration of hapten on the outside of the bag from that on the inside.

By determining the concentration of bound-hapten as a function of the free-hapten concentration, analysis of the data reveals total hapten binding capacity, and the average intrinsic association constant of the interaction between antibody and hapten can be determined (57,58). This value is of importance in elucidating the nature of the antibody and antigen combining sites and the kinetics involved in their union. The data obtained may be evaluated in several ways, and the mathematical basis for determining the association constant has recently been reviewed in detail by Pinckard and Weir (59).

A major limitation is that with the membranes currently available, equilibrium dialysis cannot be used for macromolecular antigens such as most serum proteins. Moreover, if the hapten binds ionically to albumin or other nonimmunoglobulin serum proteins, a purified antibody preparation must be used.

Ultracentrifugation to separate antigen-antibody complexes. This test is based on the principle that soluble antigen-antibody complexes sediment more rapidly than free-antigen molecules in an ultracentrifugal field. Using an I^{131}-labeled antigen, the different sedimentation characteristics of antigen and antigen-antibody complexes have been shown to be a sensitive means of detecting and measuring the interaction between antigen and antibody. Using the preparative ultracentrifuge, this method has been described in detail using I^{131}-BSA as antigen. It has also been effective where the antigen was bovine gamma globulin (BGG), an antigen difficult to study by most other primary tests, and should be applicable for other protein antigens (60).

A limitation of this test is that results are expressed as the serum dilution required to reach a selected end point rather than in terms of the amount of antigen or antibody bound at equilibrium. Also, the experimental errors are somewhat larger than observed with other less complicated quantitative primary tests and the method loses some of its desirable characteristics when the test antigen is heavier than 7S IgG or when the antibody population is a mixture of IgG and IgM.

Gel filtration. The basis for this method is that bound antigen can be separated from free antigen according to their molecular sizes and to their elution characteristics from a Sephadex column. Providing there is sufficient difference between the molecular size of the antigen-antibody complex and that of antigen alone, I^{131}-labeled antigen-bound antibody will elute from a Sephadex column ahead of free antigen. The particular size of the gel to be selected for a given antigen should exclude the larger antigen-antibody complexes and retain or retard the smaller unbound antigen (61).

Although there has not been extensive experience with this method, it appears to be a dependable system for assaying insulin and/or anti-insulin and is deserving of further application (62). The limitations of the method can be expected to be similar to those indicated for the ultra-centrifugation test described above.

Tests Dependent on the Adsorption of Antigen to Inert Surfaces

This group of procedures takes advantage of the observation that some hapten and protein antigens adsorb to certain inert surfaces such as paper or glass. Antigen-antibody complexes do not have this characteristic, and it is then possible with the aid of isotope labels to separate antibody-bound antigen (B) from free antigen (F) in an antiserum. Immunologic tests based on this principle were originally developed to fulfill a need for sensitive and specific assay procedures to detect small amounts of circulating hormones (63).

The immunoassay is based on the reaction between the isotope-labeled hormone in question and a standard, specific, and avid antiserum, usually from a guinea pig. This results in a labeled antigen-antibody complex and permits the study of competitive inhibition by varying concentrations of unlabeled hormone. In such a system, unlabeled hormone competes with labeled hormone for specific antibody, reduces the formation of labeled hormone-antibody complexes, and favors the separation of free labeled hormone from antibody-bound hormone. In practice a "standard curve" is obtained by plotting B/F ratios versus varying concentrations of unlabeled hormone using the same antiserum. Hormone concentrations in unknown sera can then be determined by substituting the unknown sera for the standard hormones and comparing the B/F ratios of the unknown solutions with the standard curve. The B/F ratio falls progressively with increase in concentration of unlabeled hormone. Details of this procedure have been described (64).

Paper chromatography. This procedure was originally described by Berson et al. (63) as a radioimmunoassay to detect small amounts of circulating insulin. The B/F determinations are based on the principle that insulin has a tendency to adsorb to paper. When I^{131}-insulin is incubated with an antiserum and the mixture separated by electrophoresis on chromatographic paper, free insulin (F) is adsorbed to paper and remains at the site of application, while the antibody-bound fraction (B) moves cationically with the serum globulins. The amount of labeled insulin in each fraction is then determined from radioactive measurements of the chromatography strips and the results expressed as the B/F ratio. The amount of unlabeled insulin in an unknown serum sample is determined from its ability to inhibit competitively the binding of I^{131}-labeled hormone to specific antibody and may be calculated from a standard curve as described above.

To obtain the desired sensitivity, it is necessary to prepare I^{131}-labeled insulin with high isotopic specificity. If antigen is damaged during labeling or if I^{131}-iodide is released in small amounts during incubation in plasma, both situations are readily distinguished from radioactivity associated with intact hormone and are not erroneously included with the bound or free fraction. Variations of the quality of the labeled hormone and subtle alterations taking place during incubation can also be recognized by abnormalities in the pattern of adsorption to paper. Inaccuracy of volumetric sampling of the incubation mixtures need not affect the precision of the assays, since the only measurement involved is the ratio of bound to free hormone on the paper strip. Other advantages of the procedure are that many accurate determinations may be carried out simultaneously, a permanent record is obtained, and the test has maintained a reputation for reliability and reproducibility over many years.

Limitations are that the volume which can be analyzed on a single strip must be less than 300 to 400 μl. Not all chromatographic papers adsorb protein or insulin equally in the presence of plasma, and among those that do, there is considerable variation. Prolonged electrophoresis may result in dissociation of antigen-antibody complexes.

This test has been applied to the measurement of other peptide hormones, such as glucagon, growth hormone, and parathyroid hormone (64).

Adsorption to silica, talcum, and Fuller's earth. This test exploits a characteristic of some peptide hormones to adsorb to glassware, whereas radiolabeled hormones bound to antibody do not (65). By employing substances similar to glass in finely divided form such as simple talcum powder (hydrated magnesium silicate); microfine particles of precipitated silica; or Fuller's earth, a complex silicate, a large surface area becomes available.

In practice, silicate in the form of powder or tablets is added directly to incubation tubes containing labeled hormone, specific antibody, and the unknown test serum. The contents are vigorously agitated, after which the tubes are centrifuged and the supernatant decanted. The radioactivity in each tube is counted and represents the unbound hormone. Knowing the total amount of labeled hormone added, one can calculate the B/F ratio. As described above, standard curves are prepared from B/F ratios using known amounts of unlabeled hormone that reacted with specific antibody. The B/F ratios in the unknown samples may then be assayed against the standard curves to determine the quantity of circulating hormone.

This test allows for the analysis of large volumes of solutions. This may be of practical value when the concentration of labeled hormone is limited because of the low concentration of endogenous hormone in plasma, as is frequently the case for ACTH, or because of the difficulty of preparing labeled hormones with high specific activity. Antigens tested with this procedure have been human growth hormone, parathyroid hormone, insulin, and ACTH (65).

Adsorption of antigen to dextran-coated charcoal. This test is based on the observation that charcoal coated with dextran will adsorb a small antigen such as insulin but will not adsorb the same antigen when it is bound to antibody.

The procedure has recently been applied to the determination of B/F ratios after separating insulin from insulin-antibody complexes using charcoal coated with dextran (molecular weight, 80,000). Advantages of this method are its simplicity and rapidity, and results of the procedure have compared favorably with those obtained by chromatographic radioimmunoassays (66–68).

Tests Dependent on the Differential Electrophoretic Mobility of Bound and Free Antigens

The basis for these tests is the separation of free from bound antigen by electrophoresis. An essential requirement is that free antigen migrate in a position so that it can be clearly differentiated from the bound antigen-antibody complex.

Disk electrophoresis in polyacrylamide gels has been employed for the separation of free from bound isotope-labeled antigen. By carrying out electrophoresis in this medium, the serum proteins and free antigen are clearly concentrated into thin lines according to their electrophoretic mobility. Free antigen can then be separated from antibody-bound antigen by cutting the gel into small segments which can be tested for radioactivity. Equipment has been developed that allows elution of the separated proteins in a liquid state, facilitating the analysis of fractions for protein concentration and radioactivity. The separation of free from antibody-bound antigen has been found to be as precise as, if not more precise than, the separation achieved with other methods described above.

Immunoassays have been made with this procedure for I^{131}-labeled thyrotropin, insulin, and human growth hormone (69,70). Assays are usually carried out as described above for the tests dependent on the adsorption of labeled antigen to inert surfaces, i.e., the use of a standard inhibition curve obtained by adding a known amount of unlabeled antigen to the predetermined isotopic-labeled antigen-antibody system.

Paper or acetate electrophoresis. Separation of free from antibody-bound antigen has been accomplished by electrophoresis of mixtures on chromatographic paper and cellulose acetate strips. Two antigens studied in this manner have been diphtheria toxoid (71) and BSA (72), both of which migrate toward the anode when free but migrate toward the cathode when bound to antibody. After electrophoresis and drying, the paper or acetate strips are cut into small sections, and their radioactivity is determined in a scintillation counter. This procedure resembles that developed by Berson et al. (63), described above, but differs in that the latter depends on adsorption of free-antigen to cellulose rather than to its natural electrophoretic properties.

Tests Dependent on the Adsorption of Specific Antibody to Polymeric Surfaces

These tests are based on the adsorption of specific antibody to polymeric surfaces and the ability of the antibody-coated polymers to bind radioactive tracer antigen.

Polypropylene and polystyrene. These tests were recently described by Catt and Tregear (73) to measure nanogram quantities of human growth hormone and placental lactogen. The interior of plastic tubes manufactured from polypropylene or polystyrene and suitable for use in a gamma scintillation counter are coated with dilutions of specific antibody. The antibody-coated tubes have capacity to bind radioactive antigen and provide a site for competitive binding of unlabeled antigen. Free labeled antigen is removed by washing the tube on completion of the immune reaction. The labeled antigen bound to the antibody on the solid phase material is then counted to quantitate the bound antigen and the B/F ratio then determined.

Advantages of this procedure are its simplicity, sensitivity, and economy. A single tube may be used for all phases of the procedure: incubation, separation of bound and free antigen, and counting of the bound antigen are all performed in one tube. The lack of broad experience with this test precludes a discussion of possible limitations which may exist.

Coupling of antibody to Sephadex. The antibody ploymer in this test is an isothiocyanate derivative of Sephadex, and the procedure was first described by Wide and Porath (74). The polymer-coupled antibodies were shown to retain their capacity to bind to specific antigen, and the procedure has been applied to assays of insulin, growth hormone, human chorionic gonadotrophin, luteinizing hormone, and IgG.

In practice, isotope-labeled hormone, the serum to be investigated, and a suspension of the antibody polymer are added to a single disposable plastic test tube and incubated for 24 hours. The bound labeled antigen is separated from free antigen by centrifugation, and the radioactivity of the antigen bound to antibody polymer particles is counted in the precipitate.

The advantages of this method are its high sensitivity, precision, and simplicity. A small amount of the antibody Sephadex is sufficient for many reactions, can be stored for long periods of time, and the entire procedure can be carried out in a single tube. Again, an evaluation of the possible limitations of this method awaits further attempts to apply it to a variety of other antigens.

Isotope-labeled Eluates

The basis for this procedure is that unlabeled antigen can be measured according to its reactivity with a specific isotope-labeled antiserum (75). It has been applied to detect and quantitate the erythrocyte Rh antigen in normal individuals (76,77). An anti-Rh-antiserum was fractionated using ammonium sulfate, and the resulting globulin preparation was labeled with I^{131}. This was then adsorbed to Rh-positive erythrocytes after which nonspecific globulin was eluted. It was then possible to calculate the amount of eluate bound to erythrocytes and the amount of unbound antibody. Isotope-labeled eluates used in this manner are powerful tools to study subtle differences in antigen concentration on cell surfaces, and the procedure may also be employed to measure the capacity of soluble unlabeled antigen or antibody to block the uptake by red cells of an I^{131}-labeled antibody.

Although the test was developed using an antiserum to red cells, it should be adaptable for antisera to other insoluble antigens and should also be applicable to purified antibody as prepared from an immunoadsorbent. A limitation of the procedure is that it is not known whether each or any of the procedures involved is exerting a selective influence in terms of antibody heterogeneity or reactivity. Another limitation is that eluates must be repeatedly prepared, and there are usually variations from one preparation to another.

Qualitative Tests that Depend Entirely on the Primary Interaction Between Antigen and Antibody

Tests Dependent on the Binding of Antigen to Insoluble Antigen-Antibody Precipitates

These procedures have been applied in many investigations to study antigen-binding characteristics of immunoglobulins and immunoglobulin subunits (15,78,79) and may be carried out by either indirect or direct methods.

Indirect radioimmunoelectrophoresis is usually carried out on microscope slides coated with agar into which wells and troughs are cut according to the needs of the experiment. The test serum, or serum component, is usually applied to one well, with an appropriate negative control sample on the same slide. After electrophoresis is carried out, agar is removed to form the troughs, which are then filled with the appropriate antiserum to precipitate the desired immunoglobulin in the test serum. The reactants are allowed to diffuse so that precipitin bands will form, after which the slides are washed and I^{131}-labeled antigen is added to the trough. After 24 hours, the slides are washed again and applied to sensitive x-ray film (e.g., Kodak Industrial Type KK) for 24 to 36 hours, after which the film is developed.

Indirect radioimmunodiffusion is similarly performed on microscope slides coated with a thin layer of agar. After application of the appropriate antigens and antisera to wells that have been cut in the agar, the slides are incubated for 24 hours, washed for 24 hours, and then I^{131}-labeled antigen is added to the center or other appropriate well. Twenty-four hours after the addition of I^{131}-antigen, the slides are washed, air-dried, and overlayed with x-ray film, as described above for 24 to 36 hours, after which the film is developed.

Direct radioimmunodiffusion and direct radioimmunoelectrophoresis may be performed using the same techniques described above, except that I^{131}-labeled protein antigen is added directly to the IgG antiserum. These procedures have previously been described in greater detail (78,80).

The extreme sensitivity of these tests was pointed out by studies using dilutions of rabbit IgG where the anti-BSA precipitating antibody had been calculated. By radioimmunodiffusion, antigen binding was noted by as little as 0.003 μg N per ml anti-BSA and by radioimmunoelectrophoresis binding was detected in preparations that contained 0.025 μg N anti-BSA per ml.

A limitation of these procedures is the occasional occurrence of nonspecific reactions. Figure 12-2 illustrates a radioimmunoelectrophoresis preparation in which a strongly positive radioactive line was associated with antibody IgG which was applied to the well above the trough and a less intense but definite radioactive line was associated with normal IgG applied to the well below the trough. Figure 12-3 indicates some nonspecific radioimmunodiffusion reactions when normal IgG was applied to wells that were adjacent to wells containing anti-BSA IgG. I^{131}-BSA binding was observed in precipitin lines produced by normal IgG as well as those produced by IgG antibody. The likely explanation for the false positive reactions is that some anti-BSA IgG molecules diffused and became a part of the immune precipitate formed by normal IgG and anti-IgG so that within the normal IgG/anti-IgG precipitin band the anti-BSA IgG molecules also formed IgG/anti-IgG complexes with the capacity to bind I^{131}-BSA. These reactions have been described in greater detail (80). Because of the apparent ease with which false-positive reactions can occur,

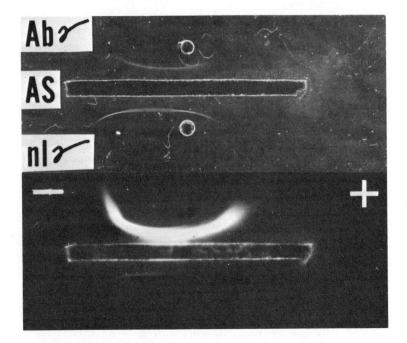

Fig. 12-2   Paired stained immunoelectrophoresis and radioimmuno-electrophoresis preparations. Immunoelectrophoresis lines are on top slide; radioimmunoelectrophoresis lines are on lower slide.   Radioactivity is associated with the normal γG/anti-γG precipitin arc below trough as well as with the precipitin arc formed by the specific antibody γG/anti-γG arc above trough.   From Minden et al. (80) with permission.

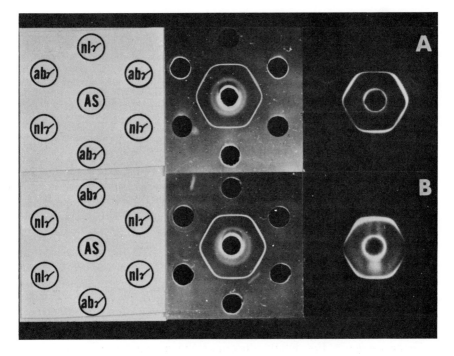

Fig. 12-3 Paired immunodiffusion and radioautograph preparations. Code is in left column. Immunodiffusion lines are in center column. Radioimmunodiffusion lines are in right column. ab γ = rabbit anti-bovine albumin (BSA) γG.
nl γ = normal rabbit serum γG devoid of anti-BSA.
AS = antiserum is duck anti-rabbit γG.
A and B demonstrate nonspecific radioactivity over precipitin lines produced by normal γG/anti-γG. From Minden et al. (80) with permission.

it is advisable that only one preparation containing specific antibodies be applied to a single slide in radioimmunoelectrophoresis and that in radio-immunodiffusion the antigen preparations not be applied in adjacent wells if they are of a cross-reacting or partially cross-reacting nature. Cross-reactions between IgG and the test antigen also limits the use of certain antigens for these procedures.

Immunofluorescence is a qualitative primary test that allows direct observation and the precise localization of the reaction between small amounts of antigen or antibody. This may be observed on or in cells and in frozen or freeze-dried tissue sections or smears. It is based on the property of fluorescein, a fluorochrome dye, to emit fluorescence when excited by ultraviolet light. Fluorescein is readily conjugated to protein such as gamma globulin, and the conjugate retains its specific immunologic reactivity. If the conjugate is layered on a tissue section containing the corresponding antigen, combination between the fluorescein-conjugated antibody molecules and antigen takes place in situ in the tissue. The uncombined conjugate is removed by washing so that on examination the sites of specific combination and hence of antigen localization appear fluorescent. This procedure may be used either with a conjugated antibody of known specific reactivity to detect antigen or with a known tissue or protein to test an unknown serum for the presence of a corresponding antibody. This test, as outlined above, was first described by Coons et al. (81) in 1941 and is frequently termed the *direct method.*

The *indirect method* was described in 1954 by Weller and Coons (82) and Gitlin et al. (83) and is based on the use of three layers. Unlabeled specific antiserum is added as a second layer to the preparation, allowed to react, and the excess removed by washing. Labeled antiglobulin prepared against the homologous species in which the unlabeled antiserum was prepared is then added as a third layer. After the proper staining time, it is removed by washing. The middle layer acts as antibody in relation to the antigen and as antigen in relation to the conjugated antiglobulin. The advantage of the indirect method is that one fluorescent antiglobulin can be used to stain a variety of homologous antisera against different antigens. For details concerning the conjugation of antisera, the choice of fluorochromes, the technical procedures of conjugation, histologic preparation, and staining, a recent complete review is recommended (84).

Immunofluorescence has been used for the visualization and identification of bacterial, viral, protozoan, helminthic, fungous, and animal tissue antigens; for the localization of antibody in tissues; and for the detection and characterization of serum antibody. Of particular interest is its frequent application to the detection of gamma globulin and complement in lesions at the site of immunologic tissue injury. This application will be referred to more fully in the section in this chapter on the role of complement. It should be mentioned that the method has a limitation in that the strength of the bond between the tissue slices and the fluorescent or nonfluorescent reactants must be sufficiently strong to withstand the subsequent washes necessary to eliminate nonspecific positive results. Figure 12-4 is an example of immunofluorescence as seen in a glomerulus from the kidney of a patient with Goodpasture's disease. The section was stained with fluorescent rabbit antihuman IgG (85).

Tests Dependent on the Differential Electrophoretic Mobility of Bound and Free Antigen

Radio gel electrophoresis. In this procedure, electrophoresis of an I^{131}-antigen-antibody complex is carried out on microscope glass slides. Radioactivity is then detected by exposing the fixed and dried preparations to

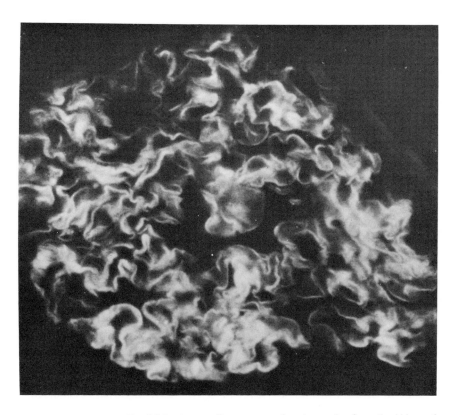

Fig. 12-4 Immunofluorescence of a glomerulus from the kidney of a patient with Goodpasture's disease. Tissue was incubated with fluorescent rabbit antihuman IgG. A linear deposit of IgG is demonstrated along the glomerular capillary walls. X350. From Lerner et al. (85) with permission.

sensitive x-ray film (Kodak Industrial type KK). This test is simple to perform, since precipitation of serum proteins in gel by antibody is not needed. An example of this procedure is seen in Fig. 12-5, where free I^{131}-labeled BSA incubated in a 1:250 dilution of normal rabbit serum migrates naturally towards the anode (A). If I^{131}-BSA is incubated in the same dilution of serum from a rabbit immunized to BSA, I^{131}-BSA-antibody complexes migrate closer to the point of application (B), although some uncombined antigen is also evident. Section C demonstrates specificity of the reaction. If the antiserum in (B) is incubated with unlabeled BSA prior to incubation with I^{131}-BSA, all the I^{131}-BSA appears in the unbound state (86). At present this test has not been developed to give information of a quantitative nature, but further investigation may make this possible.

Free boundary electrophoresis is performed by placing microgram amounts of antigen in the buffers over an antiserum in a Tiselius type of

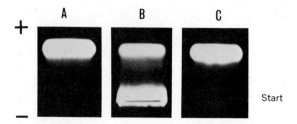

+

A   B   C

Start

−

Fig. 12-5 Radio gel electrophoresis radioautographs of 1:250 dilutions of rabbit anti-BSA antiserum in 1:10 dilutions of normal rabbit serum. (A) I^{131}-BSA after incubation in dilution of normal rabbit serum migrates toward anode. (B) I^{131}-BSA after incubation in dilution of anti-BSA rabbit serum migrates as I^{131}-BSA-antibody complex closer to point of application; some uncombined I^{131}-BSA is also evident. (C) When antiserum used in B was incubated with unlabeled BSA prior to incubation with I^{131}-BSA, all the I^{131}-BSA migrates toward the anode in the unbound state. From Minden et al. (86) with permission.

free boundary electrophoresis cell. When a primary interaction occurs between antigen and trace amounts of antibody, well-defined boundary disturbances are created that can be detected visually.

In practice, the reactant is put in the buffer over both the ascending and descending limbs of the cell. If an interaction takes place between the serum in the cell and the reactant, a boundary disturbance associated with the particular serum component involved results because the mobility of the new reactant-protein complex is different from that of the serum component alone.

The method is sensitive and will detect as little as 0.1 μg of antigen per ml. It has been used with unlabeled antigens such as BSA, bovine gamma globulin (BGG), *Pneumococcus* polysaccharide, the Boivin-type antigen from *E. coli* (87), and ragweed pollen (88). A limitation is that the nonspecific B boundary disturbance is frequently encountered, and control studies to distinguish between this phenomenon and an antigen-antibody reaction is essential for each antigen used. The B boundary disturbance can be eliminated from the descending limb of the electrophoretic pattern by the addition of as little as 1 percent normal homologous albumin or 1 percent whole serum.

COMPARISON OF SECONDARY AND TERTIARY TESTS WITH PRIMARY TESTS

The importance of separating primary, secondary, and tertiary antibody tests was pointed out in a study performed on sera from 15 humans and 2 rabbits with antibodies directed toward a protein in cow's milk, bovine

354

serum albumin (BSA) (15). These observations will be discussed in some detail because they illustrate that the separation of primary, secondary, and tertiary antibody measurements is not merely of academic interest but has important practical implications. Table 12-5 lists the data obtained when a battery of seven tests were performed on 15 selected human sera. The ammonium sulfate test and radioimmunoelectrophoresis are primary binding tests; the P-80, hemagglutination, and gel diffusion are secondary tests; passive cutaneous anaphylaxis (PCA) and the Prausnitz-Küstner passive transfer test (P-K) are tertiary tests.

As discussed previously, the ammonium sulfate test measures the antigen-binding capacity of the sera and provides quantitative information in terms of the μg I*BSA bound per ml of undiluted serum when tested with a standard antigen concentration of 0.02 μg N per ml. Radioimmunoelectrophoresis, the other primary test, is a qualitative test that indicates which of the immunoglobulins are responsible for the binding. In this study, the ammonium sulfate test was positive in all the sera because this was the criterion for choosing them. As to be expected for another primary test of nearly equal sensitivity, radioimmunoelectrophoresis confirmed that each of the 15 human sera contained antibodies capable of binding I^{131}-BSA. All of the sera showed I^{131}-BSA-binding associated with IgG, and in five cases it was also associated with IgA.

Antigen Precipitating Capacity (P-80)

The capacity of antisera to precipitate BSA was measured using a variation (14) of the technique described by Talmage and Maurer (10) in which a constant amount of I^{131}-BSA was added to serial dilutions of antiserum. After 6 days of incubation the tubes were centrifuged, the supernatant decanted, and the amount of I^{131}-BSA in the specific antigen-antibody precipitate measured. The end point selected was that dilution of antiserum at which 80 percent (P-80) of I^{131}-labeled antigen was precipitated. The P-80 values were then expressed as the μg I^{131}-BSA N spontaneously precipitated per ml of undiluted serum.

The P-80 data indicated no detectable precipitating anti-BSA in 7 of the 14 sera so studied. Of the remaining 7 sera, 3 (numbers 2, 4, and 5) reached the P-80 end point, and 4 had only trace amounts of precipitating activity. There was poor correlation between the amount of circulating anti-BSA as measured by the ammonium sulfate test and the amount of antigen precipitating capacity measured by the P-80 test. In fact, the serum (number 1) with the highest I^{131}-BSA binding capacity had no detectable precipitating activity.

TABLE 12-5

Comparison of Methods for Determination of Antibody in Human and Rabbit Sera

	HUMAN SERA, NUMBER															RABBIT SERA[a]	
	1	2	3	4	5	6	7	8	9	10	11	12	13	14	15	a[b]	b[c]
ABC-33 at 0.02μg I*BSA N/ml	11.6	6.07	5.02	4.62	2.77	1.52	1.24	0.96	0.96	0.77	0.66	0.45	0.37	0.34	0.31	3.83	5.94
Radioimmuno-electrophoresis																	
Anti-whole serum	+	+	+	+	+	+	+	+	+	+	+	+	+	+	+	+	+
Anti-γ A	+	+	+	+	–	–	–	–	–	–	+	–	–	–	–	?	?
Anti-γ M	–	–	–	–	–	–	–	–	–	–	–	–	–	–	–	?	?
Anti-γ G	+	+	+	+	+	+	+	+	+	+	+	+	+	+	+	+	+
% antigen precipitated	–	>80	36.4	>80	>80	–	63.3	32.9	–	46.4	–	–	–	–	>80	>80	>80
P-80 at 0.02μg I*BSA N/ml	–	0.70	–	1.28	0.32	–	–	–	–	–	–	–	–	*d	–	0.67	2.24
P-80/ABC-33	–	0.11	–	0.28	0.12	–	–	–	–	–	–	–	–	–	–	0.17	0.38
Hemagglutination	1/64	1/32	1/256	1/512	1/256	1/16	0	1/32	1/64	1/32	1/128	0	0	0	0	γ/4096	1/2048
Gel diffusion	–	–	–	+	*d	–	–	–	–	–	–	–	–	–	–	+	+
PCA	–	–	–	–	–	–	–	–	–	–	–	–	–	–	–	+	+
P-K	+	*d	+	+	–	–	–	–	*d	–	–	*d	+	–	–	*d	*d
Age	17	17	8	18	6	10	39	3	61	46	3	44	34	8	78		
Diagnosis[e]	1	1,2	1	1	1	3	4	3	5	3	3	6	1,3	1,3	4		

[a] Diluted 1:10.
[b] Immunized by IV route.
[c] Immunized by oral route.
[d] Asterisk indicates not examined.
[e] Diagnosis of patients with symptoms unrelated to milk and beef: 1 = allergic rhinitis, 2 = regional enteritis, 3 = bronchial asthma, 4 = neurodermatitis, 5 = hypertension 6 = functional bowel disorder.
SOURCE: From Minden et al. (14).

Antigen Precipitating Efficiency

It is convenient to express the antigen precipitating efficiency of an anti-serum by the P-80/ABC-33 ratio, which is obtained by dividing the P-80 value (antigen precipitating capacity) by the ABC-33 value (antigen binding capacity). Since this ratio can be calculated only when there is a P-80 value, and only three of the antisera had enough precipitating capacity to reach this end point, it appears that most samples of human anti-BSA have lower precipitating efficiencies than either of the two rabbit antisera presented in Table 12-5 or most of several hundred additional samples of rabbit anti-BSA previously studied in this respect. An occasional human antiserum (number 4) appeared to have a high antigen precipitating efficiency comparable to most rabbits and, as previously reported (6), some rabbits may have low antigen precipitating efficiencies comparable to most human anti-BSA. Low precipitating efficiency may be a characteristic of the human species, not limited to the BSA-anti-BSA system, because Grey (29) also observed low precipitating efficiency in a human antiserum where the antigen was I^{131}-labeled M-12 streptococcal extract.

Gel Diffusion

Gel diffusion demonstrated a precipitin (89) in only the one human serum (number 4) with the high precipitating efficiency. These findings indicate that gel diffusion is a less sensitive method for detecting human precipitating antibody than the P-80 test and suggest that high precipitating efficiency may favor the formation of precipitin lines in gel.

Hemagglutination Studies

These were performed with a microtechnique described by Sever (90) with sheep erythrocytes prepared according to Stavitsky (91). The titers were expressed as the highest dilution which gave grossly positive agglutination. Specific antibodies to BSA were detected by hemagglutination in 10 of the 15 sera. Specificity was established in each case by the successful inhibition of the reaction upon the addition of BSA to the antiserum prior to its interaction with BSA-coated cells. As is evident in Table 12-5, the hemagglutination results did not correlate with the other methods used. This is especially noteworthy when comparing the high hemagglutination titers of the rabbit antisera to the relatively low titers obtained with the human sera, even though the binding capacity of some of the human sera were higher than those of the rabbit antisera.

The lack of correlation between hemagglutinating titers and other methods of detecting antibodies are caused in part by differences in hemagglutinating efficiencies among different populations of antibody. Grey (19) compared hemagglutination, the ammonium sulfate test, and spontaneous precipitation in a rabbit antiserum by examining 19S and 7S anti-BSA as separated by sucrose gradient ultracentrifugation. On day 11 hemagglutinating capacity was greatest in the 19S antibody fraction, whereas binding capacity (ABC-33) and precipitating capacity (P-80) were greatest in the 7S fraction. These studies suggested that the hemagglutinating efficiency of rabbit 19S antibody is relatively high as compared to that of 7S antibodies. Subsequent studies have suggested similar conclusions (92).

Passive Cutaneous Anaphylaxis (PCA)

PCA was performed using a variation of the technique described by Ovary (93). Guinea pigs were given duplicate 0.1-ml injections of the test sera, the rabbit anti-BSA control sera, and human serum that contained no detectable anti-BSA. The guinea pigs were injected intravenously with a BSA-Evans blue dye solution 16 hours after application of the test sera. The injection sites were observed for 45 minutes, and when interpretation of results was in doubt, the guinea pigs were killed and the skin removed for examination of the undersurface. None of the 14 human sera examined showed PCA activity, but both rabbit antisera tested gave strongly positive reactions.

P-K Passive Transfer Tests

These tests were performed on 12 of the 15 human antisera using 1 mg/ml of crystallized BSA in saline as a test antigen. A 0.1-ml aliquot of test serum was injected intradermally into skin-test-negative recipients, the antigen was applied 48 hours later, and results were read 20 minutes after the test dose of antigen. As seen in Table 12-5, none of these 4 serum donors had detectable clinical symptoms after ingestion of either milk or beef, the most probable sources of antigen for the stimulation of anti-BSA in humans (28). It has been previously demonstrated that an immunologically specific positive wheal and erythema immediate type of skin reaction to a given antigen is not always associated with a symptomatic state of allergy (94,95).

Table 12-6 is a summary of the detailed results presented in Table 12-5. The data demonstrate that secondary tests were frequently negative when primary tests were positive and that tertiary tests, which are farthest removed from the primary interaction, were equally uninformative in telling whether antibodies were or were not present. Even when the sec-

TABLE 12-6
Comparison of Primary Tests with Secondary and Tertiary Manifestations

	Number studied	Number positive
Primary binding tests		
Ammonium sulfate test	15	15
Radioimmunoelectrophoresis	15	15
Secondary manifestations		
P-80	14	3
Gel diffusion	15	1
Hemagglutination	15	10
Tertiary manifestations		
PCA	14	0
P-K	12	4
Clinical symptoms after drinking milk	15	0

ondary and tertiary tests were positive, the results did not correlate with the amount of antibody present. This is another indication that the quality as well as the quantity of antibody was important with respect to the secondary tests and that host factors plus the quality of antibody were important to the tertiary tests.

The complexity of the variables which control secondary and tertiary antibody tests, especially the tests' failure to sometimes detect large amounts of antibody when present in human antisera, suggests that under ideal circumstances an experimental protocol should include at least one test which measures the primary interaction. This is particularly true if the purpose of the experiment is to look for the presence or absence of antibody and to measure the total antibody content.

THE ROLE OF COMPLEMENT IN SECONDARY AND TERTIARY ANTIGEN-ANTIBODY REACTIONS

The complement system consists of a set of serum factors which, together with some but not all populations of antibody, has long been recognized to have the capacity of causing lysis of erythrocytes and a large variety of mammalian and bacterial cells. In recent years complement has been found to play a role as an effector of the immune response other than its role in immune cytolysis. When these responses are observed as isolated events in vitro, they represent secondary tests; when they occur in the more complicated biologic milieu in vivo to cause protection and/or tissue injury, they represent tertiary manifestations of the primary interaction between antigen and antibody.

It has lately become apparent that the complement system consists of at least 11 discrete protein substances, some of which have been isolated in highly purified form (96). These 11 components, which are designated C'1q, C'1r, C'1s, C'2 through C'9, together with some of their physicochemical properties as they occur in human serum, are listed in Table 12-7. The system is even more complex when it is considered that many or possibly all components are subject to the activity of inhibitors.

Erythrocyte lysis requires all the known components of complement and begins with the attachment of the first component (C'1q, C'1r, C'1s) to antibody on the cell surface. In the presence of calcium all these subunits become attached, and C'1s, the proesterase, is converted into the active esterase C'1a. After a series of reactions that involve the sequential participation of all the components of complement, immune cytolysis ends with a damaged site at the cell surface and, in the case of the erythrocyte, with hemolysis and the release of hemoglobin. The intermediate steps of this entire reaction and the stages at which certain nonhemolytic types of reactions take place are schematically outlined in Fig. 12-6. For a more detailed analysis of these steps, several complete and recent reviews are recommended (97,98).

The noncytolytic immunologic reactions mediated by complement, unlike the hemolytic reaction, require some but not all of the complement components. Those that appear to be of biologic significance and which may be involved directly or indirectly in secondary or tertiary manifestations of the primary antigen-antibody interaction will be discussed below.

Immunoconglutination

This is the agglutination of complement-coated cells by auto-, iso-, or hetero-IgM antibodies directed against hidden groups on C'3 and C'4 which become accessible or altered during the fixation of complement (99). These antibodies, or immunoconglutinins, are present in low titer in the serum of many apparently healthy humans. Higher levels of immunoconglutinins arise in humans in response to immunization and to certain acute and chronic bacterial diseases. Although their biologic significance is obscure, there is some evidence that they enhance the tertiary manifestations of host resistance to infection (100).

Immune Adherence

This refers to the ability of antigen-antibody-complement complexes to adhere to the surface of nonsensitized particles, such as red cells, leukocytes, platelets, and starch granules. C'1, C'4, C'2, and C'3 are involved

TABLE 12-7
Properties of Human Complement Components

	C'1q	C'1r	C'1s	C'2	C'3	C'4	C'5	C'6	C'7	C'8	C'9
Serum concentration (μg/ml)	100–200	—	22	<5	1,200	430	75	—	—	—	1–2
Sedimentation rate	11.1S	7S	4S	5.5S	9.5S	10S	8.7S	5–6S	5–6S	8S	4S
Approximate mol. wt	500,000	—	—	115,000	200,000	230,000	—	—	—	—	—
Electrophoretic mobility	γ_2	β	α_2	β_2	β_1	β_1	β_1	β_2	β_2	γ_1	α
Carbohydrate concentration (%)	30	—	—	—	2.7	14	19	—	—	—	—
Reactive SH	—	—	—	1 or more	2	—	—	—	—	—	—

SOURCE: From Müller-Eberhard (98) with permission.

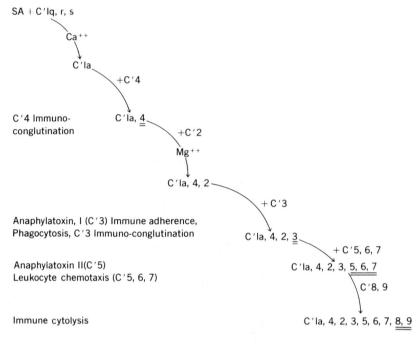

SA + C'lq, r, s
　　Ca++
　　C'la
　　　+C'4

C'4 Immuno-　　C'la, 4
conglutination
　　　　　+C'2
　　　　Mg++
　　　C'la, 4, 2
　　　　　+C'3

Anaphylatoxin, I (C'3) Immune adherence,
Phagocytosis, C'3 Immuno-conglutination　　C'la, 4, 2, 3
　　　　　　　+C'5, 6, 7

Anaphylatoxin II(C'5)　　C'la, 4, 2, 3, 5, 6, 7
Leukocyte chemotaxis (C'5, 6, 7)
　　　　　　　C'8, 9

Immune cytolysis　　C'la, 4, 2, 3, 5, 6, 7, 8, 9

Fig. 12-6 The sequence of action of the individual complement components leading to immune cytolysis is represented schematically as a cascade reaction similar to that proposed for the coagulation system. A total of 11 proteins constitute the 9 components. All components are required for immune cytolysis. On the left the non-cytolytic complement dependent biologic reactions are indicated which are mediated by discrete portions of the entire system. S represents an antigen site on a cell membrane (red blood cell, bacterium) and A, a specific antibody to the site. Modified from Kohler and ten Bensel (117) with permission.

in this reaction. Immune adherence of bacteria and viruses have been shown to promote the tertiary manifestations of phagocytosis in vivo (101). It is also the principle behind a number of sensitive in vitro secondary tests to detect antibody to many microorganisms (102).

Chemotaxis and Inflammation

Antigen-antibody complexes per se fail to attract polymorphonuclear leukocytes in vitro but do so in the presence of complement. This activity has been shown to depend on an activated complex of C'5, C'6, and C'7 (103). This function of complement is essential for the full expression of antibody-induced inflammatory lesions mediated by the release from leukocytes of proteolytic enzymes and other permeability factors. As discussed elsewhere in this section the complement system is also involved in most of the other parameters of the immune inflammatory responses, e.g., potentiation of phagocytosis, opsonification, immune adherence, increased vascular permeability due to anaphylatoxin, and some forms of histamine release. Hence, the complement system plays an essential part in the complex immunologic lesions of the Arthus phenomenon, of glomerulonephritis caused by soluble antigen-antibody complexes or nephrotoxic antibody, and of the arteritis of serum sickness (104). Figure 12-7 is an outline of the present understanding of the mechanisms that lead to the observed injury in acute nephrotoxic nephritis, the arteritis of serum sickness, and Arthus vasculitis, three lesions that have been thoroughly investigated using experimental models. The same system may also be responsible for a variety of other lesions.

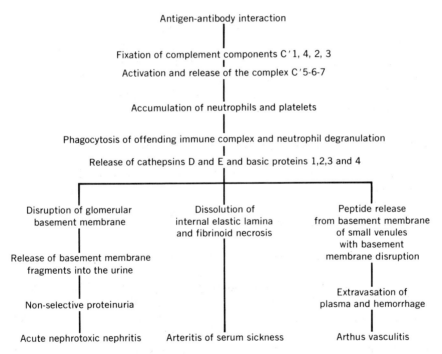

Fig. 12-7 Schematic outline of events that may follow a primary antigen-antibody interaction. Using experimental models, the complement system is directly involved in the production of three immunologic lesions. From Cochrane (104) with permission.

Phagocytosis

The response of phagocytic cells for foreign matter may be divided into three stages: (1) chemotaxis or the migration of phagocytes towards the particles, an effect for which complement is an absolute requirement; (2) the actual phagocytosis of particles, an event for which complement components are sometimes required, depending on the nature of the surface of the particle to be ingested; and (3) the digestion of particles within the phagocyte, a process for which complement is not required at all.

For erythrophagocytosis, the presence of C'1, C'4, C'2, and C'3 are essential. For phagocytosis of bacteria the same components are required in some instances and in others antibody alone is sufficient. The titration of antibody by observing its effect on phagocytosis may also be considered a secondary manifestation of a primary antigen-antibody reaction.

Anaphylatoxin I and II

When fresh serum is treated with antigen-antibody complexes, histamine-releasing substances are produced which have been called *anaphylatoxins*. They are derived from the complement system and are believed to represent small split products from C'3 (anaphylatoxin I) and C'5 (anaphylatoxin II) (98). They have the potential of inducing smooth muscle contraction and increasing vascular permeability.

Noncytotoxic Complement-dependent Histamine Release

Rat mast cells possess a natural coat of rat gamma globulin. Treatment of these cells with an antibody to rat gamma globulin results in histamine release, if complement is present. Components C'1 through C'5 are required for such histamine release (105).

Immunologic Phenomena Associated with Human Diseases

These may also be considered tertiary manifestations of an antigen-antibody reaction. In this respect, there is much interest currently in the possible relationship between complement and renal disease. Lowered complement titers have been observed in acute nephritis, some forms of chronic nephritis and congenital nephrosis, in systemic lupus erythematosus and in plasma cell hepatitis associated with kidney damage, and in rejection of renal homografts (106–112). Moreover, complement as well as host gamma globulin has been found deposited in lesion sites in the glomeruli of acute poststreptococcal glomerulonephritis (113), lupus erythematosus (114), in hypersensitive vasculitis, and in the vessels of some cases of cryoglobulinemia (115).

Recently developed techniques for immunochemical quantitation of four complement system proteins (C'1q, C'3, C'4, C'5) have been shown to be sensitive and convenient procedures (116). When serial determinations of serum C'1q, C'3, C'4, and C'5 were carried out in patients with acute glomerulonephritis and systemic lupus erythematosus, subjects with these two disease states manifested distinctly different component alterations (117). In acute glomerulonephritis the concentration of C'1q was normal and that of C'4 was depressed only during the initial phase of illness. More prolonged depression of C'3 and C'5 occurred which paralleled the whole complement titers. The finding of normal complement levels usually preceded spontaneous resolution of disease. In contrast, subjects with active systemic lupus erythematosus had normal C'5 and decreased C'1q, C'3, and especially C'4. It appears that serial measurements of complement components may prove to be of important diagnostic and prognostic value in these and possibly other clinical conditions.

Hereditary Deficiency of Complement and Complement Inhibitors

A selective hereditary deficiency of C'2 has been reported in healthy individuals and appears to be transmitted as an autosomal recessive characteristic. Although the bactericidal and immune adherence activity of the serum from these individuals was markedly reduced, some residual activity persisted because total lack of C'2 would be expected to result in serious health impairment, especially with regard to resistance to infection (118,119).

Patients with hereditary angioneurotic edema have been shown to lack the serum α_2-globulin inhibitor of C'1a esterase. This condition is characterized by a recurrent, acute, circumscribed, and transient subepithelial edema of the skin and mucosa of the gastrointestinal and upper respiratory tracts. During clinical attacks, uninhibited C'1a elicits the reaction of angioedema, presumably by generation of an as yet unidentified vasoactive peptide (120). Purified C'1 esterase (C'1a) has been shown to cause increased vascular permeability in guinea pig skin (98).

In rabbits, a genetically controlled deficiency of C'6 has been demonstrated (121). The sera of these animals lack hemolytic and bactericidal action and are unable to generate the C'567 complex necessary for chemotaxic activity (122).

Studies of these hereditary complement deficiencies in humans and animals have yielded significant information regarding the biology of the respective components and will undoubtedly contribute to complement research in the future.

Experimentally Induced Complement Deficiencies

The possibility of inhibiting complement activity in order to suppress the consequences of an untoward immune response and to manipulate inflammation is an approach which promises to shed light on complement function in vivo and may ultimately be of therapeutic value. It has been demonstrated that cobra venom inactivates C′3 (123), and it is likely that anticomplementary factors exist elsewhere in nature. Such factors should facilitate the study of complement in vivo and provide better understanding of the role of complement in the immune response, a role that until now has been almost confined to observations necessarily made in vitro.

CONCLUDING STATEMENT

Some of the methods currently employed to detect and measure the interactions between antigen and antibody have been reviewed and considered in three general categories: primary, secondary, and tertiary. Although emphasis has been placed on information obtained from primary tests, it should be stressed that data derived from secondary and tertiary tests are also of great importance. The purpose of this emphasis on primary binding tests is to point out the value of having primary binding data to compare with the secondary and tertiary manifestations. Such comparisons are needed to clarify which immunologic and nonimmunologic factors are critical to the control of the secondary and especially the tertiary manifestations of tissue injury and/or protection.

REFERENCES

1. Springer, G. F., Williamson, P., and Brandes, W. C.: *J. Exp. Med.*, **113**: 1077, 1961.
2. Kim, Y. B., Bradley, S. G., and Watson, D. W.: *J. Immunol.*, **97**:52, 1966.
3. Rothberg, R. M., Kraft, S. C., and Farr, R. S.: *J. Immunol.*, **98**:386, 1967.
4. Kabat, E. A., and Mayer, M. M.: in "Experimental Immunochemistry," 2d ed., Charles C Thomas, Springfield, Ill., 1961.
5. Forsgren, A., and Sjöquist, J.: *J. Immunol.*, **97**:822, 1966.
6. Farr, R. S.: *J. Infect. Dis.*, **103**:239, 1958.

7. Grey, H. M.: *J. Immunol.*, **91**:90, 1963.
8. Mulligan, J. J., Jr., Osler, A. G., and Rodriguez, E.: *J. Immunol.*, **96**:324, 1966.
9. Osler, A. G., Mulligan, J. J., Jr., and Rodriguez, E.: *J. Immunol.*, **96**:334, 1966.
10. Talmage, D. W., and Maurer, P. H.: *J. Infect. Dis.*, **92**:288, 1953.
11. Altemeier, W. A., III, Robbins, J. B., and Smith, R. T.: *J. Exp. Med.*, **124**:443, 1966.
12. Ishizaka, T., Ishizaka, K., Salmon, S., and Fudenberg, H.: *J. Immunol.*, **99**:82, 1967.
13. Talmage, D. W., Freter, G. G., and Taliaferro, W. H.: *J. Infect. Dis.*, **98**:300, 1956.
14. Minden, P., and Farr, R. S.: in "Handbook of Experimental Immunology," D. M. Weir (ed.), F. A. Davis Company, Philadelphia, 1967.
15. Minden, P., Reid, R. T., and Farr, R. S.: *J. Immunol.*, **96**:180, 1966.
16. Linscott, W. D.: *Science*, **142**:1170, 1963.
17. Lidd, D., and Farr, R. S.: *J. Allergy*, **34**:48, 1963.
18. Talmage, D. W.: *J. Infect. Dis.*, **107**:115, 1960.
19. Grey, H. M.: *Immunology*, **7**:82, 1964.
20. McCarter, J. H., and Farr, R. S.: *Federation Proc.*, **21**:30, 1962.
21. Farr, R. S.: *Federation Proc.*, **16**:412, 1957.
22. Weigle, W. O., and Dixon, F. J.: *J. Immunol.*, **79**:24, 1957.
23. Dixon, F. J., Vazquez, J. J., Weigle, W. O., and Cochrane, C. G.: *AMA Arch. Pathol.*, **65**:18, 1958.
24. Dixon, F. J.: *Harvey Lecture Series*, **58**:21, 1962–63.
25. Weigle, W. O.: *J. Immunol.*, **87**:599, 1961.
26. Weigle, W. O.: *J. Immunol.*, **88**:9, 1962.
27. Weigle, W. O., and McConahey, P. J.: *J. Immunol.*, **88**:121, 1962.
28. Rothberg, R. M., and Farr, R. S.: *J. Allergy*, **36**:450, 1965.
29. Grey, H. M.: *J. Exp. Med.*, **115**:671, 1962.
30. Lidd, D., and Farr, R. S.: *J. Allergy*, **33**:45, 1962.
31. Lidd, D., and Connell, J. T.: *J. Allergy*, **35**:289, 1964.
32. Freter, R.: *J. Infect. Dis.*, **111**:25, 1962.
33. Kibler, R. F., and Barnes, A. E.: *J. Exp. Med.*, **116**:807, 1962.
34. Wold, R. T., Young, F. E., Tan, E. M., and Farr, R. S.: *Federation Proc.*, **27**:260, 1968.
35. Gupta, J. D., and Reed, C. E.: *J. Immunol.*, **98**:1093, 1967.
36. Cerottini, J. C.: *J. Immunol.*, **101**:433, 1968.
37. Grodsky, G. M., and Forsham, P. H.: *J. Clin. Invest.*, **39**:1070, 1960.
38. Grodsky, G. M., and Forsham, P. H.: *J. Clin. Invest.*, **40**:799, 1961.
39. Odell, W. D., Wilber, J. F., and Paul, W. E.: *J. Clin. Endocrinol.*, **25**:1179, 1965.
40. Feinberg, R.: *Federation Proc.*, **15**:586, 1956.
41. Skom, J. H., and Talmage, D. W.: *J. Clin. Invest.*, **37**:787, 1958.
42. Schalch, D. S., and Parker, M. L.: *Nature (London)*, **203**:1141, 1964.
43. Anthony, B. F.: Unpublished observations, 1968.

44. Fink, J. N., Patterson, R., and Pruzansky, J. J.: *J. Allergy*, **38**:84, 1966.
45. Farr, R. S., and Bloch, H.: *Amer. Rev. Resp. Dis.*, **82**:687, 1960.
46. Eisen, H. N., and Siskind, G. W.: *Biochemistry*, **3**:996, 1964.
47. Velick, S. F., Parker, C. W., and Eisen, H. N.: *Proc. Nat. Acad. Sci. U.S.*, **46**:1470, 1960.
48. Parker, C. W.: in "Handbook of Experimental Immunology," D. M. Weir, (ed.), F. A. Davis Company, Philadelphia, 1967.
49. Winkler, M.: *J. Mol. Biol.*, **4**:118, 1962.
50. Yoo, T. J., Roholt, O. A., and Pressman, D.: *Science*, **157**:707, 1967.
51. Dandliker, W. B., Schapiro, H. C., Meduski, J. W., Alonso, R., Feigen, G. A., and Hamrick, J. R., Jr.: *Immunochemistry*, **1**:165, 1964.
52. Dandliker, W. B.: in "Methods in Immunology and Immunochemistry," vol. III, M. W. Chase and C. A. Williams (eds.), in preparation, Academic Press, Inc., New York, 1968.
53. Dandliker, W. B., Schapiro, H. C., Alonso, R., and Williamson, D. E.: *Proc. San Diego Symp. Biomed. Eng., Session* **IV**: 1963.
54. Dandliker, W. B., and Levison, S. A.: *Immunochemistry*, **5**:171, 1968.
55. Dandliker, W. B., Halbert, S. P., Florin, M. C., Alonso, R., and Schapiro, H. C.: *J. Exp. Med.*, **122**:1029, 1965.
56. Marrack, J., and Smith, F. C.: *Brit. J. Exp. Pathol.*, **13**:394, 1932.
57. Eisen, H. N., and Karush, F.: *J. Amer. Chem. Soc.*, **71**:363, 1949.
58. Nisonoff, A., and Pressman, D.: *J. Immunol.*, **80**:417, 1958.
59. Pinckard, R. N., and Weir, D. M.: in "Handbook of Experimental Immunology," D. M. Weir, (ed.), F. A. Davis Company, Philadelphia, 1967.
60. Rothberg, R. M., and Farr, R. S.: *J. Immunol.*, **98**:792, 1967.
61. Hunter, W. M., and Greenwood, F. C.: *Biochem. J.*, **91**:43, 1964.
62. Genuth, S., Frohman, L. A., and Lebovitz, H. E.: *J. Clin. Endocrinol.*, **25**:1043, 1965.
63. Berson, S. A., Yalow, R. S., Bauman, A., Rothschild, M. A., and Newerly, K.: *J. Clin. Invest.*, **35**:170, 1956.
64. Yalow, R. S., and Berson, S. A.: *Methods Biochem. Analy.*, **12**:69, 1964.
65. Rosselin, G., Assan, R., Yalow, R. S., and Berson, S. A.: *Nature (London)*, **212**:355, 1966.
66. Herbert, V., Lau, K., Gottlieb, C. W., and Bleicher, S. J.: *J. Clin. Endocrinol.*, **25**:1375, 1965.
67. Lau, K., Gottlieb, C. W., and Herbert, V.: *Proc. Soc. Exp. Biol. Med.*, **123**:126, 1966.
68. Meyer, V., and Knobil, E.: *Endocrinology*, **80**:163, 1967.
69. Fitschen, W.: *Immunology*, **7**:307, 1964.
70. Heideman, M. L.: *Ann. N.Y. Acad. Sci.*, **121**:501, 1964.
71. Weir, R. C., and Porter, R. R.: *Biochem. J.*, **100**:69, 1966.
72. Minden, P., and Farr, R. S.: Unpublished observations, 1968.
73. Catt, K., and Tregear, G. W.: *Science*, **158**:1570, 1967.
74. Wide, L., and Porath, J.: *Biochim, Biophys. Acta*, **130**:257, 1966.
75. Talmage, D. W., and Freter, G. G.: *J. Infect. Dis.*, **98**:277, 1956.

76. Masouredis, S. P.: *J. Clin. Invest.*, **39**:1450, 1960.
77. Barnes, A. E., and Farr, R. S.: *Blood*, **21**:429, 1963.
78. Yagi, Y., Maier, P., Pressman, D., Arbesman, C. E., and Reisman, R. E.: *J. Immunol.*, **91**:83, 1963.
79. Terry, W. D., and Fahey, J. L.: *Science*, **146**:400, 1964.
80. Minden, P., Grey, H. M., and Farr, R. S.: *J. Immunol.*, **99**:304, 1967.
81. Coons, A. H., Creech, H. J., and Jones, R. N.: *Proc. Soc. Exp. Biol. Med.*, **47**:200, 1941.
82. Weller, T. H., and Coons, A. H.: *Proc. Soc. Exp. Biol. Med.*, **86**:789, 1954.
83. Gitlin, D., Landing, B. H., and Whipple, A.: *J. Exp. Med.*, **97**:163, 1953.
84. Holborow, E. J., and Johnson, G. D.: in "Handbook of Experimental Immunology," D. M. Weir (ed.), F. A. Davis Company, Philadelphia, 1967.
85. Lerner, R. A., Glassock, R. J., and Dixon, F. J.: *J. Exp. Med.*, **126**:989, 1967.
86. Minden, P., Anthony, B. F., and Farr, R. S.: *J. Immunol.*, **102**:832, 1969.
87. Farr, R. S., Campbell, D. H., and Vinograd, J.: *J. Immunol.*, **90**:619, 1963.
88. Bookman, R., and Shen, J.: *Proc. Soc. Exp. Biol. Med.*, **107**:542, 1961.
89. Ouchterlony., Ö.: *Progr. Allergy*, **5**:1, 1958.
90. Sever, J. L.: *J. Immunol.*, **88**:320, 1962.
91. Stavitsky, A. B.: *J. Immunol.*, **72**:360, 1954.
92. Benedict, A. A., Brown, R. J., and Ayengar, R.: *J. Exp. Med.*, **115**:195, 1962.
93. Ovary, Z.: *Progr. Allergy*, **5**:459, 1958.
94. Lindblad, J. H., and Farr, R. S.: *J. Allergy*, **32**:392, 1961.
95. Connell, J. T., and Sherman, W. B.: *J. Allergy*, **34**:409, 1963.
96. Müller-Eberhard, H. J., Nilsson, U. R., Dalmasso, A. P., Polley, M. J., and Calcott, M. A.: *Arch. Pathol.*, **82**:205, 1966.
97. Polley, M. J., and Müller-Eberhard, H. J.: *Progr. Hematol.*, **5**:2, 1966.
98. Müller-Eberhard, H. J.: *Advan. Immunol.*, **8**:1, 1968.
99. Lachmann, P. J., and Coombs, R. R. A.: in "Complement," G. E. W. Wolstenholme and J. Knight (eds.), Little, Brown and Company, Boston, 1965.
100. Coombs, R. R. A., Coombs, A. M., and Ingram, D. G.: in "The Serology of Conglutination and its Relation to Disease, Blackwell Scientific Publications, Oxford, 1961.
101. Nelson, D. S.: in "Complement," G. E. W. Wolstenholme and J. Knight (eds.), Little, Brown and Company, Boston, 1965.
102. Nelson, R. A., Jr.: in "The Inflammatory Process," B. W. Zweifach, L. Grant, and R. T. McCluskey (eds.), Academic Press, Inc., New York, 1965.

103. Ward, P. A., Cochrane, C. G., and Müller-Eberhard, H. J.: *Immunology*, **11**:141, 1966.
104. Cochrane, C. G.: *Advan. Immunol.*, **9**:97, 1968.
105. Becker, E. L., and Austen, K. F.: *Immunochemistry*, **3**:495, 1966.
106. Lange, K., Graig, F., Oberman, J., Slobody, L., Ogur, G., and LoCasto, F.: *Arch. Intern. Med.*, **88**:433, 1951.
107. Wedgwood, R. J. P., and Janeway, C. A.: *Pediatrics*, **11**:569, 1953.
108. West, C. D., Northway, J. D., and Davis, N. C.: *J. Clin. Invest.*, **43**: 1507, 1964.
109. Morse, J. H., Müller-Eberhard, H. J., and Kunkel, H. G.: *Bull. N.Y. Acad. Med.*, **38**:641, 1962.
110. Gewurz, H., Pickering, R. J., Muschel, L. H., Mergenhagen, S. E., and Good, R. A.: *Lancet*, **II**:356, 1966.
111. Gewurz, H., Page, A. R., Pickering, R. J., and Good, R. A.: *Int. Arch. Allergy*, **32**:64, 1967.
112. Rapp, H. J., and Borsos, T.: *J. A. M. A.*, **198**:1347, 1966.
113. Koffler, D., and Paronetto, F.: *J. Clin. Invest.*, **44**:1665, 1965.
114. Koffler, D., Schur, P. H., and Kunkel, H. G.: *J. Exp. Med.*, **126**:607, 1967.
115. Miescher, P. A., Paronetto, F., and Koffler, D.: in "Immunopathology," IVth International Symposium, P. Grabar and P. A. Miescher (eds.), Grune and Stratton, Inc., New York, 1965.
116. Kohler, P. F., and Müller-Eberhard, H. J.: *J. Immunol.*, **99**:1211, 1967.
117. Kohler, P. F., and ten Bensel, R.: *Clin. Exper. Immunol.*, **4**:191, 1969.
118. Klemperer, M. R., Woodworth, H. C., Rosen, F. S., and Austen, K. F.: *J. Clin. Invest.*, **45**:880, 1966.
119. Müller-Eberhard, H. J.: in "Bacterial and Mycotic Infections of Man, R. J. Dubos and J. G. Hirsch (eds.), Lippincott, Philadelphia, 1965.
120. Donaldson, V. H., and Evans, R. R.: *Amer. J. Med.*, **35**:37, 1963.
121. Rother, K., Rother, U., Müller-Eberhard, H. J., and Nilsson, U. R.: *J. Exp. Med.*, **124**:773, 1966.
122. Ward, P. A., Cochrane, C. G., and Müller-Eberhard, H. J.: *J. Exp. Med.*, **122**:327, 1965.
123. Klein, P. G., and Wellensiek, H. J.: *Immunology*, **8**:590, 1965.

13
Immunologic Protection

A principal function of the immune response is protection of the host against injurious foreign materials. Rigorous proof of this assertion is difficult, but there is no other ready explanation of the evolutionary development and persistence of a system which must involve a large number of genes and several unique genetic mechanisms (see Chap. 11). Most of the foreign materials are infectious organisms (bacteria, viruses, etc.) or their products (toxins). Humoral antibodies play the dominant role in protection against these agents. The system of cellular immunity, which may have delayed hypersensitivity as one of its manifestations, appears to play a subsidiary role. Another role for cellular immunity, the suppression of the genetically altered and thus presumably antigenically foreign cells that grow as malignant tumors, has been proposed. Therefore, a section on tumor immunology is included in this chapter.

Immunity, in the broadest sense, encompasses all the host's mechanisms of resistance. Thus, it encompasses much more than the system of humoral and cellular antibodies. In this chapter, the antibody system will be referred to as the *immune response* or as *specific acquired immunity*, in contrast to the broader term, *immunity*.

The general phenomena which will be examined in studying the protective effects of the immune response include

1. Specific acquired immunity—exposure of an animal to an injurious agent such as an infectious agent, toxin, or a transplantable tumor often results in an enhanced ability of the animal to resist a second challenge by the agent.

2. Immunization—specific acquired immunity can be produced artificially. Active immunity is produced by exposing the animal to the agent, which is often altered to make it less injurious (tetanus toxoid is produced by treating the toxin with formaldehyde, making it nontoxic but not affecting its antigenicity). Passive immunity results from the transfer of serum or globulin from an immune animal into a nonimmune one. It occurs naturally in the transfer of antibody from mother to offspring across the placenta or in colostrum.

3. Recovery from an infectious disease may correlate with the appearance of specific antibodies in the serum.

4. In vitro reactions of antibody with injurious agents are capable of neutralizing many agents. Neutralization of viruses, inactivation of toxins, lysis of some bacteria, and enhancement of phagocytosis of others are examples.

The interaction of host and parasite is a complex and changing one (see Chap. 1). It is influenced by a large number of factors in addition to the immune response, involving both the host and the parasite. The interplay of these factors, and thus the outcome of infection, varies with the nature of the host, the nature of the parasite, and the conditions of infection. In view of this interaction of numerous, often poorly understood factors, it is difficult to evaluate the role of the immune response in protection, and each combination of host and parasite must be considered separately. For example, immunization against anthrax provides protection for a variety of species, including sheep and mice. However, different antigens of the bacillus induce immunity in these two species, and the mechanism of protection is presumably also different (1). A large amount of work has defined many of these factors for a number of diseases in the past 50 years, but several other factors, and particularly many mechanisms of resistance and virulence, are still unclear.

Raffel (1) has proposed three criteria that should be met before resistance to an agent is attributed to the immune response. (1) Specific antibodies must be present in the blood of the immune animal. (2) Since many antibodies are known not to confer resistance to the organism inducing them, it must also be shown that serum from an immune animal can protect a previously nonimmune one. (3) Finally, the factor in the serum conferring this passive immunity should be shown to be antibody. If absorption of the serum, with the organism in question, removes the protective effect of the active factor, this can be assumed to be specific antibody. These criteria can be satisfied for many diseases, but the chain of evidence is not complete for many others in which the immune response is felt to play a role.

MECHANISMS OF IMMUNOLOGIC PROTECTION

While it is often difficult to confirm the protective role of the immune response in a particular disease, it is usually much more difficult to define the mechanism of this protection. From in vitro reactions of antibodies and injurious agents a number of potential mechanisms are apparent. Some of these can be shown to operate in vivo. For others the evidence is less convincing.

Phagocytosis

Since several of these mechanisms are effective by promoting the activity of phagocytes, a brief consideration of phagocytosis is included here.

The body normally rids itself of particulate foreign material by phagocytosis and subsequent lysosomal digestion. Phagocytosis is a specialized form of pinocytosis, the mechanism by which both fluids and particles are taken into cells for absorption (e.g., fat by the lining cells of the small intestine), nutrition, etc. Phagocytosis is performed by polymorphonuclear leukocytes (PMLs) and macrophage cells; the latter include monocytes in the bloodstream; the lining cells of the sinusoids of the liver, bone marrow, lymph nodes, and spleen; histiocytes within the various tissues; and mononuclear cells within the body cavities and the alveoli of the lungs. PMLs are brought into contact with foreign particles either directly in the bloodstream or more usually through a complex process of passage through vessel walls and attraction to the foreign substance. Changes in vessel walls permitting emigration of PMLs are a poorly understood part of the local inflammatory response to injury (2). The stimulation of nonrandom ameboid movement of phagocytes toward particles to be engulfed is called *chemotaxis*. The mechanism of chemotaxis is unknown, but the effect is produced on PMLs by a great variety of agents, including antigen-antibody complexes (3). Macrophages are often fixed and material is presented to them through the flow of blood or lymph, but migration of mononuclear cells into areas of tissue injury is also seen. Macrophages respond to somewhat different chemotactic stimuli than PMLs and at a different rate (4).

The actual engulfment of particles is similar in both macrophages and PMLs. The phagocyte, after making contact with the particle, enfolds it with cytoplasmic pseudopods. The membranes of these pseudopods then fuse to form a continuous membrane about the particle, thus enclosing it in a vacuole within the cytoplasm (2).

Following engulfment, lysosomes, which carry the hydrolytic enzymes needed for the degradation of organic materials and which are characteristic cytoplasmic features of phagocytes, fuse membranes with the vacuole containing the phagocytosed particle. Thus the particle is exposed to the lytic action of the enzymes (5). The exact mechanism of intracytoplasmic killing of bacteria is not clear. Some but not all phagocytes contain substances such as phagocytin and lysozyme which can kill bacteria, but which of these operate in vivo, and under what conditions, is not known.

Not all microorganisms are equally susceptible to phagocytosis, and once engulfed, not all are equally susceptible to lysis. Resistance offers an organism a great survival advantage, thereby enhancing its virulence. Several of the immunologic mechanisms discussed in the following paragraphs permit the host to overcome resistance to phagocytosis or intracellular killing, restoring the advantage to the phagocyte.

Opsonization

Humoral substances which promote phagocytosis are called *opsonins*, and the most important opsonins (but not the only ones) are specific antibodies (6). These play their most important role in infections by organisms with capsules which make them ordinarily resistant to phagocytosis. The capsules of virulent strains of pneumococci, streptococcci, klebsiella, and other bacteria prevent engulfment of the bacteria by phagocytes; the physicochemical mechanisms of this effect are unknown, but the property is an important virulence factor for these organisms. Strains that do not produce capsules are rapidly phagocytosed and killed; thus they are avirulent. Antibodies directed against the capsular antigens change the surface properties of the bacteria so that phagocytosis occurs readily. Opsonization is not limited to organisms which have capsules known to be important virulence factors; specific antibody enhances phagocytosis of numerous other organisms such as *E. coli* and the *Salmonella*.

The mechanism of opsonization by specific antibody is unknown. Extremely small amounts of antibody are effective, indicating that the whole organism does not have to be coated. IgM antibodies are much more effective than IgG; Rowley and Turner (7) have shown that 8 or fewer IgM molecules per bacterium will enhance phagocytosis of *Salmonella adelaide*, while about 2200 molecules of IgG are needed to produce the same effect. Complement mediates the opsonizing effect of specific antibody in at least some instances, but even without complement some opsonizing effect may still be retained (8).

After phagocytosis has occurred, organisms such as pneumococci and most streptococci are killed by lysosomal digestion. Other organisms such as mycobacteria, some staphylococci, brucellas, and salmonellas may survive and even reproduce and kill the phagocyte. Specific antibody appears to promote lysosomal destruction and prevent intracellular reproduction of at least some of these organisms (6,9). This effect is distinct from the enhancement of phagocytosis. Its mechanism is unknown. Another mechanism potentiating intracellular killing of these organisms, the acquired cellular immunity manifested by macrophages, complicates these studies and is discussed below.

In addition to promoting the actual engulfment of foreign material by phagocytes and enhancing lysosomal killing of organisms, antibody may play a further role in phagocytosis through chemotaxis, the nonrandom movement of phagocytes toward foreign materials. Antigen-antibody complexes have a strong chemotactic effect, mediated by the activation of complement (3,10).

Bactericidal and Bacteriolytic Actions of Antibody

In the presence of specific antibody, complement, lysozyme, and perhaps other serum factors many strains of gram-negative bacteria of the genera *Vibrio, Escherichia, Salmonella, Proteus, Shigella, Neisseria, Hemophilus* and *Brucella* are killed and subsequently lysed. The antibodies involved are directed against the somatic antigens of the organism (11), and only small amounts of antibody are needed (12). In many respects this process is similar to immune hemolysis (see Chap. 12); it is dependent on complement. Electron microscopic studies of lysed bacteria show holes in their walls essentially identical to the holes seen in lysed erythrocytes (12). Bacterial killing (i.e., inhibition of reproduction) is accomplished by antibody and complement and is probably enhanced by lysozyme. Under usual conditions in the in vitro studies summarized here lysis is accomplished by lysozyme present in the serum used (13). In the absence of lysozyme, lysis still occurs but is considerably delayed (12). The mechanism of killing and lysis, and the interaction of the factors involved, are poorly understood.

The bactericidal and bacteriolytic action of antibody would appear to be an ideal mechanism of host resistance, but it is extremely difficult to document its role in natural infections. Several considerations suggest its role may be limited. First, gram-positive bacteria and mycobacteria are not killed and lysed by antibody and complement. Second, the more virulent strains of the enteric organisms are often also resistant; those cultured from the blood of patients with gram-negative infections are nearly always so (14). Third, many infections by susceptible organisms are limited to the lumen of the intestine, where complement fixing antibodies may not be present and where complement may be unavailable or inactivated. Finally, at least in cholera, adsorption of the anti-O antibody, which possesses the lytic activity, from immune serum does not remove its protective effect (15).

Agglutination

Agglutination has been discussed in Chap. 12 as an in vitro method for the measurement of antibody titer. There is considerable evidence that it plays a role in vivo in the defense against infectious agents. Antibodies which confer protection by passive transfer against many organisms, both gram-positive and gram-negative, cause agglutination of the organisms. Both plague bacilli (*Pasteurella pestis*) and pneumococci injected into the skin of immune hosts remain localized instead of spreading as they do in nonimmune animals. They continue to multiply, however, and phagocytosis is required for their destruction and the clearing of the infection (16,17).

Inactivation of Toxins

Many biologic products are toxic to animals and man, often in very small amounts. The most important toxins are the exotoxins and endotoxins of many strains of bacteria. Other toxins include snake and bee venoms and toxins produced by various strains of fish. Most of these substances are proteins and are good antigens. Their toxic effects are neutralized by specific antibodies. That is, incubation of toxin and antitoxin before injection into a susceptible animal will protect the animal from an otherwise lethal dose of toxin.

The mechanism of this in vitro neutralization of toxin by specific antibody appears to be a direct result of the primary antigen-antibody reaction, not requiring precipitation or the action of complement (18,19). It does not involve irreversible alteration of toxin molecules, since toxic activity is regained after dissociation of the toxin-antitoxin complexes. In some cases, antibody may combine directly with the active site, but the evidence for this mode of action is poor. In at least some instances the antigenic site on the toxin molecule is clearly distinct from the active site. The two sites can be separated by trypsinization of the toxin of *Clostridium botulinum* (20). The inhibition of *C. welchii* lecithinase by antibody in the presence of substrate is noncompetitive (19). If the antigenic and toxic sites were identical, competitive inhibition would be expected. In these cases the antibody may change the configuration of the toxin molecule enough to inactivate the active site or it may prevent the toxin molecule from attaching to or entering its target cells.

The importance of fixation of toxin molecules to cells is illustrated by the failure of diphtheria antitoxin to prevent injury if it is added to cells in tissue culture after addition of diphtheria toxin (21). The same amount of antitoxin has an easily demonstrable neutralizing effect if it is added before or concurrently with the toxin.

The most dramatic actions of antitoxins are against the exotoxins of several gram-positive bacteria that produce disease almost exclusively by the action of the toxins they elaborate. Diphtheria, tetanus, and botulism are examples of these diseases. Immunization produces essentially complete protection in these cases, and passive immunity is conferred by administration of antisera. However, once the disease is manifest in a non-immune host, antisera are less effective and must be used in much greater amounts. This indicates that through fixation to cells or some other mechanism toxins rapidly become relatively resistant or inaccessible to antitoxins. Other enzymes elaborated by a variety of gram-positive bacteria, such as the fibrinolysins, are antigenic and are inactivated by specific antibodies. It seems likely that these substances play a role in the pathogenesis of disease, and therefore the antitoxic antibodies might be expected to provide protection (22). However, direct demonstrations of a pathogenic role for these enzymes or of a protective effect of antibodies to them are lacking.

Another important group of bacterial toxins are the endotoxins (see Chap. 9) which are released upon the death of many gram-negative bacteria. These substances are complex antigens and have multiple effects, both toxic and protective (23). In the intact bacterium they form the somatic or O antigens, and antibodies against them are often protective. Most studies, however, indicate that the isolated endotoxins, although they combine readily with specific antibodies, are not detoxified by them. Perhaps the antibodies do not combine with the toxic moieties of the endotoxin molecule (24). This paradoxical situation is further complicated by recent careful studies which demonstrate neutralization of several toxic effects of endotoxin from one strain of bacteria by specific antibody (25).

Virus Neutralization

The interaction of antibody with virus particles resulting in virus neutralization has been studied extensively. In order to discuss the subject meaningfully, we must first define the initial steps in the infection of a cell by a virus. Initially, virus particles are adsorbed onto the cell membrane. This is a specific combination between sites on the viral surface and receptors on the cell membrane. Next, virus penetration into the cell occurs by a process similar to pinocytosis or phagocytosis. The cell membrane extends about the virus and the resulting vesicle with its enclosed virus is released into the cytoplasm. Uncoating of the viral nucleic acid so that it can function in replication is then accomplished partially within the vesicle by lysosomal enzymes and apparently, in some cases, free in the cytoplasm after dissolution of the vesicle (26).

Neutralizing antibodies are directed against the viral envelope or coat proteins; antibodies are also formed against internal viral proteins but they play no known role in immunity (22). In the presence of an excess of antibody, adsorption is prevented by masking the sites on the virus which combine with the cell receptors. At lower antibody concentrations adsorption is not prevented, but neutralization still occurs (27). In poliomyelitis virus and in several others penetration does not occur (28). In vaccinia virus penetration occurs, but uncoating is delayed and accompanied by a loss of infectivity as a result of the degradation of viral DNA (26).

Kinetic analysis of the neutralization reaction of poliomyelitis and western equine encephalomyelitis viruses reveal one-hit kinetics (28). That is, one virus particle can be inactivated by a single antibody molecule. Despite this apparent simplicity, the interaction of neutralizing antibody with virus is a complex one. In some cases neutralization is potentiated by complement (29). Initially the antibody-virus complex formed is easily dissociated; later, dissociation is still possible but is much more difficult (30). This sequence probably reflects the combination of first one and then the second combining site of the antibody molecule to the virus. The attachment of both ends of antibody molecules to viruses has been shown by electron microscopy; the usually straight, rodlike antibody molecules are bent to permit the attachment (31). After dissociation of even firmly held antibody-virus complexes, viral infectivity is regained; the action of antibody apparently does not alter animal viruses irreversibly (32). Finally, a small fraction of a virus inoculum treated with neutralizing antibody forms a complex with the antibody but retains its infectivity (22). The significance of these findings in the pathogenesis of viral disease is not known.

Cellular Immunity

Cellular immunity is used here to denote the acquired capacity of macrophages to kill phagocytosed bacteria of strains that would resist intracellular killing in a nonsensitized host. The term must be defined, since it has also been used to denote the cellular mechanism involved in anti-tissue immunity (homograft and tumor rejection and possibly autoimmunity) and sometimes is used synonomously with the term *delayed hypersensitivity*. These three phenomena are closely related and may all be manifestations of a single basic process. But until this is demonstrated, a careful definition of terms is desirable. The relationship of cellular immunity and delayed hypersensitivity is discussed briefly below. Anti-tissue immunity is mentioned in the section on tumor immunology and discussed in greater detail in Chap. 14.

When an animal is infected with an organism which resists intracellular killing and can multiply within macrophages, such as *Mycobacterium tuberculosis, Brucella abortus, Listeria monocytogenes,* or *Salmonella typhimurium,* the animal's macrophages become activated and multiply and are subsequently able to kill the sensitizing organisms (6,33,34). There is a latent period of 4 days or more between infection and activation. This effect is a nonspecific one, for macrophages activated by one organism are resistant to a wide variety of organisms in addition to the one used to produce sensitization. Activation appears to result from an increase in lysosomes and lysosomal enzymes and, possibly, the development of new enzymes (35). The activated state persists as long as the inciting bacteria are present and disappears soon after they are destroyed. The mechanism by which the macrophages become sensitized is unknown.

Although activation itself is nonspecific, there is a highly specific anamnestic response which indicates the immunologic nature of the phenomenon (see Chap. 8). That is, after an animal has been sensitized and has recovered from an infection by one organism, a challenge with the same organism gives a much more rapid recurrence of resistance than occurred after the initial infection. Further, although resistance in both the primary and the secondary responses is nonspecific, the secondary response can be elicited only by the organism used to produce the primary response. While the primary response can be evoked only by injection of living organisms (except in the case of *M. tuberculosis*), the secondary response can be produced by killed organisms as well.

Many parallels between this form of cellular immunity and delayed hypersensitivity have been observed. Both can be transferred by cells but not by serum (6). This observation, plus the nonspecificity of the activated macrophages, eliminates the possibility that humoral antibody plays a role in the process. Delayed hypersensitivity is always demonstrable in the diseases characterized by cellular immunity, and the two phenomena develop at the same time (34). These and other similarities indicate a close relationship, and many observers believe cellular immunity and delayed hypersensitivity are different expressions of the same underlying response (36). However, no direct demonstration of this identity has been made, and differences between the two phenomena have also been observed. Lymphocytes are clearly involved as mediators of delayed hypersensitivity. They have not been shown to play a role in cellular immunity. Delayed hypersensitivity is very long-lasting, while the anamnestic period in cellular immunity is remarkably short. The relationship between delayed hypersensitivity and cellular immunity is not yet clear.

PROTECTION AGAINST BACTERIAL INFECTION

It is apparent from the discussion of mechanisms of protection that the nature of antibody defense against bacterial infection will depend on the nature of the particular organism and the pathogenesis of the disease it produces. Thus opsonization will hardly be effective in botulism, where the organism which produces the lethal toxin never enters the host. Nor will the course of tuberculosis be altered by an antitoxin, since the tubercle bacillus produces no toxins. Further, since our understanding of the pathogenesis of many bacterial diseases is incomplete, it is not surprising that the mechanisms of immunologic defense are often equally poorly understood. The following paragraphs will consider the current knowledge of protective mechanisms in several groups of infectious diseases.

A broad generalization that soon becomes apparent is that protective antibodies are often directed against virulence factors. All bacteria contain a number of antigenic substances and many elaborate antigenic products. The host forms antibodies against many of these antigens, but only a few of the antibodies provide protection. Most virulent organisms have one or more specific characteristics which cause injury or permit them to overcome the host's defense mechanisms. These virulence factors are often specific parts or products of the bacterium, such as the polysaccharide capsules of pneumococci which hinder phagocytosis or the neurotoxin of tetanus. The antibodies which provide protection in these and many other diseases are directed against these substances.

Four groups of bacterial diseases, each with different sets of virulence factors, will be discussed. These are (1) acute diseases, usually caused by gram-positive organisms, which are readily killed following phagocytosis and which possess capsules or other surface components which inhibit phagocytosis. Diseases caused by pneumococci, streptococci, and meningococci are examples. (2) Diseases in which toxins are the primary or sole virulence factors. These include tetanus, botulism, diphtheria, and gas gangrene. (3) Diseases caused by gram-negative enteric bacilli, such as typhoid fever, cholera, and shigellosis. The virulence factors of many of these organisms are poorly understood. Surprisingly, a role for endotoxins, which all of these organisms possess and which have such potent toxic properties, has not been clearly established. (4) Diseases caused by organisms which can survive and multiply within phagocytes. Tuberculosis is the most important disease in this group.

Pneumococcal pneumonia is the best studied of the acute diseases in group 1. Antibodies against the type-specific pneumococcal capsular polysaccharides provide protection on passive transfer and cause both agglutination and opsonization of the organisms (37). Unencapsulated pneumococci are avirulent, and antibodies against components of the organism other than the capsule do not confer immunity (1). In vitro studies show anticapsular antibodies are needed for phagocytosis of pneumococci in a fluid medium, although phagocytosis without opsonization will occur when the organism is "trapped" on a solid surface or against an adjacent cell (38). Finally, an animal depleted of leukocytes rapidly succumbs to pneumococcal infection despite prior immunization sufficient to protect normal animals (17). In experimental pneumococcal pneumonia the alveoli in the advancing margin of the lesion are filled with edema fluid containing proliferating organisms but few or no neutrophils. Later, neutrophils enter these alveoli and, when their concentration is great enough, trap the organisms against each other or against the alveolar walls and ingest them, even in the absence of opsonizing antibody (39). Meanwhile, the infection has spread by passage of pneumococci in the edema fluid through the pores of Cohn into adjacent alveoli. In immunized animals, the organisms in this advancing margin are clumped together and adhere to the alveolar walls, presumably through the action of agglutinating antibody, and spread of the lesion is slowed (39). The organisms are eventually killed by phagocytes.

This kind of proof of the roles of opsonization and agglutination is lacking in most other infectious diseases, even though opsonization and agglutination can be demonstrated in vitro. This does not mean that they (or other mechanisms) are not important in these diseases; rather, it reflects an incomplete understanding of the complex, interrelated factors that determine the course of most infections.

Anticapsular antibodies also protect against meningococcal infections through opsonization and possibly agglutination. Lysis of meningococci by antibody and complement occurs in vitro, but its role in infection has not been demonstrated (22). Streptococci have antigenic, antiphagocytic surface components. In the group A streptococci these are called *the M proteins*; antibodies against them confer immunity, while antibodies against other cell components do not (40).

Antitoxic immunity is highly effective against the second group of diseases. No other antibody defense mechanism can be effective against botulism, in which only the toxin enters the host. Problems in treatment arise because the disease is so uncommon that mass immunization is impractical. Passive immunity by means of antitoxins must be given early in the course of the disease to be effective. The three strains of toxin are antigenically distinct, so that antisera to all three must be used (41). The organisms of diphtheria, gas gangrene, and tetanus are all present in the affected host, but antitoxic immunity alone is sufficient to control the diseases. In the first two local injury from the toxins is needed for the continued growth of the organisms in tissue. There is some evidence, however, that in diphtheria antibacterial as well as antitoxic antibodies can provide a degree of protection (42).

The gram-negative enteric bacilli all have lipopolysaccharide antigens, termed O antigens, which form a part of the endotoxin molecule released when the bacilli die. In general, antibodies against the O antigens promote phagocytosis, cause bacteriolysis in the presence of complement, and induce agglutination. They provide protection on passive transfer. Some strains also have a capsular polysaccharide, the Vi antigen, which also induces protective antibodies. The antibodies formed against the H, or flagellar, antigens possessed by some of the enteric bacilli are not protective. The mechanisms of protection provided by anti-O and anti-Vi antibodies are not known. Among the problems involved are the correspondence of antibody levels in the serum and the intestinal contents where many of the infections occur and the determination of the activity of both antibody and complement in the intestine. Although the anti-O antibodies are directed against a portion of the endotoxin molecule and are protective, it is questionable if the protection results from inactivation of endotoxin. First, the role of endotoxin in the pathogenesis of the enteric diseases has not been established, and second, most investigators have found that antibodies against O antigens inactivate endotoxin only slightly or not at all (43). The problem of immunity to *Salmonella typhosa* is complicated by its ability to survive lysosomal digestion by macrophages. The protection from humoral antibody which the *Salmonella* attains in this fashion is probably countered by the cellular immunity developed by the macrophage (44).

Diseases caused by bacteria which can survive and multiply within phagocytes tend to be chronic, perhaps because of the protected environment the organisms adopt. Mechanisms of both pathogenesis and of immunity have been difficult to study, and there is much conflicting evidence and opinion. Tuberculosis is the most important, most studied, and most controversial of these diseases. Only a few broad conclusions from a vast literature can be presented here, and it should be emphasized that while most of them are generally accepted, most are also challenged vigorously by at least a few investigators. First, and without question, acquired immunity develops following a first exposure to the tubercle bacillus (45). A wide variety of humoral antibodies are formed against the organism, but these have not been shown to be protective, and immunity cannot be transferred by serum (46). The cellular immunity provided by activation of macrophages is induced by tubercle bacilli and is paralleled by the development of delayed hypersensitivity (36). If, as many believe, cellular immunity and delayed hypersensitivity are two aspects of the same phenomenon, the role of cellular immunity in tuberculosis is open to question because desensitization can abolish delayed hypersensitivity, both local and systemic, without abolishing tuberculoimmunity. However, the phenomena might be dissociated in desensitization or they may not be that closely related. Cellular immunity remains the best available explanation for acquired immunity in tuberculosis. It is also the most likely mechanism of immunity in the other bacterial diseases in this group (and, incidentally, in many fungus diseases), although humoral antibodies also appear to play a role in diseases such as typhoid fever and probably, brucellosis.

To conclude the discussion of immunity in bacterial diseases, we must consider the extent and duration of immunity and the efficacy of vaccination. Immunity is complete and long lasting, and vaccination is highly effective, in the "toxin" diseases such as diphtheria and tetanus. Immunity is much less complete in a number of diseases including tuberculosis; both prior tuberculous infection and vaccination with an avirulent strain of tubercle bacilli (BCG) fail to protect a significant proportion of those exposed (47). The large number of antigenically different strains of organisms such as pneumococci and streptococci, in which the antigens in question are the ones which induce protective antibodies, make acquired immunity against all pneumococcal or streptococcal organisms virtually impossible. Further, while immunity against a given strain of streptococci appears to be very long lasting, immunity against pneumococci lasts only a few months.

It is clear that generalizations about immunity in bacterial disease are hazardous, and the reasons for the dramatic variations cited above are obscure.

PROTECTION AGAINST VIRAL INFECTION

The fact that lifelong immunity is conferred by a single attack of many virus diseases has long been known. Human diseases in which this nearly absolute protection is found include smallpox, poliomyelitis, chicken pox, measles, and many others. Similar long-term immunity can be induced by immunization against many of these diseases, and most of the highly effective vaccines available today are for viral diseases. Other viruses, such as influenza, herpes simplex, and cold viruses, induce only partial or short-term immunity, and vaccines against them are of limited effectiveness.

To examine the nature and mechanism of protection against viral diseases, we must consider several features of virus infections. First, viruses are intracellular parasites and are accessible to attack by antibodies only before penetration of the cell or after release of virus progeny from it. Further, many viruses are usually confined to the cells of mucosal surfaces (influenza, adenoviruses), where they are relatively protected from anti-bodies in the blood. They are exposed, however, to IgA immunoglobulins, which are secreted by the salivary glands and the respiratory and gastro-intestinal mucosa. Other viruses spread from a portal of entry to target organs elsewhere in the body, with one or two viremic phases while they are spreading. Fenner (48) has shown this most elegantly for ectromelia, a disease of mice caused by a virus similar to that of herpes and smallpox. The mousepox virus enters through a break in the skin, multiplies locally, and spreads to the regional lymph nodes. It is next released into the bloodstream (primary viremia) and spreads to the visceral organs. A secondary viremia then occurs, followed by localization of the virus in the skin, the appearance of a rash, and the clinical onset of disease. The time between the introduction of virus and the clinical onset of disease is called the *incubation period*. Finally, some viruses can persist in tissues for very long periods of time without producing any overt symptoms of disease.

Although the data are not always complete or convincing, viral immunity appears to be the result of the induction of circulating antibodies. The evidence for this includes the following: (1) Antiviral antibodies are usually present in the blood of immune animals, and the titer usually corresponds roughly with the degree of immunity. (2) Antibodies from immunized animals will neutralize viruses; that is, antibodies directed against a given virus will render it noninfectious if the antibody is mixed with the virus prior to introduction of the virus into a susceptible host (or tissue culture preparation). (3) Passive transfer of antibody by the injection of serum or gamma globulin from an immune animal to a susceptible one provides protection against subsequent viral infection (1).

The protective role of cellular immunity is much less well established.

Many viral infections induce delayed hypersensitivity, and in some cases the time of onset or the intensity of the hypersensitivity reaction correlates better with the level of immunity than does the level of serum antibody. Also, patients with agammaglobulinemia, who do not respond to antigenic stimulation with detectable levels of serum antibodies but who do manifest delayed hypersensitivity, usually recover from viral illnesses as readily as normal subjects do and rarely have recurrent attacks of the virus diseases known to confer lifelong immunity (49). This rather surprising finding certainly casts doubt on the role of circulating antibodies in resistance to viruses, but it cannot be taken as more than suggestive evidence for a role for cellular immunity. "Agammaglobulinemics" have very small amounts of globulin in their serum, and it is possible that they give an antibody response which is too feeble to be detected (50).

Thus there is strong evidence that protection against a second attack of a viral disease has an immunologic basis. In contrast, the role of these immunologic mechanisms in the recovery from viral infections is much less clear. In an established infection viruses are protected from antibody by their intracellular location. Further, they can spread from cell to cell by way of intercellular bridges without being exposed to the extracellular environment (51). While recovery and fall in virus titer parallel the appearance of serum antibody in some instances, in others, such as influenza, recovery is well underway before antibody can be detected. This recovery is presumably mediated by interferon and other nonantibody protective mechanisms. Such mechanisms must also account for recovery from viral infections in tissue cultures (52).

We are now in a position to consider the different patterns of immunity in different viral diseases. Although there are exceptions, some of which we will discuss below, there are three pertinent differences between virus diseases which induce long-lasting immunity and those which do not. First, antibody titers persist much longer following the infections that give long-lasting immunity. Second, most of these diseases are characterized by viremia and dissemination of virus to target organs distant from the point of introduction of the virus, while the viral infections which induce only short-term or partial immunity are usually localized to a mucosal surface, such as the respiratory tract, and do not disseminate. Third, the induction period is longer for the diseases giving lasting immunity (53).

The persistence of antibody titers for years after an original infection implies continued antigenic stimulation. In diseases like chickenpox, which are endemic in the community, this might come from exposure to infected individuals. In nonendemic diseases, such as yellow fever, however, it is more reasonable to postulate latent viral infection. Such latent infection has been demonstrated for adenoviruses and herpes simplex, as well as many tumor viruses (22). Adenoviruses were first discovered in explants of human adenoid tissue grown in tissue culture (54,55). By this technique they can now be demonstrated in up to 85 percent of those individuals tested. The virus is present in the adenoids, but in some fashion its growth is suppressed so that it is not producing disease; in tissue culture this suppression is released, and viral replication and cytopathic changes result. Antiviral antibodies may play a role in the suppression of viral replication resulting in some latent viral infections, but this has not been clearly demonstrated.

In localized viral infections without a viremic phase the virus is less exposed to antibody before it penetrates the cells of the target organ than is the virus in a disseminated virus disease such as measles. Such localized infections may also provide less intense antigenic stimulation in the initial infection. IgA immunoglobulins are secreted onto the mucosal surfaces, which are the sites of most localized infections, and probably play a major role in controlling them (56). Almost all people have latent infections from herpes simplex and have specific antibodies against the virus; in some persons the latent virus is activated to produce "cold sores" or "fever blisters" by various kinds of stresses. Susceptible individuals appear to have lower IgA antibodies for herpes simplex than nonsusceptible individuals (57).

The incubation period in viral infections that produce lasting immunity is a long one, usually lasting from 7 to 21 days. In this period the virus is being disseminated by the bloodstream from the point of entry to the target organs. If it can be neutralized by antibody during this time, recurrent infection might be prevented. With a long incubation period, there is sufficient time for a previously sensitized host to mount a secondary response and attain an adequate antibody titer. On the other hand, most of the localized viral diseases which produce only short-term immunity have short incubation periods of from 2 to 4 days. This is not long enough to produce the necessary secondary response before the virus has entered the cells of the target organs and is thus protected against the action of antibody. A final factor influencing patterns of immunity to viral diseases is the tendency for some viruses to change their antigenic composition by mutation. This is a particularly striking property of influenza virus (58). These various hypotheses to explain the different patterns of immunity to viral diseases are not mutually exclusive, and probably several different mechanisms operate in different diseases.

The protective effect of antiviral antibody probably comes from its virus-neutralizing capacity. Other possible modes of action, such as agglutination of viral particles, could conceivably play a role, but these have not been studied adequately. Phagocytosis of influenza virus by mouse leuko-cytes is enhanced by the presence of immune serum, indicating that viral antibodies can act as opsonins. Infective influenza virus is cleared more rapidly from the peritoneal cavity in immune than nonimmune mice (59), but this may be the result of virus neutralization or of cellular immunity rather than opsonization.

TUMOR IMMUNOLOGY

In the past decade tumor specific antigens, that is, antigens present in tumor cells but not in the tissues of the tumor-bearing host, have been shown conclusively in a wide variety of tumors in experimental animals. The nature of these antigens and of the host response to them, the mecha-nism of tumor rejection, and the significance of these phenomena in carcinogenesis have become areas of active investigation (60).

Tumor antigens were first shown by the ability of a sensitized animal to reject a transplanted tumor. Briefly, if a malignant tumor, induced in an animal of a highly inbred strain, is transplanted into an animal of the same strain that previously has been sensitized to the tumor, the sensitized host may reject the transplanted tumor (61,62). This is an immunologic phenomenon comparable to homograft rejection. It suggests that im-munologic mechanisms may play a role in host defenses against cancer. In addition to these "transplantation" antigens, other tumor antigens have been demonstrated in virus-induced tumors by techniques such as com-plement fixation and immunofluorescence (63).

Studies in the early part of this century demonstrated rejection of transplanted tumors by sensitized recipients and aroused optimism about the possibility of a "cancer vaccine." Subsequently, however, these results were shown to be caused by differences in histocompatibility antigens be-tween the normal tissues of the donor and recipient animals rather than a reaction to tumor specific antigens (64). What was thought to be specific rejection of tumors was simply homograft rejection. Thus the demonstra-tion of tumor antigens awaited the development of inbred strains of ani-mals, in which the genetic (and thus the antigenic) identity of donor and host animals eliminated the overriding effect of histocompatibility antigens. This problem has prevented the conclusive demonstration of tumor anti-gens in human cancers, although there is no reason to doubt their existence.

Tumor-specific antigens have been found in nearly every experimental tumor in which they have been sought. This includes spontaneously aris-ing tumors as well as those induced by chemical carcinogens and viruses (60). An important distinction must be drawn between the virus-induced tumors and those induced by chemical carcinogens. Different tumors, even tumors induced in different species, have common antigens if they are induced by the same virus. Different tumors induced by chemical carcinogens, even tumors induced by the same carcinogen in the same animal, have distinctive antigens that do not cross-react with each other.

The antigens of carcinogen-induced tumors have been detected by the rejection of transplanted tumors and thus are referred to as *transplantation antigens*. They presumably reside on the cell surface. Their chemical nature is unknown. The diversity of transplantation antigens in carcinogen-induced tumors is indicated not only by their failure to cross-react, but also by the great variation in antigenicity exhibited by different tumors. Although sensitization with cells of some tumors produces a high degree of immunity to subsequent challenge with the tumor, cells from other tumors have little or no immunizing capacity (65). Tumors that have a short latent period, i.e., a short time between application of the carcinogen and development of the tumor, may be strongly or weakly antigenic. On the other hand, tumors with a long latent period are uniformly weakly antigenic. This is probably evidence of immunoselection by the host; all the chemical carcinogens are also immunosuppressive agents, and the tumors which arise rapidly while the host is less responsive may be either strongly or weakly antigenic. Tumors arising later are all weakly antigenic, since those with strong antigens are eliminated in an incipient stage by the now fully reactive host (66).

Antigens in virus-induced tumors, in contrast to those caused by carcinogens, are specific for the inducing virus. In addition to transplantation antigens, other (or possibly the same) cell surface antigens can be demonstrated by the lysis of leukemia cells on incubation with complement and the serum of immunized animals (67). Intracellular antigens can be shown by complement fixation, precipitation in gel, and by immunofluorescence in solid tumors induced by viruses (63). Since they are specific for the inducing virus, antigens in these tumors are probably coded for in the viral genome. They are not part of the virus particle, however.

The immune response mounted against a tumor by the host animal may be manifold. The capacity to reject transplanted solid tumors can be transferred by lymphoid cells from a sensitized animal, but not by serum. Although there have been suggestions that humoral antibodies may play an ancillary role in the rejection process, cellular immunity clearly plays the predominant role, and a humoral response to the carcinogen-induced neoplasms has not been demonstrated. In the RNA virus–induced lymphomas, however, where sensitized animals have been shown to produce antibody which is cytolytic in the presence of complement, humoral antibody appears to play the major role in the rejection process (60). The serum antibodies formed against intracellular antigens of virus-induced tumors have not been shown to play a role in rejection.

The primary host, that is, the animal in which the tumor arose, can be shown to mount an immune response to his tumor (68). Even in highly antigenic tumors, however, the response is not sufficient to cause regression of the tumor. If a sarcoma induced by a carcinogen is excised from the primary host, the animal will subsequently resist a challenge by his tumor. This resistance is relative and can be overcome if the challenge dose of tumor cells is very large. If the tumor is not excised it will continue to grow and will eventually kill the host.

The possibility remains, however, that animals (and man) reject incipient tumors, which are never detected. Only tumors which can overcome the host's immunologic defenses grow to detectable size, and these may represent only a small fraction of both experimentally induced and spontaneous tumors. The low antigenicity of carcinogen-induced tumors with a long latent period, interpreted above as evidence of immunoselection, is consistent with this hypothesis. On serial transplantation, similar tumors become less antigenic, presumably through immunoselection of less antigenic clones of tumor cells (66). Further support for the hypothesis comes from the study of polyoma virus tumors. Newborn mice infected with the virus develop tumors, while older mice with a fully developed immune mechanism do not (69). The infected older mice are more resistant to transplanted polyoma tumors than noninfected mice, however, suggesting that the infection has given rise to tumor specific antigens which have sensitized the mice, even though detectable tumors have not developed. Neonatal thymectomy increases the susceptibility of older mice and of mice from several relatively resistant strains to tumor induction by polyoma virus (70).

In summary, tumor-specific antigens have been found in experimental animals and probably are present in human tumors. The host organism mounts an immunologic response similar to homograft rejection against the tumor. This response is insufficient to control fully established tumors, but may suppress many tumors in incipient stages of development.

REFERENCES

1. Raffel, S.: "Immunity," 2d ed., Appleton Century Crofts, New York, 1961.
2. Hirsch, J. G.: *Annu. Rev. Microbiol.*, **19**:339, 1965.
3. Boyden, S.: *J. Exp. Med.*, **115**:453, 1962.
4. Ward, P. A.: *J. Exp. Med.*, **128**:1201, 1968.
5. Zucker-Franklin, D., and Hirsch, J. G.: *J. Exp. Med.*, **120**:569, 1964.

6. Suter, E., and Ramseier, H.: *Advan. Immunol.*, **4**:117, 1964.
7. Rowley, D., and Turner, K. J.: *Nature (London)*, **210**:496, 1966.
8. Rowley, D., Thöni, M., and Isliker, H.: *Nature (London)*, **207**:210, 1965.
9. Li, I. W., and Mudd, S.: *J. Immunol.*, **97**:41, 1966.
10. Ward, P. A., Cochrane, C. G., and Müller-Eberhard, H. J.: *Immunology*, **11**:141, 1966.
11. Muschel, L. H.: in "Complement," G. E. W. Wolstenholme and J. Knight (eds.), Little, Brown and Company, Boston, 1965.
12. Glynn, A. A., and Milne, C. M.: *Immunology*, **12**:639, 1967.
13. Glynn, A. A., and Milne, C. M.: *Nature (London)*, **207**:1309, 1965.
14. Roantree, R. J., and·Pappas, N. C.: *J. Clin. Invest.*, **39**:82, 1960.
15. Burrows, W., Mather, A. N., Elliott, M. E., and Havens, I.: *J. Infect. Dis.*, **81**:157, 1947.
16. Meyer, K. F.: *J. Immunol.*, **64**:139, 1950.
17. Rich, A. R., and McKee, C. M.: *Bull. Johns Hopkins Hosp.*, **54**:277, 1934.
18. Marrack, J. R.: *Int. Arch. Allergy*, **2**:264, 1951.
19. Cinader, B.: *Annu. Rev. Microbiol.*, **11**:371, 1957.
20. Sugiyama, H., von Mayerhauser, B., Gogat, G., and Heimsch, R. C.: *Proc. Soc. Exp. Biol. Med.*, **126**:690, 1967.
21. Lennox, E. S., and Kaplan, A. S.: *Proc. Soc. Exp. Biol. Med.*, **95**:700, 1957.
22. Davis, B. D., Dulbecco, R., Eisen, H. N., Ginsberg, H. S., and Wood, W. B., Jr.: "Microbiology," Harper & Row, New York, 1967.
23. Freedman, H. H., and Sultzer, B. M.: *Ann. N.Y. Acad. Sci.*, **133**:580, 1966.
24. Neter, E., Westphal, O., Lüderitz, O., Gorzynski, E. A., and Eichenberger, E.: *J. Immunol.*, **76**:377, 1956.
25. Radvany, R., Neale, N. L., and Nowotny, A.: *Ann. N.Y. Acad. Sci.*, **133**:763, 1966.
26. Dales, S.: *Progr. Med. Virol.*, **7**:1, 1965.
27. Fazekas de St. Groth, S.: *Advan. Virus Res.*, **9**:1, 1962.
28. Dulbecco, R., Vogt, M., and Strickland, A. G. R.: *Virology*, **2**:162, 1956.
29. Heineman, H. S.: *J. Immunol.*, **99**:214, 1967.
30. Lafferty, K. J.: *Virology*, **21**:76, 1963.
31. Lafferty, K. J., and Oertelis, S.: *Virology*, **21**:91, 1963.
32. Mandel, B.: *Virology*, **14**:316, 1961.
33. Mackaness, G. B., and Blanden, R. V.: *Progr. Allergy*, **11**:89, 1967.
34. Mackaness, G. B.: *Brit. Med. Bull.*, **23**:52, 1967.
35. Saito, K., and Suter, E.: *J. Exp. Med.*, **121**:727, 1965.
36. Mackaness, G. B.: *Amer. Rev. Resp. Dis.*, **97**:337, 1968.
37. Wood, W. B., Jr.: *The Harvey Lectures, Ser.* **47**:72, 1951–52.
38. Wood, W. B., Jr., Smith, M. R., and Watson, B.: *Science*, **104**:28, 1946.
39. Wood, W. B., Jr.: *J. Exp. Med.*, **73**:201, 1941.
40. McCarty, M.: in "Bacterial and Mycotic Infections of Man, 3d ed. R. J. Dubos (ed.), J. B. Lippincott Company, Philadelphia, 1958.

41. Lamanna, C.: *Science*, **130**:763, 1959.
42. Frobisher, M., Jr., and Parsons, E. I.: *Amer. J. Hyg.*, **52**:239, 1950.
43. Kim, Y. B., and Watson, D. W.: *Ann. N.Y. Acad. Sci.* **133**:727, 1966.
44. Blanden, R. V., Mackaness, G. B., and Collins, F. M.: *J. Exp. Med.*, **124**: 585, 1966.
45. Rich, A. R.: "The Pathogenesis of Tuberculosis," 2d ed., Charles C Thomas, Springfield, Ill., 1951.
46. Raffel, S.: in "Experimental Tuberculosis," Ciba Foundation Symposium, Little, Brown and Company, Boston, 1955.
47. Aronson, J. D., and Aronson, C. F.: *JAMA*, **149**:334, 1952.
48. Fenner, F.: *Lancet*, **II**:915, 1948.
49. Gitlin, D., Janeway, C. A., Apt, L., and Craig, J. M.: in "Cellular and Humoral Aspects of the Hypersensitive States," H. S. Lawrence (ed.), Harper & Row, New York, 1959.
50. Baron, S., Nasou, J. P., Friedman, R. M., Owen, G. M., Levy, H. B., and Barnett, E. V.: *J. Immunol.*, **88**:443, 1962.
51. Baron, S.: *Advan. Virus Res.*, **10**:39, 1963.
52. Glasgow, L. A., and Habel, K.: *J. Exp. Med.*, **115**:503, 1962.
53. Hale, J. H.: *Advan. Immunol.*, **1**:263, 1961.
54. Hilleman, M. R., and Werner, J. H.: *Proc. Soc. Exp. Biol. Med.*, **85**:183, 1954.
55. Rowe, W. P., Huebner, R. J., Gilmore, L. K., Parrott, R. H., and Ward, T. G.: *Proc. Soc. Exp. Biol. Med.*, **84**:570, 1953.
56. Hobson, D.: *Mod. Trends Immunol.*, **2**:53, 1967.
57. Tokumaru, T.: *J. Immunol.*, **97**:248, 1966.
58. Andrewes, C. H.: *Advan. Virus Res.*, 4:1, 1957.
59. Hanson, R. J., Kempf, J. E., and Boand, A. V., Jr.: *J. Immunol.*, **79**:422, 1957.
60. Smith, R. T.: *New Engl. J. Med.*, **278**:1207, 1268, 1326, 1968.
61. Foley, E. J.: *Cancer Res.*, **13**:835, 1953.
62. Prehn, R. T., and Main, J. M.: *J. Nat. Cancer Inst.*, **18**:769, 1957.
63. Old, L. J., and Boyse, E. A.: *Med. Clinics N. Amer.*, **50**:901, 1966.
64. Klein, G.: *Cancer Res.*, **19**:343, 1959.
65. Globerson, A., and Feldman, M.: *J. Nat. Cancer Inst.*, **32**:1229, 1964.
66. Prehn, R. T.: *Cancer Res.*, **28**:1326, 1968.
67. Sjögren, H. O.: *Progr. Exp. Tumor Res.*, **6**:289, 1965.
68. Klein, G., Sjögren, H. O., Klein, E., and Hellström, K. E.: *Cancer Res.*, **20**:1561, 1960.
69. Hattler, B., Jr., and Amos, B.: *Mongr. Surg. Sci.*, **3**:1, 1966.
70. Ting, R. C., and Law, L. W.: *Progr. Exp. Tumor Res.*, **9**:165, 1967.

14
Immunologic Injury

As discussed in Chap. 13, acquired antibodies have a protective action and are effective in combating viral and bacterial diseases.

The study of human and animal pathology has disclosed, however, many disease states and pathological entities which are mediated by immune reactions. The allergic manifestations of hay fever and asthma are brought about by antigen-antibody reactions, with secondary neurohumoral events leading to cell injury and inflammatory processes. Necrotic lesions due to vascular injury follow delayed hypersensitivity reactions in which cell-bound antibodies become important. Finally, a host of disease processes have been described which appear to be related to the effect of antibodies on cells and tissues. These include the so-called autoimmune diseases, involving a large number of tissues, organs, and systems; both humoral antibodies and cell-bound antibodies appear to play a role in their etiology and pathogenesis.

This chapter is a brief discussion of some of these processes and of what is known of their underlying mechanisms.

IMMEDIATE HYPERSENSITIVITY

The term *anaphylaxis* was first described in 1902 by Portier and Richet (1), who had been studying antitoxic immunity in dogs. They found that some dogs previously immunized with an extract of sea anemones exhibited severe symptoms and died when they were reinjected with a sublethal dose of poison. Since this phenomenon was contrary to immunity, in which animals are in a prophylactic state, they called the phenomenon *anaphylaxie*.

The anaphylactic state can be induced in many experimental animals, such as guinea pigs, rabbits, dogs, rats, and mice, by immunization (sensitization) with antigen. For example, guinea pigs receiving an injection of antigen exhibit anaphylactic shock when the same substance is reinjected intravenously 10 days to 3 weeks later. The interval between the first and second injection necessary for the induction of anaphylaxis is correlated with the time of antibody formation. In rats and mice, the interval is shorter when antigens are injected along with certain adjuvants. As will be described below, the short interval is due to a transient formation of anaphylactic antibodies in the animal species in the early stages of immunization. Anaphylaxis can also be induced passively by the administration of antiserum. The anaphylactic state induced by active sensitization of animals by antigen is called *active anaphylaxis* and that obtained by the administration of antibody is called *passive anaphylaxis*. In active anaphylaxis, the first injection of antigen is called the *sensitizing injection* and the second injection is named the *shocking dose*. After receiving a sublethal shocking dose of antigen, sensitized animals become specifically refractory to the antigen used. This phenomenon, called *desensitization*, is due to neutralization of antibody.

In passive anaphylaxis, antibody is administered to animals and is followed by an intravenous injection of antigen 24 to 48 hours later. As will be described later, anaphylactic shock can be elicited by the injection of antigen followed by antibody within a day when antigen is IgG-immunoglobulin from certain animal species. This type of reaction is called *reversed passive anaphylaxis*.

Allergic reactions are now classified into immediate- and delayed-type reactions. Anaphylaxis and Arthus-type reactions are immediate-type allergies. An important difference between immediate- and delayed-type reactions is that an immediate type of allergic state can be transferred passively by serum from a sensitized animal (both anaphylactic and Arthus-type), whereas the passive transfer of delayed-type reactions requires lymphoid cells from sensitized animals and cannot be achieved by their serum. Originally, anaphylaxis comprised those types of allergic reactions of which the manifestations began within a few minutes after the combination of antigen with antibody in vivo. Therefore, it included a variety of allergic reactions with respect to the mechanisms involved. However, the typical anaphylaxis, represented by the reactions in guinea pigs, is different from Arthus-type reactions in many respects. Immunologically, anaphylactic reactions are induced by a combination of antigen with cell-bound antibody, and therefore, the sensitization process involves "fixation" of antibodies to certain cells. Even though the same reactions can be elicited experimentally by preformed antigen-antibody complexes, there is evidence that the complexes combine to the same cells through antibody molecules. Sensitization in Arthus-type reactions does not involve the fixation of antibodies to these cells. Since most of the previous work on anaphylaxis has been carried out in guinea pigs using rabbit IgG antibodies, which elicit both anaphylactic and Arthus-type reactions, differentiation of the two reactions is difficult. However, recent studies clearly show that the properties of antibodies required for anaphylaxis and Arthus reactions are different and that anaphylactic antibodies in homologous animal species are different from those responsible for Arthus-type reactions with respect to the immunoglobulin class. It is now apparent that anaphylaxis and Arthus-type reactions are elicited by entirely different mechanisms.

So-called reaginic hypersensitivity reactions in humans have been classified independently. As will be described later, however, evidence has been accumulated that the immune mechanisms involved in reaginic hypersensitivity are similar to those of anaphylaxis in experimental animals. Therefore, both anaphylaxis and reaginic hypersensitivity will be discussed in this section.

Systemic and Local Anaphylaxis

Anaphylactic shock may be provoked in numerous animal species, including man. Manifestations of the shock are different depending on the animal species. Guinea pigs show a very rapid and severe response, characterized by restlessness, rubbing of the nose and ears, dyspnea, and convulsion. Decrease of blood pressure and body temperature are also characteristic symptoms. The predominance of asphyxial signs in the guinea pig is considered to be due to contraction of the smooth muscles of the bronchi. In the rabbit, breathing becomes irregular and then rapid. Finally, nystagmus becomes evident, and the animals collapse as a result of right heart failure. Anaphylaxis in the dog is characterized by restlessness, vomiting, defecation, and urination. Both the vomit and feces may be bloody, and the animal becomes comatose. The major cause of the symptoms is hepatic congestion due to contraction of the smooth muscles of the hepatic venous tree.

In all species examined the shock symptoms are based on (1) an increased permeability of capillaries and small vessels, and (2) contraction of smooth muscles. Therefore, anaphylactic reactions can be observed locally by measuring these responses. One type of local anaphylaxis commonly utilized in experiments is cutaneous anaphylaxis (2). If antigen is injected intracutaneously into actively or passively sensitized guinea pigs and followed by an intravenous injection of Evans blue, the dye accumulates at the skin sites. The reaction is due to an increased permeability resulting from antigen-antibody interaction at the skin site. Cutaneous anaphylaxis is also observed when the skin sites are passively sensitized with antibody and a mixture of antigen and Evans blue is injected intravenously 3 to 6 hours later. A similar reaction can be observed when the challenging antigen is injected into a skin site which had previously received antibody and the dye is then injected intravenously. These reactions are called *passive cutaneous anaphylaxis* (PCA) regardless of which method is used. The PCA reaction is also observed in mice and rats. The reactions in the guinea pig reach a maximum within 15 to 20 minutes after the injection of antigen. In rats and mice, a maximal reaction is not reached until 30 minutes after treatment.

The so-called Prausnitz-Küstner (P-K) reactions in humans probably correspond to PCA reactions in experimental animals. If serum samples taken from atopic patients are injected intracutaneously into a normal individual and the skin sites are challenged 24 to 48 hours later by allergen to which the patient is sensitive, the sites show an erythema-wheal-type reaction. The reactions become maximal within 15 to 20 minutes after injection of allergen. The allergic reaction by human reaginic serum and allergen can be observed in the monkey by the same procedure as that of PCA reactions in the guinea pig (3). Evidence has been obtained that the same antibody in the patient's serum is involved in P-K reactions in humans and PCA reactions in the monkey (4). However, the minimal dose of the antibody required for the induction of the reaction in monkeys (*Macaca mulatta* or *Macaca irus*) is 10 to 30 times more than that required for a positive P-K reaction in humans.

Another representative anaphylactic reaction is contraction of isolated uterus or ileum from sensitized animals on contact with antigen (Schultz-Dale reaction). In this reaction, the intestinal or uterine strips from either actively or passively sensitized animals are suspended in a Dale bath containing Tyrode solution at 37°C. Oxygen is continuously bubbled in the bath, and antigen solution is added to the bath. The strips contract upon contact with the antigen. Passive sensitization of isolated guinea pig ileum can be accomplished in vitro by incubating the isolated ileum from normal guinea pigs with antibody in Tyrode solution (5). By the same procedure, monkey ileum can be sensitized with serum from atopic patients (6).

Local anaphylaxis can also be observed in lung tissues. Chopped lung from a sensitized guinea pig is suspended in Tyrode solution and incubated with antigen (7). The intensity of the anaphylactic reaction is determined by measuring the quantity of histamine liberated. In vitro sensitization of normal guinea pig lung with antibody has also been achieved (7,8). The same technique was recently applied to human reaginic serum (9). Lung tissues from normal monkey can be sensitized with the patient's serum for histamine release by allergen.

Anaphylactic reactions can also be observed at the cellular level. Vasoactive amines such as histamine and 5-hydroxytryptamine are chemical mediators of anaphylactic reactions. These amines are present in granules of mast cells. Mota (10) has reported that mast cells of the isolated mesenteries of sensitized guinea pigs were damaged by antigen and released histamine. Release of histamine from rat mast cells has been observed by Mota (11) as well as by Austen et al. (12). Barbaro and Zvaifler (13) observed histamine release from rabbit platelets and leukocytes as a result of an antigen-antibody reaction. Histamine release from leukocytes by antigen was also observed in humans. Lichtenstein and Osler (14) incubated allergen with leukocytes from atopic patients and detected histamine in the medium. Recently, Levy and Osler (15) succeeded in sensitizing normal human leukocytes with reaginic sera for histamine release. The ability of the patients' sera for passive sensitization paralleled their skin-sensitizing activity.

Active Sensitization and Anaphylactic Antibodies

Guinea pigs are actively sensitized with various kinds of foreign protein antigens but not with haptens. The sensitization can be achieved with as little as 0.05 μg of crystalline ovalbumin. In most experiments, however, a single injection of 0.1 to 1 mg of protein antigen or repeated injections at 3- to 4-day intervals are used. Sensitization has been effected by inhalation of antigen as well (16). Sensitivity in the guinea pig usually persists for several months.

Mice and rats may be actively sensitized for anaphylactic shock. For mice 1 mg of bovine serum albumin (BSA), 0.05 to 0.25 mg of alum-precipitated BSA (17), or 0.1 mg of the antigen included in Freund's complete adjuvant are optimal sensitizing doses (18). In these cases, anaphylactic shock can be obtained by injecting 1 to 2 mg of the antigen 24 to 35 days later. If the immunizing antigen is mixed with *H. pertussis* vaccine, active sensitization can be induced in mice with a single injection of a minute amount of antigen (19,20). The maximal effect is obtained by an intraperitoneal injection of 250 million phase-one pertussis vaccine. The same effect of the vaccine is observed in the rat. In addition to the adjuvant effect, *H. pertussis* vaccine also increases the susceptibility of mice to passive anaphylaxis (21), histamine (22), and serotonin (23). However, the increased susceptibility to passive anaphylaxis disappears at the time when histamine and serotonin sensitivity are still present (24).

Since most of the immunologic studies on anaphylactic reactions were carried out in guinea pigs using rabbit IgG antibodies, it was generally believed that IgG antibodies were also responsible for anaphylaxis in homologous animal species. Benacerraf et al. (25) first detected γG_1 and γG_2 immunoglobulins in guinea pigs and subsequently found that γG_1 antibodies, but not γG_2 antibodies, induced anaphylactic reactions in homologous species (26). In normal guinea pigs, γG_1 globulin is a minor component, but the concentration in serum increases upon immunization. Antibodies associated with this protein sensitize guinea pigs for anaphylactic shock and for PCA reactions. Guinea pig lung may be sensitized by the γG_1 antibodies but not by γG_2 antibodies in vitro. The lung, sensitized with γG_1 antibodies, releases histamine and slow-reacting substance of anaphylaxis (SRS-A) upon exposure to antigen (27). Similar findings were found in mice. Mouse γG_1 antibodies but neither γG_2 nor IgM antibodies will sensitize a homologous animal (28).

Human reaginic antibodies are associated with IgE but none of the other four immunoglobulins. Skin-sensitizing activity in atopic patients' sera is correlated with the concentration of IgE antibody as measured by antigen binding activity (29). Reaginic antibodies have been precipitated with antibodies specific for IgE but not with those specific for other immunoglobulins (30). Subsequently, IgE fraction was obtained from reaginic serum. The fraction containing only IgE antibodies but none of the IgG, IgA, or IgM antibodies had high skin-sensitizing activity (31). These observations indicate that reaginic antibodies belong to IgE. However, human IgE is different from guinea pig γG_1 in both physicochemical and immunologic properties. For example, IgE is a glycoprotein with a carbohydrate content which is significantly higher than that of IgG (11 percent versus 2.6 percent). It has a sedimentation constant of 8.1S and a molecular weight of about 200,000 (32). The sedimentation coefficient of guinea pig γ_1 globulin is 6.6S, and carbohydrate content of the protein is comparable to that of γ_2 (33). The sensitizing activity of IgE antibodies is lost either by heating at 56°C for 4 hours or by reduction and alkylation (34), whereas γG_1 antibodies in both guinea pigs and mice are heat-stable and resistant to the reduction-alkylation procedure (35). Another important difference is that sensitization of human skin with IgE antibodies lasts for a long period of time, whereas sensitization of guinea pig skin by γG_1 antibodies begins to diminish within 24 hours after sensitization. Reaginic antibodies, similar to human IgE antibodies, have been detected in dogs (36), rabbits (37), rats (11,38), and mice (39). All of them are heat-labile, and passive sensitization of homologous animals' skin by the antibodies lasts for a long time. There is a similar indication that the molecular weight of reaginic antibodies in rabbits and dogs is also higher than that of their respective IgG immunoglobulins (36,37). Evidence has been obtained that the skin-sensitizing antibodies of the rat are also not found in the IgG, IgA, or IgM immunoglobulins (12). The reaginic-type antibodies in mice are neither γG_1 nor γG_2 immunoglobulin (39). However, the immunoglobulin class to which the reaginic antibody belongs has not been identified in the rabbit, rat, or mouse. The distribution of reaginic antibodies after fractionation of sera strongly suggests that they belong to a unique immunoglobulin class corresponding to human IgE. The properties of skin-sensitizing antibodies in different animal species are summarized in Table 14-1.

Reaginic-type antibodies in the rat, mouse, and rabbit are only detected in the early stages of immunization and not in hyperimmune sera (11,38,39). The antibodies are detected in serum 1 week to 12 days after a single injection of antigen and disappear within 2 to 3 weeks. Booster injections do not increase the concentration of reaginic antibodies. It was also found in the rat and mouse that active sensitization with *H. pertussis* vaccine enhanced the formation of the reaginic antibodies. This may be related to the fact that an injection of *H. pertussis* vaccine with antigen results in the sensitization of these animals. It was also found that parasitic infection resulted in the formation of reaginic antibodies in rats and rabbits (40,41). This finding may be related to the fact that reaginic antibodies are readily formed in normal individuals upon infection with *Ascaris*.

Anaphylactic antibodies in homologous species are duplicated in rats and mice. As already described, both γG_1 antibodies and reaginic antibodies in mice induce anaphylactic reactions. Rats also form two types of antibodies; one is a reaginic antibody formed early in immunization or upon parasitic infection and the other is the one detected in hyperimmune sera. The physicochemical properties of these two types are different. It was also found that reaginic antibodies sensitize mast cells for histamine release upon exposure with antigen (12). The antibodies of the second type do not sensitize mast cells. The chemical mediator responsible for anaphylactic reactions induced by the antibodies is probably SRS-A (27). Heterogeneity of skin-sensitizing antibodies with respect to the immunoglobulin class has not been established in humans, guinea pigs, or rabbits.

TABLE 14-1

Anaphylactic (Reaginic) Antibodies in Homologous Species

Species	Immuno-globulin	Electro-phoretic mobility	Sedimenta-tion coefficient	Sensitivity to 56°C	Latent period (hr)†	Persistence of sensitiza-tion
Guinea pig	γG1	Fast γ	7S	Stable	3–5	2 days
Mouse	γG1	Fast γ	7S	Stable	0.5–1	5–6 hrs
	Unidentified	n.d.§	n.d.	Labile	48–72	1 week
Rat	IgG‡	Fast γ	7S	Stable	1¶	10–20 hr¶
	Unidentified	Fast γ	7–19S	Labile	24–48	4 weeks
Dog	Unidentified	Slow β	7–19S	Labile	24	2 weeks
Rabbit	Unidentified	Slow β	7–19S	Labile	24–48	2 weeks
Man	IgE	Fast γ	8S	Labile	18–24	2 weeks

† The period after sensitization to the maximal sensitivity.
‡ Probably a subclass of IgG.
¶ Tested by release of slow reacting substance from peritoneal cells.
§ Not done.

Passive Sensitization

Latent Period and Persistence of Sensitivity

In passive anaphylaxis, an interval between the sensitizing and shocking injections is required. This latent period is a function of the sensitizing dose of antibody when the shocking dose of antigen is constant. In the guinea pig, Benacerraf and Kabat (42) have studied this relationship, using ovalbumin and rabbit IgG antibody. When the shocking dose was 1 mg of ovalbumin, an interval of 5 hours was necessary for anaphylactic death when guinea pigs received 30 μg of rabbit antibody N. With 2 mg N of antibody, fatal shock occurred without a latent period. A similar relationship has been observed in PCA reactions. Ovary and Bier (43) have shown that skin sites receiving 0.01 μg of rabbits antibody N did not give positive reactions if antigen was injected 30 minutes after the sensitization, but did so if the antigen was injected 1 to 3 hours later. However, the skin site which received 1 μg antibody N showed a positive reaction after only a 30-minute interval. These findings imply that the anaphylactic manifestations are caused by the reaction of cell-fixed antibody with antigen and that a certain time interval is required for the fixation of the antibody to target cells. In fact, Halpern et al. (5) found the requirement of a sensitizing period in the passive sensitization of guinea pig ileum in vitro. Only 0.25 μg of antibody N per ml of Tyrode solution was sufficient to sensitize guinea pig ileum if the ileum was incubated in the solution for 120 minutes. However, as much as 16 μg of antibody N per ml was required to sensitize the ileum within 15 minutes incubation. The relationship between the reciprocal of the time of incubation and the antibody concentration for sensitization was linear in their experiments.

Persistence of the sensitized state is limited in passive anaphylaxis. In the guinea pig, sensitivity following intravenous injections of 30 μg of rabbit antibody N for anaphylactic shock persisted for 8 days but disappeared by 12 days. PCA sensitivity with 0.025 μg of antibody N disappeared within 24 hours after sensitization of the skin. When 10 times as much antibody was injected, the skin site gave a positive reaction at 24 hours but not at 48 hours after the sensitization (2).

The time course of passive sensitization was different when animals were sensitized with homologous anaphylactic antibodies. Fatal anaphylaxis of guinea pigs occurred 28 days after an intravenous injection of 30 μg of guinea pig antibody nitrogen (44). Passive sensitization persisted 2 to 3 days after local injection of 0.03 μg of guinea pig antiovalbumin. Since these experiments were done before γG_1 and γG_2 immunoglobulins were identified, the effective dose of antibody ($G\gamma_1$) injected would be less. The persistence of mouse γG_1 antibody in a homologous skin site is much shorter. Maximal sensitization of the skin site is achieved within 1 hour, and sensitization disappears within several hours (45).

The time course of passive sensitization with reaginic antibodies is quite different from γG_1-type antibody. In all species, i.e., human, rat, rabbit, dog, and mouse, the maximal sensitization with reaginic antibodies is achieved at 24 to 48 hours after passive sensitization of their skin, and the sensitization persists for 1 to 2 weeks (Table 14-1). The long persistence of reaginic antibodies may be related to the fact that the antibodies belong to a minor component of immunoglobulins.

Nature and Quantities of Antibody for Passive Sensitization

In passive sensitization of guinea pigs with antibodies from heterologous animal species, it has been shown that rabbit, dog, human, and monkey antibodies, but none of the horse, cow, goat, rat, or chicken antibodies, cause either PCA or Schultz-Dale reactions (2,46). All of the antibodies giving the positive PCA reactions belong to IgG immunoglobulins (47). Rabbit IgM and human IgM and IgA antibodies failed to sensitize guinea pigs (48,49). Kabat and Boldt (50) showed that 30 μg of rabbit anti-ovalbumin N was sufficient to sensitize guinea pigs for fatal anaphylaxis. Intravenous injection of 1 mg of ovalbumin 48 hours after the passive sensitization resulted in anaphylactic shock to death. On the other hand, sensitization with 6 to 25 μg of antibody N resulted in anaphylactic shock which was not always fatal even with a large amount of antigen for challenge. In PCA reactions in the guinea pig, 0.003 to 0.01 μg of the rabbit antibody N, followed by an intravenous injection of 1 mg ovalbumin 3 to 6 hours after the passive sensitization, induced a definite skin reaction. Human IgG antibodies have less sensitizing activity than rabbit antibodies. In PCA reactions 0.1 to 0.2 μg antibody N was required for the positive reaction (2).

The sensitizing activity of guinea pig γG_1 antibodies is comparable to that of rabbit IgG antibodies. For PCA reactions in guinea pigs, 0.003 to 0.01 μg of the guinea pig antibody is required. The dose of human reaginic antibody required to give a positive P-K reaction was estimated to be 10^{-5} to 10^{-6} μg N (29). Since the immunoglobulin class of the reaginic antibodies in experimental animals is not yet identified, the dose of the antibody required to give anaphylactic reactions cannot be estimated. However, the dose should be very little, probably comparable to human IgE antibody, because this immunoglobulin is almost at an undetectable level in antisera.

Molecular Basis of Passive Sensitization

The requirement of a certain time interval between passive sensitization and the shocking dose, as well as local anaphylaxis, indicates that an antigen-antibody interaction in tissues rather than in the circulation is responsible for anaphylaxis. Although the specific cells involved in anaphylaxis are unknown, it is generally accepted that antibody is "fixed" to some tissue constituent or cell and that anaphylactic reactions are induced by the combination of antigen to the fixed antibody. This idea is supported by reversed passive anaphylaxis with γ-globulin antigens. Anaphylactic reactions are generally observed when antibody is present in vivo before the shocking dose of antigen. No anaphylaxis is observed if antigens, such as ovalbumin, hemocyanin, and polysaccharide, etc., are injected and followed by homologous antibody within a day. However, reversed passive anaphylaxis can be observed in the guinea pig when human or rabbit IgG is used as antigen. Bier and Siqueira (51) produced cutaneous anaphylaxis by intracutaneous injections of rabbit IgG followed by an intravenous injection of guinea pig antirabbit IgG antibody. In this case, the nature of the antibody is not important. Even horse, chicken, or sheep antisera induced reversed passive anaphylaxis so long as the antigen was human or rabbit IgG (52). As described previously, these antibodies were unable to sensitize the guinea pig skin directly; passive sensitization with one of these antibodies followed by IgG antigen injection did not give a positive reaction. Reversed PCA reactions in guinea pigs cannot be demonstrated with goat, cattle, or chicken γ-globulin as antigen. Only the IgG-globulin of a species whose IgG antibodies can passively sensitize the guinea pig can induce reversed passive anaphylaxis regardless of the sensitizing activity of the antibodies used. Recently, Terry (53) reported that three subclasses of human IgG, i.e., γG_1, γG_3, and γG_4, gave reversed PCA reactions, whereas γG_2 did not. It was also found that both human IgM and IgA failed to cause reversed PCA reactions (54). These findings are in agreement with the fact that neither IgM nor IgA antibody cause direct PCA reactions.

The correlation between the antigens causing reversed passive anaphylaxis and the antibodies giving direct passive anaphylaxis indicates that the same mechanisms are involved in passive sensitization in both reactions and suggests that both antibody and nonantibody IgG can be fixed to target cells. This idea suggests the possibility that nonantibody IgG may compete with antibody for passive sensitization. In fact, the sensitizing activity of antiserum does not parallel its antibody content. With weak antisera, a large amount of antibody is required for sensitization. For example, Ovary and Bier (55) found that 0.05 μg of rabbit antiovalbumin N was required for minimal PCA sensitization when the antiserum was diluted with normal rabbit serum. When the same antiserum was diluted with saline, only 0.01 μg of antibody N was sufficient to give a comparable reaction. Human serum also has this blocking effect. The blocking activity in these sera is associated with IgG immunoglobulin. Other serum proteins, including IgA and IgM, did not block the passive sensitization (56). Biozzi et al. (57) studied the quantitative relationship between the amount of antibody required for sensitization and the amount of normal IgG required for blocking the passive sensitization and found that 16 to 20 μg of normal rabbit IgG per ml was required to block PCA sensitization with 0.1 μg of rabbit antibody N per ml. They also found that horse, cattle, and chicken γ-globulin cannot block the sensitization with rabbit antibody. Systemic anaphylaxis and in vitro sensitization of the isolated guinea pig ileum were also inhibited by normal human and rabbit IgG.

The blocking of passive sensitization by the immunoglobulin, to which the sensitizing antibody belongs, is a universal phenomenon. Guinea pig γG_1 but not γG_2, showed the blocking effect in PCA reactions in guinea pigs (26). In humans passive sensitization with reaginic antibodies for P-K reactions was blocked by nonantibody IgE but not by any of the other immunoglobulins (58).

Correlation among (1) the sensitizing activity of antibodies belonging to certain immunoglobulin classes, (2) sensitizing activity of the same immunoglobulins in reversed passive anaphylaxis, and (3) the blocking activity of the same proteins on passive sensitization indicates that IgG immunoglobulins from certain animal species have affinities for guinea pig tissues (target cells) and suggests that these proteins have structures essential for "fixation" to target cells. This idea has been supported by several findings. When rabbit IgG antibodies are digested by either pepsin or papain, either Fab or (Fab')$_2$ fragments containing antibody combining site(s) do not sensitize guinea pigs for PCA reactions. Both of these fragments failed to induce reversed PCA reactions and to block passive sensitization with intact rabbit antibodies. On the other hand, the Fc fragment obtained by papain digestion gave reversed PCA sensitization and blocked passive sensitization with rabbit antibodies (59,60). These findings show that Fc fragments, but neither Fab nor (Fab')$_2$, have structures essential for the fixation of rabbit IgG to guinea pig tissues. Similarly, the Fc fragment of human IgG subclasses γG_1, γG_3, and γG_4 gave reversed PCA sensitization, whereas the fragment of γG_2 did not (61). Since γG_2 itself does not give reversed PCA and fails to block passive sensitization, it is clear that the structures of human IgG essential for passive sensitization are present in the Fc portion of the molecule.

Induction of Anaphylactic Reactions

The antigens eliciting anaphylactic reactions are not necessarily immunogenic. For example, Kabat and Landow (62) showed that pneumococcus polysaccharide, which is not immunogenic in guinea pigs, can cause anaphylactic reactions in guinea pigs passively sensitized with rabbit antiserum against pneumococcus. Polyvalent hapten can also induce anaphylaxis in guinea pigs. The only antigens which are incapable of giving anaphylactic reactions are simple haptens having only one antigenic determinant group. If the haptens are injected into sensitized animals shortly before challenge with multivalent antigen, anaphylactic reactions are inhibited. Ovary and Karush (63) showed that 85 μg of lactose administered 20 minutes before 5 μg N of lactose–human fibrinogen prevented PCA reactions in the sites previously sensitized with antilactate antibody. It was also found that ϵ-dinitrophenyl (DNP) lysine did not induce PCA reactions whereas ϵ,α-DNP-lysine did (64). These findings indicate that the presence of two or more antigenic determinants in the antigen molecule are an essential property for a challenging antigen. Since ϵ,α-DNP-lysine does not give a precipitin reaction with anti-DNP antibody, it seems that an antigen need not be able to give a precipitin reaction in order to induce an anaphylactic reaction. Similar observations were obtained by Levine (65) using a benzyl penicilloyl (BPO) haptenic system. He has compared univalent, divalent, and multivalent BPO haptens with regard to their ability to elicit PCA reactions in guinea pigs which have been sensitized by intravenous injection of rabbit anti-BPO sera. His results clearly showed that divalent and multivalent haptens evoked equally intense PCA reactions in the animals sensitized with antibodies of comparatively high affinity, whereas univalent haptens did not.

The amount of antigen needed to induce anaphylactic responses depends on the antigen-antibody system and molecular weight of antigen. If the number of moles of antigen required to induce the response was calculated in many antigen-antibody systems when animals were sensitized with an equal level of antibody, the number of antigen molecules fell approximately within the same range (66). Levine (67) has confirmed these findings using anti-BPO rabbit sera and BPO haptens of a different size and valency. In his experiments, it was clearly shown that equimolar concentrations of the divalent and multivalent haptens were equally effective in the induction of PCA reactions. This situation is entirely different from passive Arthus reactions evoked by the same antibody and haptens. His results showed that equal weight concentrations of multivalent haptens were equally effective in the induction of passive Arthus reactions and that the divalent hapten was incapable of giving the reactions. Similar experiments were carried out on human reaginic hypersensitivity to penicillin. It was reported that trivalent BPO haptens with optional distances of separation of the haptenic groups were most effective for the induction of erythema-wheal-type reactions. Divalent haptens were capable of eliciting the reaction but they were not maximally effective elicitors. Monovalent haptens failed to induce the reaction (68).

Immune Mechanisms of Anaphylactic Reactions

Anaphylactic reactions are caused by an antigen-antibody combination which results in a disturbance of the cells to which antibodies are fixed. Failure of univalent hapten to elicit anaphylactic reactions indicates that the combination of antigenic determinants to antibody combining sites is not sufficient for the initiation of cellular disturbances. This suggests the possibility that antigen-antibody complexes formed on the cells may have a biologic activity which is lacking for either antigen or antibody alone or for univalent hapten-antibody complexes and therefore that the formation of such complexes may induce allergic reactions. In fact, Germuth and McKinnon (69), Trapani et al. (70), and Ishizaka and Campbell (71) have established that the soluble antigen-antibody complexes formed in excess antigen can induce anaphylactic shock, cause contraction of isolated ileum from normal guinea pigs, and increase the permeability of guinea pig skin capillaries in a manner similar to that obtained in PCA. The amount of antigen and antibody contained in the minimal skin reactive dose of preformed soluble complexes is of the same order of magnitude as the threshold amount of these reagents required to elicit a skin reaction when they are injected without a latent period (72).

Subsequent experiments showed that the skin-reactivity of the soluble complexes depend on the nature of the antibodies involved. Rabbit IgG antibodies form skin-reactive complexes with antigen, irrespective of whether the antigen is protein, polysaccharide, or synthetic multivalent hapten, whereas both horse and chicken antibodies fail to form skin-reactive complexes (73). Pepsin-digested rabbit IgG antibody, i.e., (Fab')$_2$, did not form the skin-reactive complexes (60). An essential property of antigen for the formation of the skin-reactive complexes is that the antigenic molecules have two or more determinant groups (73). The nature of antigen and antibody required for the formation of skin-reactive complexes in vitro is in agreement with those required for eliciting PCA reactions and suggests that PCA reactions are provoked by the formation of skin-reactive complexes in vivo. In connection with this idea, it was found that a skin reaction with soluble antigen-antibody complexes is inhibited by the presence of normal human or rabbit IgG in the complex preparation.

The blocking of the skin reaction by normal IgG indicates a competition between soluble complexes and the IgG for fixation to animal tissues. The competition between soluble complexes and IgG was confirmed by the inhibition of PCA sensitization by heterologous antigen-antibody complexes. When rabbit diphtheria antitoxin was diluted with BSA-anti-BSA complexes instead of saline and used for passive sensitization, the PCA reactions by the diphtheria toxin-antitoxin system were inhibited. Soluble complexes lacking the blocking effect on PCA sensitization did not have skin reactivity (74). It seems that fixation of soluble complexes with tissues is one of the necessary processes in the skin reaction.

It was also found that a complex composed of two antigens and one antibody, i.e., Ag_2Ab, did not have skin reactivity, but the complexes containing two or more antibody molecules did, indicating that two antibody molecules are necessary for the formation of skin-reactive complexes (72). If one assumes that biologic activity of antigen-antibody complexes is based on structures of the molecules involved, one might speculate that the molecular configuration of the antibody molecule is changed to a toxic configuration when two or more antibody molecules combine with the antigen and the skin reaction is caused by combination of such altered antibody molecules with target cells. The necessity of at least two antibody molecules for the formation of skin-reactive complexes suggests the possibility that two or more antibody molecules combining with the same antigen may then interact with each other so as to produce structural changes in the antibody molecules which result in the production of skin reactivity. This idea has been supported by the fact that optical rotation changes occur as the result of the formation of skin-reactive complexes (75,76). If this idea is correct, then the role of antigen in the formation of skin-reactive complexes is merely to bring antibody molecules in close proximity for antibody-antibody interaction. This suggests the possibility that interaction of human and rabbit IgG molecules induced by reagents other than specific antigen might also be accompanied by the development of skin reactivity. In fact, nonspecifically aggregated human and rabbit IgG molecules have induced skin reactions in normal guinea pigs, and the minimal skin-reactive dose of the aggregated IgG is comparable to that of soluble antigen-antibody complexes (77). As is the case with antigen-antibody complexes, the skin-reactivity of aggregated IgG depends on the species from which the IgG immunoglobulin is obtained. Aggregated horse, cattle, and chicken IgG did not induce skin reactions (78). Aggregated human IgM and aggregated IgA also failed to give the reaction (79) (Table 14-2). Subsequent studies showed that structures in aggregated IgG essential for the induction of the skin reaction are present in the Fc portion of the molecule. When the Fab and Fc fragments of rabbit IgG were aggregated by coupling with bis-diazotized benzidine, the aggregated

Fc gave a skin reaction whereas the aggregated Fab did not (60) (Table 14-2). Recently, Henney and Ishizaka (80) analyzed the antigenic structure of aggregated IgG and found that new antigenic determinants were revealed by nonspecific aggregation of human IgG. The guinea pig antibodies specific for the determinants reacted with antigen-IgG antibody complexes as well as aggregated Fc. These findings indicate that common structural changes actually occurred in the Fc portion of the IgG (antibody) molecule upon the formation of antigen-antibody complexes and by nonspecific aggregation. These observations support the hypothesis that induction of skin-reactive properties may be due to some structural changes in the antibody molecules involved.

Since most of the work on soluble antigen-antibody complexes and aggregated IgG-globulins were carried out with rabbit and human IgG (antibody), the possibility remained that the skin reactions by the immune or nonspecific aggregates may be induced by mechanisms different from that of anaphylactic reactions. It has been shown that rabbit IgG antibodies induce anaphylactic as well as Arthus-type reactions in the guinea pig and fix complement (C') with antigen. Nonspecifically aggregated rabbit and human IgG-globulin also fixed C' and gave Arthus-type reactions in normal guinea pigs, when 30 to 100 μg N of the aggregates was injected intracutaneously (81). This suggests the possibility that the skin reactions may be induced by anaphylatoxins which are produced by fixation of C'

TABLE 14-2

Skin-reactive and Complement-fixing Properties of Immunoglobulins and IgG Fragments and of Their Aggregated Products

Species	Immuno-globulin	Aggrega-tion	Minimum skin-reactive dose	$C'F_{50}$[†]
Human	IgG	—	>20	>800
		+	1.0	8
	IgA	—	>20	>800
		+	>20	>800
	IgM	—	>16	>800
		+	>10	70
Rabbit	IgG	—	32	600
		+	1.0	6
	F_c[‡]	—	15	140
		+	2.0	8
	F_{ab}[‡]	—	>40	>800
		+	>40	>800

[†] Quantity of protein N required to inactivate 50 $C'H_{50}$ out of 100.
[‡] Papain fragments of rabbit IgG.

components to aggregates, whereas real anaphylactic reactions may be elicited by entirely different mechanisms. The possibility cannot be excluded in some cases. For example, aggregated human γG_4-immunoglobulin did not give a skin reaction or fix C′, although the original protein fixed to guinea pig skin tissues (80). However, recent observations on antigen-antibody complexes composed of homologous anaphylactic antibodies support the view that skin reactions by antigen-antibody complexes and PCA reactions would be elicited by common mechanisms. Soluble antigen–guinea pig γG_1 antibody complexes gave skin reactions in normal guinea pigs, although the complexes did not fix C′. The complexes composed of γG_2 antibodies, which fix C′, also gave skin reactions, however minimal dose of γG_2 antibody complexes for eliciting the skin reaction was more than 100 times as much as the γG_1 antibody complexes which gave a comparable reaction. It was also found that ragweed allergen–human IgE antibody complexes gave erythema-wheal reactions in nonsensitive individuals, whereas complexes composed of IgG or IgA antibodies failed to do so. Analysis of the allergen-IgE antibody complexes strongly suggests that two or more IgE antibody molecules are necessary for the formation of a skin-reactive complex (82). The theoretical consideration obtained in guinea pigs may also be applied to the mechanisms of reaginic hypersensitivity in humans.

In summarizing the information obtained on antigen-antibody complexes and the molecular basis of passive sensitization, one might speculate about the mechanisms of anaphylactic and reaginic hypersensitivity reactions as follows: Antibody molecules are fixed on target cells through a region of the Fc portion of the molecules. As a result of the combination of the cell-fixed antibodies with antigen, antigen-antibody complexes will be formed on the cells, and antibody molecules combining with the same antigen may interact with each other. Structural alteration in the Fc portion of the antibody molecules may occur as the result of the antibody-antibody interaction. Biochemical processes from the formation of the toxic configuration through release of chemical mediators such as histamine and SRS-A are not known. In view of complement-fixation by antigen-antibody complexes but not by either antigen or by antibody alone, however, it is conceivable that certain enzymes in or near the cell membrane may be activated by the altered antibody and consequently result in release of chemical mediators from the cells.

Arthus Reaction

In 1903 Arthus (83) reported a hemorrhagic, necrotic reaction that occurred a few hours after he injected an immunized animal subcutaneously with the specific immunizing antigen. This reaction has been called the Arthus reaction. In recent years the pathogenesis of this lesion has been investigated and shown to depend on four factors: antigen, antibody, complement, and polymorphonuclear leukocytes. The reaction of all four of these components causes a local vasculitis. The vascular basement membrane and endothelium is damaged, causing local hemorrhage and thrombosis. In strong reactions necrosis may also occur. In the following discussion the contribution of each of the above components will be described.

First it can be shown that the reaction depends on specific antigen and antibody. For example, an animal immunized with antigen A may be induced to give an Arthus reaction to antigen A but not to a non-cross-reacting antigen, antigen B.

The dependence of the reaction on the quantity and quality of antibody was reported by Benacerraf and Kabat (84). Using passive transfer of a known amount of antibody, they showed that the intensity of the reaction was dependent on the amount of precipitating antibody. An equal quantity of nonprecipitating antibody did not cause the Arthus reaction. More recently the immunoglobulin types that are able to elicit the Arthus reaction have been studied. IgG and IgM are effective, but IgA does not induce the reaction (85). The ability of these immunoglobulins to elicit the Arthus reaction is probably dependent on their ability to fix complement.

Antigen and antibody have both been observed in the skin site of the Arthus reaction. Using the fluorescent antibody technique, antibody and antigen have been observed in the vascular wall (86). When ferritin was used as antigen so that it could be observed in the electron microscope, antigen was found across the basement membrane between the endothelial cells and perivascular cells (87,88). Presumably antibody was also present. Discontinuity of the vascular basement membrane was also observed in these studies.

When sites of the Arthus reaction were stained with anti-β1C, the third component of complement, it was also found to be present (86). However, its presence at the site of the reaction did not prove it was required for the development of the reaction. Ward and Cochrane (89) investigated this problem by attempting to induce the Arthus reaction in immunized animals that had lowered complement levels. Macroscopic Arthus reactions were absent or markedly reduced in animals having reduced complement levels. However, using the fluorescent antibody technique, antigen was shown to be present in the injection sites regardless of the complement level. On the other hand, complement was not observed in the injection site. It is important to note that the absence of complement in the site was correlated with the absence of polymorphonuclear leukocytes and the absence of a macroscopic Arthus reaction.

By depleting an animal of polymorphonuclear leukocytes by agents such as nitrogen mustard, the macroscopic features of the Arthus reaction can be eliminated (90–92). In fact, there is a positive correlation between the number of circulating polymorphonuclear leukocytes and the severity of the reaction (93). Antigen, antibody, and complement have been detected in these depleted animals in the same location in the vascular wall as in a full-blown Arthus reaction (94,95). However, damage to the blood vessel was not detected histologically or grossly. Thus, there is good evidence that all four components (antigen, antibody, complement, and polymorphonuclear leukocytes) are necessary for the Arthus reaction to occur.

The role of complement in the Arthus reaction is to attract polymorphonuclear leukocytes (96–98). When antigen, antibody, and complement are placed on one side of a porous filter and polymorphonuclear leukocytes on the other, the cells migrated across the filter. When complement was absent, the cells did not migrate. Thus, complement is necessary for the generation of chemotactic factor. The major chemotactic factor formed has now been shown to be a complex of C'5, 6, and 7 (98,99).

It is probably lysosomal enzymes in the polymorphonuclear leukocytes that cause the actual damage to the basement membrane. In fact, cathepsins D and E are capable of digesting basement membrane in vitro (100). Since these enzymes are not active at neutral pH, they do not cause vascular injury when injected into the skin of a normal animal. The local pH at the site of an Arthus reaction, however, is probably not neutral, since the polymorphonuclear leukocytes at the site in the process of phagocytizing the antigen-antibody complexes release lactic acid (101).

Other lysosomal components may also contribute to the lesion (102–105). For example, Janoff (104) has described a neutral protease derived from leukocyte granules which causes immediate vascular injury. In addition, several basic proteins that increase vascular permeability have been obtained from leukocyte granules (105).

In summary, the Arthus reaction proceeds after an antigen-antibody complex activates the complement system. A concentration gradient of chemotactic factor, C'5, 6, 7, is generated, resulting in an accumulation of polymorphonuclear leukocytes between the endothelial cells and the basement membrane. The cells phagocytize the antigen-antibody complexes, which in turn causes a local reduction in pH, which reduces the stability of the lysosomal membrane. Some of the components released from the lysosomes destroy the basement membrane, resulting in a local vasculitis, hemorrhage, and thrombosis.

Serum Sickness

Serum sickness became a problem during the period when diseases such as pneumococcal pneumonia were treated with antisera produced in other species. In 1 to 2 weeks after treatment with foreign sera some individuals became very ill with systemic disease characterized by rashes, fevers, pain in the joints, and glandular swelling. The disease is caused by production of antibody to the foreign proteins in serum. These antibodies react with the remaining antigen causing the allergic disease. Since in humans it is likely that several types of hypersensitivity are induced, the following discussion will be limited to the experimental disease that can be induced using a purified protein.

When a foreign protein such as bovine serum albumin is injected intravenously into a rabbit and its rate of clearance from the circulation studied, this antigen disappears from the circulation rapidly during the first 1 to 2 days as it equilibrates with the extravascular space (Fig. 14-1). Following the initial equilibration, it disappears from the circulation more slowly with a half-life characteristic of the protein antigen used. When antibody is produced, it complexes with the antigen and rapidly removes it

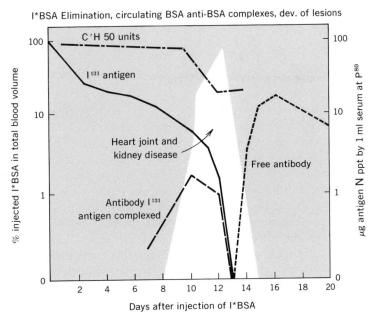

Fig. 14-1 Immunologic and morphologic events transpiring after the injection of 1^{131}-labeled bovine serum albumin (BSA) into a rabbit. From Dixon (106) with permission.

from the circulation. At this time, as is shown in Fig. 14-1, circulating antigen-antibody complexes are detected, the circulating complement level is depressed, and signs of serum sickness appear (106). The signs disappear shortly after the antigen and antigen-antibody complexes have been eliminated and free antibody appears in the circulation. During the acute phase of the disease antigen, antibody, and complement are detected in the kidney (106). This experimental disease shows the fundamentals of serum sickness; that is, the antigen-antibody complexes formed at the beginning of antibody synthesis caused the hypersensitivity. In this experimental case it appears that the circulating antigen-antibody complexes were deposited in organs such as the kidney. In these sites a hypersensitivity was initiated that probably followed the pathogenesis described above for the Arthus reaction. It is of interest that some of the manifestations of human diseases, such as acute glomerular nephritis (107) and lupus erythematosus (108), are thought to be caused by similar mechanisms.

In the human being given foreign antiserum, serum sickness may persist for some time. This is easy to visualize if one considers that the serum contains many antigens, each of which may induce antibody at a different time. Thus, one would have a family of curves similar to that shown in Fig. 14-1. In addition, several different types of hypersensitivity may arise, resulting in a considerably more complex disease than that seen in the experimental disease.

DELAYED HYPERSENSITIVITY

Delayed hypersensitivity is a topic that has both fascinated and frustrated immunologists for many years. As early as 1890 Koch (109) observed that subcutaneous injection of tubercle protein into a tuberculous animal resulted in a generalized fever as well as local induration and erythema at the injection site. In subsequent years investigators found that similar reactions could be induced using a variety of antigens. The reaction was thought to be similar to the immediate hypersensitivities but, unlike them, could not be passively transferred with immune serum. A major breakthrough in the understanding of delayed hypersensitivity occurred when Landsteiner and Chase (110) and Chase (111) reported that delayed-type hypersensitivities could be passively transferred with peritoneal exudate cells. Thus, delayed hypersensitivity was found to be intimately associated with cells of the lymphoid series.

In the following general discussion of delayed hypersensitivity, the emphasis will be on the similarities of the several kinds of delayed hypersensitivity, i.e., bacterial, contact, homograft, rather than on their differences.

Time for Elicitation of Response in an Immunized Animal

In contrast to the rather rapid response that occurs when antigen is injected into an animal having a form of immediate hypersensitivity, the reaction in an animal having delayed hypersensitivity is rather slow, hence the name *delayed hypersensitivity.*

If tuberculin is injected intradermally into a sensitized guinea pig, no gross reaction is observed at the skin site for several hours. At 12 to 24 hours erythema and induration can be seen at the injection site. The reaction continues to progress and peaks at 48 to 72 hours. At this time there is induration in the center of the site, surrounded by erythema. On some occasions, in highly sensitive animals, the center becomes necrotic (112,113).

Histology of Lesion of Delayed Hypersensitivity

Histologically, evolution of the skin reaction begins much earlier than the gross signs. The histology varies somewhat in different types of delayed hypersensitivity and in different animal species. However, the general features are the same. This means the same cell types infiltrate the lesion but at different times and in different proportions when the conditions are varied.

The initial cells to infiltrate a skin test site are polymorphonuclear leukocytes (114,115,116). The peak infiltration of these cells usually occurs 4 to 6 hours after the skin test. Some authors (115) feel that this initial infiltration is nonspecific and due, therefore, to the trauma of the injection and the toxicity of the antigen.

The specific portion of the cellular reaction begins about 8 to 12 hours after injection. At this time, mononuclear cells, both lymphocytes and macrophages, begin to infiltrate the site. The cells appear to collect in perivascular islands in the dermis. Infiltration of mononuclear cells continues and reaches a peak at 24 to 48 hours (113,115,116). When the lesion is macroscopically resolving, epithelial cells and giant cells may be observed in the site. Giant cells have been observed in the skin site as late as 14 days after injection (117). These cells may be a response to the fat and muscle necrosis that occurs as a result of the allergic reactions (118,119).

Changes in the epidermal cells have also been observed by some authors. As early as 12 hours after skin testing, pyknotic nuclei and vacuolated cytoplasm have been reported. In addition, acanthosis has been observed in the epidermis of the guinea pig (113).

In general, the reaction in a skin test site in delayed hypersensitivity may be regarded as a degenerative inflammatory change. The predominant infiltrating cells are mononuclear cells, both lymphocytes and macrophages. The roles of both these cells and ideas as to the pathogenesis of the evolution of the reaction will be discussed in a later section.

Induction of Delayed Hypersensitivity

The types of immune response that are obtained after injection of antigen are dependent, in part, on the method of injection. For example, if particulate antigen is injected intravenously, antibody synthesis occurs almost entirely in the spleen (120). However, intravenous injection of antigen seldom, if ever, induces delayed hypersensitivity (121). In fact, intravenous injection of antigen may inhibit the development of delayed hypersensitivity (122). Delayed hypersensitivity is usually induced in the laboratory by incorporation of the antigen in complete or incomplete Freund's adjuvant (123,124,125). Complete adjuvant induces a longer lived and more intense hypersensitivity than the incomplete adjuvant (124,125). For best induction of delayed hypersensitivity, this material should be injected intradermally or into the footpads of an experimental animal (126). It is not known why these routes are best for the induction of delayed hypersensitivity.

Lymphatic drainage for 16 to 24 hours after application of a contact sensitizer is necessary for the induction of delayed hypersensitivity (127, 128). In fact, if a chemical contact sensitizer is placed on a skin fragment that is surgically isolated from the surrounding tissue but is maintained by a vascular pedicle that has no lymphatic drainage, sensitization does not occur (129). In addition, excision of the local draining lymph nodes of intact guinea pigs 3 days after sensitization blocked sensitization to a chemical contact sensitizer (128). On the other hand, Freund and Lipton (130) found that induction of tuberculin sensitivity was not inhibited when the intradermal injection site was excised only 1 hour after injection. However, they observed tubercle bacilli in oil droplets in the draining lymph nodes within 1 hour of injection.

Thus, cells in the regional lymph node draining the injection site are probably the cells induced to produce the "antibody" that causes delayed hypersensitivity. Because the hypothetical antibody of delayed hypersensitivity has not been characterized, methods similar to the fluorescent antibody technique for identification of the cells synthesizing this hypothetical antibody have not been developed. Therefore, the cells involved have not been positively identified by direct methods. However, large pyroninophilic cells that probably differentiated from small lymphocytes have been observed in the lymph nodes draining the site of application of several different antigens that induce delayed hypersensitivity (124,128, 131,132). Later in the response these pyroninophilic cells may return to a form morphologically similar to the small lymphocyte (132).

Ultrastructurally, the cells involved in delayed hypersensitivity appear to be somewhat different from the cells that synthesize humoral antibody (133). They appear to be lymphoid cells but do not have the abundance of endoplasmic reticulum that is observed in cells producing humoral antibody. They contain many ribosomes but lack an endoplasmic reticulum. Thus, they do not look like secretory cells, although under the electron microscope they appear to have many of the structures necessary for protein synthesis. One is tempted to speculate that the association of delayed hypersensitivity with cells is related to the lack of secretory organelles.

Specificity of the Reaction

The specificity of delayed hypersensitivity appears to be somewhat different from that described for humoral antibodies. While humoral antibodies may discriminate between an ortho and meta substitution on a determinant group (134), the delayed hypersensitivity skin test often will not do so. For example, if a guinea pig is immunized with a hapten protein complex, at least some of its circulating antibodies will be specific for the hapten. However, when delayed hypersensitivity is induced by the same antigens in the same species, the specificity is usually directed to the carrier protein-hapten complex (135,136) although some hapten-specific delayed hypersensitivities are known (137). Indeed, when the specificity of delayed hypersensitivity reactions was shown to be directed to a hapten-protein complex, cross-reactions with antigens consisting of the same protein but different haptens were observed (136). In addition, studies utilizing synthetic polypeptides substituted with a hapten have shown that the determinant necessary to elicit a delayed reaction is larger than that required to react with humoral antibodies (138,139).

Passive Transfer of Delayed Hypersensitivity

As stated previously, delayed hypersensitivity, unlike anaphylaxis and the Arthus reaction, cannot be transferred with serum. Instead, lymphoid cells or, in the human, lysed peripheral blood cells are capable of transferring delayed hypersensitivity. Before discussing the situation in humans, however, the same problem will be considered in experimental animals.

In 1921 immediate hypersensitivity was shown to be transferable by a serum factor (140). It was not until 1942 that Landsteiner and Chase (110) reported the passive transfer of contact hypersensitivity with viable peritoneal exudate cells. Since then, passive transfer of bacterial and contact hypersensitivity has been accomplished with lymphoid cells taken from many sources including spleen, lymph node, thymus, and peripheral blood leukocytes (111,141,142), but has not been transferred with serum (143,144). In general, the ease of passive transfer in experimental animals depends on the degree of hypersensitivity of the donor animal and on the source and number of cells transferred (111). Many investigators have tried to characterize the cellular material that caused the reaction. Although there are occasional reports of transfer of delayed hypersensitivity in animals with cell-free extracts (145,146), most investigators find live cells are required (110,111,144,148). Thus, the factor that mediates the reaction directly has not been described.

The characteristics of transfer of delayed hypersensitivity in humans are, however, somewhat different from those in experimental animals. In the absence of active sensitization, hypersensitivity in experimental animals does not persist (149). On the other hand, it may extend for months in humans (150,151). In addition, cell-free extracts from human lymphoid cells are capable of transferring delayed hypersensitivity (151). Although these materials (transfer factor) have been partially characterized and are specific for the antigen to which the donor was hypersensitive, they have not been isolated.

The extracts are usually derived from peripheral leukocytes which are lysed and digested with DNase (151). Thus the active fraction probably is not DNA. However, neither RNase nor trypsin destroy the activity (151). The material is known to have a fairly low molecular weight since it is dialyzable (152).

It is difficult to explain the mechanism of action of the transfer factor. If it were simply a passive transfer of an antibody or antibody-like molecule, one would expect hypersensitivity to wane after a few weeks. Some authors have postulated that antigen or antigen fragments are transferred with the cell extract with the host taking an active role in the process (153). Thus the host cells are actively sensitized resulting in prolonged hypersensitivity.

In Vitro Tests for Delayed Hypersensitivity

Because skin tests may vary from person to person due to variations in the physiology of the individual's skin as well as in the degree of hypersensitivity, many investigators have tried to develop an in vitro test of delayed hypersensitivity. Unfortunately, the criterion for an in vitro test representing delayed hypersensitivity is that it correlates with the skin test. Several tests, however, have been described, and study of these in vitro reactions has contributed to an understanding of the pathogenesis of the in vivo reaction. This discussion will be limited to only two of the in vitro tests which have recently been under active investigation.

Migration Inhibition

Early investigators reported that migration of cells from buffy coat or spleen explants of hypersensitive animals did not occur in the presence of specific antigen (154). This test has been utilized with cells from a variety of sources. A form of this test frequently utilized is described by George and Vaughan (155). The cell suspension to be analyzed is placed in a capillary tube which is then sealed and centrifuged. After centrifugation, the capillary tube is broken at the cell-medium interface, and the portion containing the cells is placed in a tissue culture chamber. In the absence of specific antigen, the cells migrate from the capillary tube in a fanlike fashion. In contrast, in the presence of antigen they fail to migrate. The test appears to be quite sensitive. If as few as 2.5 percent of the cells in the reaction mixture are obtained from a hypersensitive animal and the rest from a normal animal, the migration does not occur (156) (Fig. 14-2).

Studies have shown that two cells are necessary for the inhibition of migration to occur, the lymphocyte and the macrophage (157,158). These

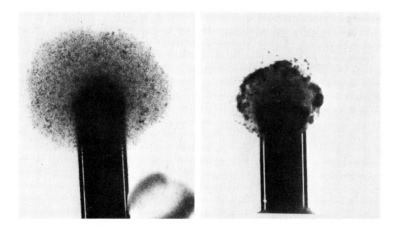

Fig. 14-2 Migration of macrophage out of capillary tubes and its inhibition by specific antigen. On the left, the normal migration of pulmonary alveolar macrophages from a tuberculin sensitive rabbit; on the right, the same macrophages exposed to 5 μg PPD/ml.

studies indicate that the lymphocyte is the cell that reacts with specific antigen, releasing a soluble material called *migration-inhibition factor*. This factor, in turn, inhibits migration of the macrophages, which are the indicator cells in this in vitro test. The factor is nondialyzable, resistant to heating at 56°C for 30 minutes, and is inactivated by RNase and DNase but not trypsin (159).

Abolition of inhibition of migration has been reported when the cells are incubated with trypsin prior to the test (160). The treated cells are capable of passively transferring delayed hypersensitivity to a normal animal, indicating that the enzyme treatment did not kill the cells. In addition, the ability of the cells to respond to the in vitro test is restored after 24 hours incubation in tissue culture in the absence of trypsin.

Inhibition of migration does not occur in the presence of puromycin or actinomycin-D (161). Thus, this test is probably dependent on an active process in which both RNA and protein are synthesized.

Studies of the size of the hapten necessary to cause inhibition of migration have also suggested that an active synthetic process occurs (162). Using an antigen, DNP-polylysine, it was found that haptens too small to induce delayed hypersensitivity did not cause inhibition of migration when incubated with sensitive cells. In contrast, DNP-polylysine molecules large enough to induce delayed hypersensitivity caused inhibition of migration.

Cytotoxic Test

Sensitized lymphocytes in the presence of specific antigen have a cytotoxic effect on indifferent tissue culture monolayers (163,164,165). This test correlates well with the skin test of delayed hypersensitivity and is unrelated to the presence of humoral antibody. The reaction is initiated by the interaction of antigen with the sensitized lymphocytes. A cytotoxic factor released from lymphocytes over a period of several hours kills the tissue culture cells. Therefore, it appears that at least two factors are released from sensitized lymphocytes upon interaction with antigen: one factor that inhibits migration of macrophages, and a second factor that exerts a cytotoxic effect on unrelated cells.

Source of the Cells in the Skin Reaction

The sequence of events in the development of the skin reaction of delayed hypersensitivity is still not completely known. However, several recent studies have contributed to our knowledge of some of the factors involved. Studies utilizing a variety of techniques have shown that most of the cells in the skin site are not those that react with the antigen. The use of the passive transfer technique has been instrumental in these studies. For example, if sensitive cells labeled with tritiated thymidine are injected into a normal recipient and the skin test examined for the presence of these cells, only about 5 percent of the exudate cells are labeled (166). In fact, just as many labeled cells were found in a skin test site to an unrelated antigen as in the specific skin test site (167). In addition, when sensitized cells from an untreated animal were injected into a normal animal that had recently been injected with tritiated thymidine, as many as 90 percent of the cells in the site were labeled. These studies suggest two characteristics of the cellular exudate of delayed hypersensitivity: (1) that only a few of the cells in the exudate are specifically sensitive to the antigen and (2) that most of the cells comprising the inflammatory exudate have recently divided.

Recently, two cells have been shown to be necessary for the generation of the skin reaction, lymphocytes, and macrophages derived from the bone marrow (168,169). If lymphocytes from a hypersensitive guinea pig are injected into a thymectomized, heavily x-radiated recipient, the recipient, unlike a normal recipient, does not become sensitized. If, however, the x-radiated recipient is injected with sensitized lymphocytes and normal bone marrow, the recipient becomes sensitized. At 24 hours the majority of the cells in the skin test site are derived from bone marrow. Thus, it appears that the lymphocyte carries the specificity for the reaction, but the bone-marrow-derived macrophage is necessary for the generation of the reaction.

It is possible that local biosynthesis of antibody occurs at the site of the skin reaction. In a study using DNP-polylysine where the length of the lysine chain was varied, it was found that only the molecules that were large enough to be immunogenic elicited the skin reaction. In contrast, molecules containing fewer lysines could account for all the binding energy of the reaction of humoral antibody and hapten (138,139).

The following is a hypothetical model of the events occurring in the development of the skin reaction.

Upon injection of antigen into the skin, a slight inflammatory reaction is initiated. In the course of this reaction, lymphocytes, some of which are sensitive, pass through the site. The sensitive lymphocytes then react with antigen and are stimulated to synthesize more "antibody," migration-inhibition factor, and cytotoxic factor. Upon damage to the tissue by cytotoxic factor, the inflammatory process is increased, a cellular exudate is induced, and the presence of migration inhibition factor in the site will prolong the inflammatory reaction. Thus, the skin reaction involves only a few specifically sensitized cells that, upon interaction with antigen, release agents which cause a prolonged inflammatory reaction.

Systemic Delayed Hypersensitivity

If tuberculin is given intraperitoneally to a tuberculin-sensitive guinea pig, a systemic reaction may occur. In mild reactions hyperthermia develops; but in severe reactions the animal may become hypothermic. Other symptoms include malaise, joint pains, and leukopenia (126).

The major autopsy findings are hemorrhagic lungs and intestines. Although humoral antibody has been implicated in causing some of the symptoms, fatal systemic reactions have been transferred passively with cells.

Contact Hypersensitivity

Contact hypersensitivity is a unique type of delayed hypersensitivity because the antigens involved are haptens which must combine with host protein to become antigenic (170,171). Hypersensitivity is induced when a hapten contacts the skin and combines with host proteins, becoming a complete antigen. The specificity of the hypersensitivity that is induced is directed both to the hapten and the carrier protein. When the hapten contacts the skin of a hypersensitive animal, it again combines with the host proteins and elicits a reaction if the hapten-protein conjugate is present at the epidermodermal junction (172). The gross appearance of the reaction varies with the animal species. The histology is similar to a tuberculin reaction in that at the peak of the reaction the predominant cells in the exudate are mononuclears.

MECHANISMS OF AUTOIMMUNE DISEASE

The mechanisms operating in autoimmune injury are immediate hypersensitivity and Arthus-type reactions with demonstrable circulating antibodies, and delayed hypersensitivities in which antibodies are of the cell-bound type. There are at least three ways in which the autoimmune process may be mediated: the antigen may be endogenous, that is it originates in the host and produces injury by being modified so that the host cannot recognize it as self and will respond to it with the production of antibodies which in turn combine with the antigen; it may be exogenous and be very similar to endogenous material or cross-react with it; or a third possibility, it may be a combination of these two mechanisms, which is also very likely and may be a frequent occurrence. The most common endogenous antigen may be one of the constituents of the host tissue.

This may be liberated by a number of injurious processes which, by modifying it slightly, render it antigenic and nonrecognizable as self. It may also be a body component which was segregated and therefore unknown to the immunologically responsive cells (e.g., thyroglobulin, sperm). A vicious circle is then initiated, with antibody response, combination of antibody with antigen, and liberation of more altered tissue constituents, which in turn starts another cycle of antibody production and ultimately leads to autoimmune disease. Many kinds of responses can occur. As indicated above there may be production of humoral antibodies which are very effective against circulating cells (for example in hemolytic anemias of autoimmune nature). There may also be a cellular antibody with the lymphoid cells penetrating tissues and organs to injure the target cells. On the other hand, the humoral and cellular responses may be combined to produce injury by both mechanisms.

Definition of Autoimmune Diseases

In discussing autoimmune diseases certain parameters are necessary to give evidence of autoimmune injury. First is the demonstration of cells or immunoglobulins which can react with the specific tissue involved in autoimmune injury and can attack this tissue. Second is the necessity to demonstrate the presence of antibodies in vitro and the transfer of the injury with this antibody, be it humoral or cell-bound. Third, the production of the injury must be possible with experimental animals by using specific tissues to immunize the animals. Autoimmune injury is a reasonably common occurrence in pathologic manifestations in humans and experimental animals, and the role of this injury in determining disease may be of different natures. The autoimmune response may be a primary causative agent of disease as outlined above when the antigen is endogenous and becomes somewhat altered. It then sets up a cycle of antibody production with consequent injury. On the other hand, tissues may combine with some injurious agent—chemical, drug, or otherwise. This may modify tissue antigens which are then capable of instituting the autoimmune injury.

Hematologic Autoimmune Diseases with Primarily Circulating Antibodies

The main group of autoimmune diseases are those comprising the autoimmune hematologic disorders: hemolytic anemias, granulocytopenia, and thrombocytopenia (173).

Hemolytic Anemias

Two types of antibodies are present in these anemias: warm antibodies and cold antibodies. The warm antibodies are incomplete and will sensitize erythrocytes for agglutination by anti-immunoglobulin serum. They can also be detected in serum by their property to agglutinate red cells treated with enzymes. Their reactivity is optimal at 37°C. On the other hand, cold antibodies can also be detected in the serum and have an optimal reactivity at 4°C. These are complete antibodies and will agglutinate red cells with very high titers or produce hemolysis. They are still reactive up to a maximum of 30°C. Complete antibodies are usually of the macroglobulin type, while the warm antibodies are of the IgG type. The mechanism of sensitization in this group of diseases is quite hard to understand. Perhaps some red cells may have reached the lymphoid system by a mechanism as yet unknown and then become somewhat modified to set up antibody production. On the other hand, the lymphoreticular system may be abnormal and react with red cells in an abnormal fashion, or there may be exogenous antigens (drugs, etc.) which combine with the erythrocytes to make them antigenic.

Granulocytopenia

Another form of hematologic disorder which may be autoimmune is the granulocytopenia. This may, in some cases, be induced by drugs or other haptenic substances, combining with white cells which then become antigenic.

Autoimmune Diseases with Circulating and Cell-bound Antibodies

In another group of well-established autoimmune diseases gamma globulins or cell constituents appear to be the main antigen. These are characterized by both circulating and cell-bound antibodies. Lupus erythematosus and rheumatoid arthritis are the main diseases in this group. Several other entities appear to be closely related, although the nature of their relationship is not very clear. These include scleroderma, dermatomyositis, polyarteritis, etc. This group of diseases is quite interesting in that one can demonstrate affinity of gamma globulin or mononuclear cells for tissue constituents by serologic methods like complement fixation, hemagglutination, antiglobulin consumption, etc. The fluorescent antibody method can also be used to demonstrate this antigen-antibody combination. Mixed tissue cultures of lymphocytes from patients that have the disease can also be employed (174). Hashimoto's thyroiditis is another well-described autoimmune disease. It is primarily mediated by thyroglobulin as the antigen; thryoglobulin may become liberated from its segregated position within the thyroid follicles and become antigenic, since it is "unknown" to the lymphoid tissue as self until it leaves the follicles. Rheumatic fever, ulcerative colitis, myasthenia gravis, and glomerulonephritis are other examples of possible autoimmune diseases. The latter is perhaps the one which has best been examined experimentally (175). The thyroiditis has also been carefully studied by several authors (176). In the case of these two diseases it is apparent that circulating antibody is produced and also that lymphoid cells are present which are capable of mediating autoimmune injury. The antibody appears to be an anti-gamma globulin in the case of the kidney, with deposition of antigen-antibody complexes on the basement membrane and perivascular mononuclear cell infiltrates. In autoimmune thyroiditis, circulating antithyroglobulin antibody can be demonstrated and lymphocytic accumulation in the gland is prominent.

Experimental Production of Autoimmune Injury

The experimental animal has been used extensively to study autoimmune diseases, and the methods of production of the disease have varied with different investigators. Autologous, homologous, or heterologous tissues have been used with or without complete or incomplete Freund's adjuvant. The result has usually been to produce both circulating immunoglobulin and sensitized cells which carry the antibody. The lesions observed have corresponded to the tissue used as an antigen in the host in which the autoimmune phenomenon has been elicited. The models that have been constructed have been compared to the human pathologic entities observed clinically. When the comparison resulted in a number of parallel findings in the experimental and clinical situation, a direct correlation was postulated in the case of human disease with autoimmune etiopathogenetic mechanisms.

Experimental allergic encephalomyelitis, experimental neuritis, experimental thyroiditis, experimental orchitis with aspermatogenesis, experimental glomerulonephritis, experimental uveitis, experimental dermatitis, arthritis, gastritis, and adrenalitis have been produced in laboratory animals by various investigators, and in many cases the similarity between these diseases and human autoimmune injury have been striking.

Experimental Allergic Encephalomyelitis (EAE)

EAE has been produced in monkeys, dogs, rabbits, guinea pigs, rats, mice, and as an accidental byproduct of vaccination with rabies vaccine in humans. The antigen has been shown to be the white matter of the central nervous system in association with myelin. The response consists of circulating antibodies toxic to myelin in vitro and also of cellular sensitivity so that the disease can be transferred by transferring lymphoid cells. The changes observed have consisted of demyelination with inflammation usually in the central nervous system. Neuritis has also been found which is very similar except that antigen is derived from the peripheral rather than the central nervous system (177).

Experimental Thyroiditis

Thyroiditis has been studied by several investigators in dogs, rabbits, guinea pigs, and rats. Thyroglobulin has usually been used as antigen, although less refined, more crude thyroid extracts have also been used. A circulating antibody has been demonstrated which usually did not follow the disease development in terms of its increase or decrease. The disease could be transferred with the serum, but cellular sensitivity which paralleled the course of the disease was observed, and the disease could definitely be transferred by lymphoid cells. The main observable injury has been the appearance of large accumulations of lymphoid cells in the thyroid with destruction of the thyroid. This is similar to Hashimoto's disease observed in humans (176).

Aspermatogenesis

The guinea pig and the rat have been used as hosts for the production of aspermatogenesis with nonprotein material from sperm (probably a lipopolysaccharide). Both cellular and humoral antibodies have been demonstrated, with inflammation of the testes of the host animal and injury of the germinal cells.

Glomerulonephritis

The glomerulonephritis which has been produced in rats and mice has usually been induced with specific antigens from the renal cortex, and the response has consisted of gamma globulin deposition in the glomeruli of the host with thickening of the glomerular basement membrane and proteinuria. The other diseases have been produced with antigen derived from the organ in question in many hosts, primates or rodents, with corresponding production of humoral and cellular antibodies and the classical infiltration of lymphoid cells into the organ in which the injury was manifested (178).

SUMMARY

This has been a very brief outline of some of the autoimmune diseases which are observed in humans and of the possible mechanisms by which these diseases may be generated, together with a short description of some of the diseases which have been produced in experimental animals by the use of either autologous or homologous antigens. We hope it has pointed to the fact that (as it has become apparent in the first part of this chapter dealing with immediate and delayed hypersensitivity) antibodies may injure as well as protect. In fact one encounters daily, in the practice of medicine and in many other areas, the injurious properties of antibodies. While one tries to control injury, at the same time the protective properties of antibodies are developed to prevent disease.

Although quite a large number of less well understood pathologic manifestations have been ascribed to autoimmune reactions, it is apparent that autoimmunity is not a wastebasket into which every unknown disease can be thrown. There are quite definitely pathologic entities which are produced by the interaction of autoantigens with the immunologically competent cells, thus leading to the production of disease. On the other hand, many so-called autoimmune diseases find their origin in the fact that injury is brought upon tissue constituents, and these are modified to act as antigens. This leads to the perpetuation of disease which is not really autoimmune in origin, since the etiologic factor is of a different nature. Be this as it may, this is an important phenomenon in immunology which is of great biologic importance and may ultimately help to explain quite a number of hitherto poorly understood pathologic entities. Recent research in this area is intensive, and new results are being presented frequently in the literature. These investigations are continually clarifying the very complex problem of self and self-recognition and its relationship to the production of disease by immune responses directed toward parts of this self which should not be ordinarily handled as foreign antigens by the immunologically competent cells.

REFERENCES

1. Portier, P., and Richet, G.: *Compt. Rend. Soc. de Biol.*, **54**:170, 1902.
2. Ovary, Z.: *Progr. Allergy*, **5**:459, 1958.
3. Layton, L. L., Lee, S., and DeEds, F.: *Proc. Soc. Exp. Biol. Med.*, **108**: 623, 1961.
4. Ishizaka, K., Ishizaka, T., and Arbesman, C. E.: *J. Allergy*, **39**:254, 1967.

5. Halpern, B. N., Liacopoulos, P., Liacopoulos-Briot, M., Binaghi, R., and Van Neer, F.: *Immunology*, **2**:351, 1959.
6. Arbesman, C. E., Girard, P., and Rose, N. R.: *J. Allergy*, **35**:535, 1964.
7. Mongar, J. L., and Schild, H. O.: *J. Physiol.*, **135**:320, 1957.
8. Baker, A. R., Bloch, K. J., and Austen, K. F.: *J. Immunol.*, **93**:525, 1964.
9. Mongar, J. L., and Schild, H. O.: *J. Physiol.*, **150**:546, 1960.
10. Mota, I.: *J. Physiol.*, **140**:6P, 1958.
11. Mota, I.: *Immunology*, **7**:681, 1964.
12. Austen, K. F., Bloch, K. J., Baker, A. R., and Arnason, B. G.: *Proc. Soc. Exp. Biol. Med.*, **120**:542, 1965.
13. Barbaro, J. F., and Zvaifler, N. J.: *Proc. Soc. Exp. Biol. Med.*, **122**:1245, 1966.
14. Lichtenstein, L. M., and Osler, A. G.: *J. Exp. Med.*, **120**:507, 1964.
15. Levy, D. A., and Osler, A. G.: *J. Immunol.*, **97**:203, 1966.
16. Chase, W,: in "Bacterial and Mycotic Disease of Man," R. J. Dubos, (ed.), J. B. Lippincott Company, Philadelphia, 1958.
17. Solotorovsky, M., and Winsten, S.: *J. Immunol.*, **71**:296, 1953.
18. Morgan, P., Sherwood, N. P., and Werder, A. A.: *J. Immunol.*, **79**:46 1957.
19. Malkiel, S., and Hargis, B. J.: *Proc. Soc. Exp. Biol. Med.*, **81**:689, 1952.
20. Malkiel, S., and Hargis, B. J.: *J. Allergy*, **23**:352, 1952.
21. Kind, L. S.: *J. Immunol.*, **79**:238, 1957.
22. Parfentjev, I. A., and Goodline, M. A.: *J. Pharmacol. Exp. Therap.*, **92**: 411, 1948.
23. Munoz, J.: *Proc. Soc. Exp. Biol. Med.*, **95**:328, 1957.
24. Munoz, J., Schuchardt, L. F., and Verwey, W. F.: *J. Immunol.*, **80**:77, 1958.
25. Benacerraf, B., Ovary, Z., Bloch, K. J., and Franklin, E. C.: *J. Exp. Med.*, **117**:937, 1963.
26. Ovary, Z., Benacerraf, B., and Bloch, K. J.: *J. Exp. Med.*, **117**:951, 1963.
27. Stechschulte, D. J., Austen, K. F., and Bloch, K. J.: *J. Exp. Med.*, **125**: 127, 1967.
28. Nussenzweig, R. S., Merryman, C., and Benacerraf, B.: *J. Exp. Med.*, **120**:315, 1964.
29. Ishizaka, K., Ishizaka, T., and Hornbrook, M. M.: *J. Immunol.*, **98**:490, 1967.
30. Ishizaka, K., Ishizaka, T., and Hornbrook, M. M.: *J. Immunol.*, **97**:840, 1966.
31. Ishizaka, K., and Ishizaka, T.: *J. Immunol.*, **99**:1187, 1967.
32. Johansson, S. G. O., and Bennich, H.: *Immunology*, **13**:381, 1967.
33. Oettgen, H. F., Binaghi, R. A., and Benacerraf, B.: *Proc. Soc. Exp. Biol. Med.*, **118**:336, 1965.
34. Ishizaka, K., Ishizaka, T., and Menzel, A. E. O.: *J. Immunol.*, **99**:610, 1967.

35. Bloch, K. J., Ovary, Z., Kourilsky, F. M., and Benacerraf, B.: *Proc. Soc. Exp. Biol. Med.*, **114**:79, 1963.
36. Rockey, J. H., and Schwartzman, R. M.: *J. Immunol.*, **98**:1143, 1967.
37. Zvaifler, N. J., and Becker, E. L.: *J. Exp. Med.*, **123**:935, 1966.
38. Binaghi, R. A., Benacerraf, B., Bloch, K. J., and Koursilsky, F. M.: *J. Immunol.*, **92**:927, 1964.
39. Mota, I.: *Immunology*, **12**:343, 1967.
40. Schoenbechler, M. J., and Sadun, E. H.: *Proc. Soc. Exp. Biol. Med.*, **127**:601, 1968.
41. Wilson, R. J. M., and Bloch, K. J.: *J. Immunol.*, **100**:622, 1968.
42. Benacerraf, B., and Kabat, E. A.: *J. Immunol.*, **62**:517, 1949.
43. Ovary, Z., and Bier, O. G.: *J. Immunol.*, **71**:6, 1953.
44. Chandler, M. H., Rosenberg, L. T., and Fischel, E. E.: *J. Immunol.*, **82**:103, 1959.
45. Munoz, J., and Anacker, R. L.: *J. Immunol.*, **83**:640, 1959.
46. Humphrey, J. H., and Mota, I.: *Immunology*, **2**:19, 1959.
47. Ovary, Z., Bloch, K. J., and Benacerraf, B.: *Proc. Soc. Exp. Biol. Med.*, **116**:840, 1964.
48. Ovary, Z., Fudenberg, H., and Kunkel, H. G.: *J. Exp. Med.*, **112**:953, 1960.
49. Ishizaka, K., Ishizaka, T., Lee, E. H., and Fudenberg, H.: *J. Immunol.*, **95**:197, 1965.
50. Kabat, E. A., and Boldt, M. H.: *J. Immunol.*, **48**:181, 1944.
51. Bier, O. G., and Siqueira, M.: *Int. Arch. Allergy*, **6**:391, 1955.
52. Ovary, Z.: *Immunology*, **3**:19, 1960.
53. Terry, W. D.: *Proc. Soc. Exp. Biol. Med.*, **117**:901, 1964.
54. Franklin, E. C., and Ovary, Z.: *Immunology*, **6**:434, 1963.
55. Ovary, Z., and Bier, O. G.: *Ann. Inst. Pasteur (Paris)*, **84**:443, 1953.
56. Ishizaka, K., Ishizaka, T., and Hornbrook, M. M.: *J. Allergy*, **34**:395, 1963.
57. Biozzi, G., Halpern, B. N., and Binaghi, R.: *J. Immunol.*, **82**:215, 1959.
58. Ishizaka, K., Ishizaka, T., and Terry, W. D.: *J. Immunol.*, **99**:849, 1967.
59. Ovary, Z., and Karush, F.: *J. Immunol.*, **86**:146, 1961.
60. Ishizaka, K., Ishizaka, T., and Sugahara, T.: *J. Immunol.*, **88**:690, 1962.
61. Terry, W. D.: *J. Immunol.*, **95**:1041, 1965.
62. Kabat, E. A., and Landow, H.: *J. Immunol.*, **44**:69, 1942.
63. Ovary, Z., and Karush, F.: *J. Immunol.*, **84**:409, 1960.
64. Ovary, Z.: *C. R. Acad. Sci. (Paris)*, **253**:582, 1961.
65. Levine, B. B.: *J. Immunol.*, **94**:111, 1965.
66. Leskowitz, S., and Ovary, Z.: *Immunology*, **5**:1, 1962.
67. Levine, B. B.: *J. Immunol.*, **94**:121, 1965.
68. Levine, B. B., and Redmond, A. P.: *J. Clin. Invest.*, **47**:556, 1968.
69. Germuth, F. G., Jr., and McKinnon, G. E.: *Bull. Johns Hopkins Hosp.*, **101**:13, 1957.

70. Trapani, I. L., Garvey, J. S., and Campbell, D. H.: *Science,* **127**:700, 1958.
71. Ishizaka, K., and Campbell, D. H.: *Proc. Soc. Exp. Biol. Med.,* **97**:635, 1958.
72. Ishizaka, K., Ishizaka, T., and Campbell, D. H.: *J. Exp. Med.,* **109**:127, 1959.
73. Ishizaka, K., Ishizaka, T., and Campbell, D. H.: *J. Immunol.,* **83**:105, 1959.
74. Ishizaka, K., and Campbell, D. H.: *J. Immunol.,* **83**:116, 1959.
75. Ishizaka, K., and Campbell, D. H.: *J. Immunol.,* **83**:318, 1959.
76. Henney, C. S., and Stanworth, D. R.: *Nature (London),* **210**:1071, 1966.
77. Ishizaka, T., and Ishizaka, K.: *Proc. Soc. Exp. Biol. Med.,* **101**:845, 1959.
78. Ishizaka, K., and Ishizaka, T.: *J. Immunol.,* **85**:163, 1960.
79. Ishizaka, T., Ishizaka, K., Salmon, S., and Fudenberg, H.: *J. Immunol.,* **99**:82, 1967.
80. Henney, C. S., and Ishizaka, K.: *J. Immunol.,* **100**:718, 1968.
81. Ishizaka, K.: *Progr. Allergy,* **7**:32, 1963.
82. Ishizaka, K., and Ishizaka, T.: *J. Immunol.,* in press.
83. Arthus, M.: *Compt. Rend. Soc. de Biol.,* **55**:817, 1903.
84. Benacerraf, B., and Kabat, E. A.: *J. Immunol.,* **64**:1, 1950.
85. Tada, T., and Ishizaka, K.: *J. Immunol.,* **96**:112, 1966.
86. Levenson, H., and Cochrane, C. G.: *J. Immunol.,* **92**:118, 1964.
87. Fernando, N. V. P., and Movat, H. Z.: *Amer. J. Pathol.,* **43**:381, 1963.
88. Cochrane, C. G., and Aikin, B. S.: *J. Exp. Med.,* **124**:733, 1966.
89. Ward, P. A., and Cochrane, C. G.: *J. Exp. Med.,* **121**:215, 1965.
90. Stetson, C. A.: *J. Exp. Med.,* **94**:347, 1951.
91. Humphrey, J. H.: *Brit. J. Exp. Pathol.,* **36**:268, 1955.
92. Humphrey, J. H.: *Brit. J. Exp. Pathol.,* **36**:283, 1955.
93. Cochrane, C. G., Weigle, W. O., and Dixon, F. J.: *J. Exp. Med.,* **110**:481, 1959.
94. Cochrane, C. G., Weigle, W. O., and Dixon, F. J.: *J. Exp. Med.,* **110**:481, 1959.
95. Cochrane, C. G., and Aikin, B. S.: *J. Exp. Med.,* **124**:733, 1966.
96. Meier, R., and Schär, B.: *Experentia,* **11**:1, 1955.
97. Boyden, S.: *J. Exp. Med.,* **115**:453, 1962.
98. Ward, P. A., Cochrane, C. G., and Müller-Eberhard, H. J.: *J. Exp. Med.,* **122**:327, 1965.
99. Ward, P. A., Cochrane, C. G., and Müller-Eberhard, H. J.: *Immunology,* **11**:141, 1966.
100. Hawkins, D., and Cochrane, C. G.: *Immunology,* **14**:665, 1968.
101. Sbarra, A. J., and Karnovsky, M. L.: *J. Biol. Chem.,* **234**:1355, 1959.
102. Seegers, W., and Janoff, A.: *J. Exp. Med.,* **124**:833, 1966.
103. Janoff, A., and Schaefer, S.: *Nature (London),* **213**:144, 1967.
104. Janoff, A.: *Federation Proc.,* **27**(2):250, 1968.

105. Ranadive, N. S., and Cochrane, C. G.: *J. Exp. Med.*, **128**:605, 1968.
106. Dixon, F. J.: *The Harvey Lectures*, **58**:21, 1962–63.
107. Unanue, E. R., and Dixon, F. J.: *Advan. Immunol.*, **6**:1, 1967.
108. Koffler, D., and Kunkel, H. G.: *Amer. J. Med.*, **45**:165, 1968.
109. Koch, R.: *Deut. Med. Wochschr.*, **16**:1029, 1890.
110. Landsteiner, K., and Chase, M. W.: *Proc. Soc. Exp. Biol. Med.*, **49**:688, 1942.
111. Chase, M. W.: *Proc. Soc. Exp. Biol. Med.*, **59**:134, 1945.
112. Mantoux, C.: *Presse Méd.*, **18**:10, 1910.
113. Dienes, L., and Mallory, T.: *Amer. J. Pathol.*, **8**:689, 1932.
114. Follis, R. H.: *Bull. Johns Hopkins Hosp.*, **66**:245, 1940.
115. Boughton, B., and Spector, W. G.: *J. Pathol. Bact.*, **85**:371, 1963.
116. Turk, J. L., Heather, C. J., and Dirngdon, J. V.: *Int. Arch. Allergy*, **29**: 278, 1966.
117. Laporte, R.: *Ann. Inst. Pasteur (Paris)*, **53**:598, 1934.
118. Kolin, A., Johanovsky, J., and Pekárek, J.: *Z. Immunitäts-Allergieforsch.*, **128**:117, 1965.
119. Kolin, A., Johanovsky, J., and Pekarek, J.: *Int. Arch. Allergy*, **26**:167, 1965.
120. Campbell, P. A., and La Via, M. F.: *Proc. Soc. Exp. Biol. Med.*, **124**: 571, 1967.
121. Lawrence, H. S.: *Amer. J. Med.*, **20**:428, 1956.
122. Crowle, A. J., and Hu, C. C.: *Clin. Exp. Immunol.*, **3**:323, 1966.
123. Coulaud, E.: *C. R. Soc. Biol.* **119**:368, 1935.
124. Uhr, J. W., Salvin, S. B., and Pappenheimer, R. M., Jr.: *J. Exp. Med.*, **105**:11, 1957.
125. Salvin, S. B.: *J. Exp. Med.*, **107**:109, 1958.
126. Crowle, A. J.: "Delayed Hypersensitivity in Health and Disease," Springfield, Ill., Charles C Thomas, Publisher, 1962.
127. Landsteiner, K., and Chase, M. W.: *J. Exp. Med.*, **69**:767, 1939.
128. Turk, J. L., and Stone, S. H.: in "Cell Bound Antibodies," B. Amos and H. Koprowski (Eds.), Philadelphia, Wistar Institute Press, 1963.
129. Frey, J. R., and Wenk, P.: *Int. Arch. Allergy*, **11**:81, 1957.
130. Freund, J., and Lipton, M. M.: *J. Immunol.*, **75**:454, 1955.
131. Scothorne, R. J., and McGregor, I. A.: *J. Anat.*, **89**:282, 1955.
132. Oort, J., and Turk, J. L.: *Brit. J. Exp. Pathol.*, **46**:147, 1965.
133. de Petris, S., Karlsbad, J. G., and Pernis, B.: *Int. Arch. Allergy*, **29**:112, 1966.
134. Landsteiner, K.: "The Specificity of Serological Reaction," Springfield, Ill., Charles C Thomas, Publisher, 1936.
135. Benacerraf, B., and Lexine, B. B.: *J. Exp. Med.*, **115**:1023, 1962.
136. Gell, P. G. H., and Silverstein, A. M.: *J. Exp. Med.*, **115**:1037, 1962.
137. Leskowitz, S.: *J. Exp. Med.*, **117**:909, 1963.
138. Schlossman, S. F., Ben-Efraim, S., Yaron, A., and Sober, H. A.: *J. Exp. Med.*, **123**:1083, 1966.

139. Schlossman, S. F., and Levine, H.: *J. Immunol.*, **98**:211, 1967.
140. Prausnitz, C., and Küstner, H.: *Zentr. Bakteriol.*, **86**:160, 1921.
141. Hauxthausen, H.: *Acta Dermato-Venerol.*, **27**:275, 1947.
142. Hauxthausen, H., *Acta Dermato-Venerol.*, **31**:659, 1951.
143. Zinsser, H., and Mueller, J. H.: *J. Exp. Med.*, **41**:159, 1925.
144. Freund, J., *J. Immunol.*, **11**:383, 1926.
145. Jeter, W. S., Tremaine, M. M., and Seebohm, P. M.: *Proc. Soc. Exp. Biol. Med.*, **86**:251, 1954.
146. Cummings, M. M., Patnode, R. A., and Hudgins, P. C.: *Amer. Rev. Tuberc.*, **73**:246, 1956.
147. Turk, J. L., and Asherson, G. L.: *Int. Arch. Allergy*, **21**:321, 1962.
148. Metaxas, M., and Metaxas-Bühler, M.: *J. Immunol.*, **75**:333, 1955.
149. Chase, M. W., and Battisto, J. R.: *J. Allergy*, **26**:83, 1955.
150. Lawrence, H. S.: *Proc. Soc. Exp. Biol. Med.*, **71**:516, 1949.
151. Lawrence, H. S.: in "Cellular and Humoral Aspects of the Hypersensitive States," H. S. Lawrence (Ed.), New York, Harper & Row (Hoeber), 1959.
152. Lawrence, H. S.: in "Cell Bound Antibodies," B. Amos and H. Koprowski (Eds.), Philadelphia, Wistar Institute Press, 1963.
153. Turk, J. L.: "Delayed Hypersensitivity," New York, John Wiley & Sons, Inc., 1967.
154. Rich, A. R., and Lewis, M. R.: *Bull. Johns Hopkins Hosp.*, **50**:115, 1933.
155. George, M., and Vaughan, J. H.: *Proc. Soc. Exp. Biol. Med.*, **111**:514, 1962.
156. David, J. R., Lawrence, H. S., and Thomas, L.: *J. Immunol.*, **93**:274, 1964.
157. Bloom, B. R., and Bennett, B.: *Science*, **153**:80, 1966.
158. David, J. R.: *Proc. Nat. Acad. Sci. U.S.*, **56**:72, 1966.
159. David, J. R.: *Federation Proc.*, **27**:6, 1968.
160. David, J. R., Lawrence, H. S., and Thomas, L.: *J. Exp. Med.*, **120**:1189, 1964.
161. David, J. R.: *J. Exp. Med.*, **122**:1125, 1965.
162. David, J. R., and Schlossman, S. F.: *J. Exp. Med.*, **128**:1451, 1968.
163. Ruddle, N. H., and Waksman, B. H.: *J. Exp. Med.*, **128**:1237, 1968.
164. Ruddle, N. H., and Waksman, B. H.: *J. Exp. Med.*, **128**:1255, 1968.
165. Ruddle, N. H., and Waksman, B. H.: *J. Exp. Med.*, **128**:1267, 1968.
166. Najarian, J. S., and Feldman, J. D.: *J. Exp. Med.*, **114**:479, 1961.
167. McClusky, R. T., Benacerraf, B., and McClusky, J. W.: *J. Immunol.*, **90**:466, 1963.
168. Lubaroff, D. M., and Waksman, B. H.: *J. Exp. Med.*, **128**:1425, 1968.
169. Lubaroff, D. M., and Waksman, B. H.: *J. Exp. Med.*, **128**:1437, 1968.
170. Landsteiner, K., and Jacobs, J. L.: *J. Exp. Med.*, **64**:625, 1936.
171. Eisen, H. N., Orris, L., and Belman, S.: *J. Exp. Med.*, **95**:473, 1952.
172. Eisen, H. N., and Tabachnick, M.: *J. Exp. Med.*, **108**:773, 1958.
173. Miescher, P. A.: in "Textbook of Immunopathology," P. A. Miescher

and H. J. Müller-Eberhard (Eds.), New York, Grune & Stratton, Inc., 1969.

174. Miescher, P. A., and Müller-Eberhard, H. J. (Eds.): "Textbook of Immunopathology," New York, Grune & Stratton, Inc., 1969.

175. Unanue, E. R., and Dixon, F. J.: *Advan. Immunol.*, **6**:1, 1967.

176. Rose, N. R., and Witebsky, E.: in "Textbook of Immunopathology," P. A. Miescher and H. J. Müller-Eberhard (Eds.), New York, Grune & Stratton, Inc., 1969.

177. Paterson, P. Y.: in "Textbook of Immunopathology," P. A. Miescher and H. J. Müller-Eberhard (Eds.), New York, Grune & Stratton, Inc., 1969.

178. Unanue, E. R., Dixon, F. J., and Feldman, J. D.: in "Textbook of Immunopathology," P. A. Miescher and H. J. Müller-Eberhard (Eds.), New York, Grune & Stratton, Inc., 1969.

15
Transplantation Immunity

Although comprehensive monographs concerning the morphological descriptions of lymphocytes and lymphoid tissues have long been available, it is only recently that the lymphocyte has been the focus of intensive experimental investigations into the mechanisms of the immune response. Much of the recently acquired knowledge of the biologic properties of the lymphocyte and many of the modern concepts of its involvement in immunity have stemmed from studies employing principles and techniques of transplantation immunology. This chapter will concern itself with some of the fundamental principles of transplantation immunology and the functional role of the lymphocyte in the development and execution of the immune response with emphasis on homograft immunity.

BASIC PRINCIPLES OF HOMOGRAFT IMMUNITY

The Homograft Reaction

Techniques for the transplantation of human tissues from one site to another in the same individual (autografts) for the purpose of surgical repair of accidental or physiological deficits have their historical origins before the birth of Christ. The literature throughout the centuries thereafter contains scattered accounts of attempts to transplant tissues, predominately skin, from different individuals (homografts) and even from different species (heterografts) (1). Although there may have been some temporary benefit to the recipients of homo- and heterografted tissues, these grafts did not remain functionally intact for more than a few days. On this basis Ehrlich concluded that innate chemical and consequent nutritional differences between the tissues of different individuals, even of the same species, accounted for the prompt rejection of foreign grafts.

In the 1940s the results of the classic experiments of Medawar (2–6) demonstrated the fallacy of this premise of innate resistance by showing that the reaction provoked by homografts of normal tissue is an actively acquired immunity. Orthotopic homografts of skin transplanted between randomly selected pairs of rabbits were accepted for a short time, became healed in, and reacquired a vascular supply in a manner similar to that of autografts. Their viability was affirmed by the growth of hair. Within a few days this grace period terminated. Unlike the autografts, homografts developed signs of inflammation, acquired an infiltrate of leukocytic cells, became necrotic, and were sloughed. This rejection of foreign tissues (the homograft reaction) was considered to be the outcome of an immunologic response by the host against alien, antigenic factors contained in the grafted tissues for the following reasons: (1) within limits this was a "dose"-dependent phenomenon; i.e., smaller grafts were destroyed at a slower rate than larger ones. (2) Second grafts from the initial donor underwent a more prompt, accelerated rejection process (the "second-set reaction"), while grafts from third-party donors underwent rejection with the tempo of a first graft (Fig. 15-1). Further evidence of the immunologic nature of the homograft reaction was provided by the findings that (3) the resistance developed to foreign tissues was systemic rather than local; that is, second grafts were rejected in a second-set manner whether placed into the original or a distant site; and (4) antibodies with specificities directed against donor red blood cells appeared in the serum of the host concomitant with the rejection of the graft. The results of Medawar's original experiments went a long way toward dispelling Ehrlich's doctrine of innate resistance and establishing the immunologic basis of the homograft reaction. This conclusion was reinforced with studies using homologous grafts of transplantable neoplastic, rather than normal, tissues (5–8).

The vector agents responsible for the homograft reaction became the subject of primary concern. Attempts to locate graft-destructive factors in the serum of sensitized animals were unsuccessful. Serum, obtained from animals that had rejected a sensitizing graft, when infused, even in large quantities, into normal animals routinely failed to curtail the survival time of test homografts on these animals (9). Instead, in some cases, test homo-

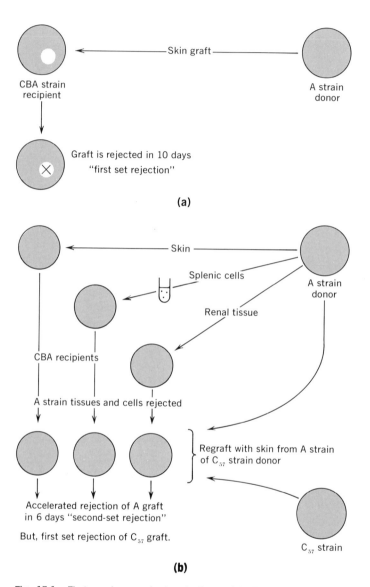

(a)

(b)

Fig. 15-1 First- and second-set rejection. (a) First-set. Skin grafted orthotopically from an A-strain mouse donor to a CBA, homologous recipient is rejected in approximately 10 days. (b) Second-set. Tissues or cells of various histologic origin from an A-strain donor transplanted to a CBA recipient are rejected as a first-set reaction. When test grafted later with skin from another donor of the A strain, this graft is rejected with an accelerated tempo (second-set rejection). If tested with skin from a third party, C57 strain donor, this graft is rejected in the first-set manner.

grafts survived longer than expected on these serum-treated hosts. This phenomenon was later attributed to an interference with primary sensitization and was described as immunologic enhancement (10). Convincing evidence for the susceptibility of grafts to antibodies has been presented only under special circumstances with transplants of leukotic tumors and certain cellular homografts (11).

Mitchison (12–14) found that homograft sensitivity could be transferred "adoptively" to otherwise normal recipients by means of living lymphoid cells from immunized donors. Furthermore, his studies established that the principal seats of host response in the homograft reaction are those regional lymph nodes which drain the site of the graft (Fig. 15-2).

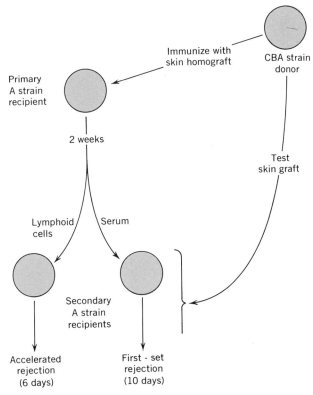

Fig. 15-2 This diagram illustrates the principle of the "adoptive" transfer of immunity. A primary A-strain recipient is immunized with a skin homograft from a CBA donor. Two weeks later a suspension of splenic or lymph node cells or serum is prepared from this primary host and transferred to secondary, isologous A-strain recipients. These are then grafted with skin from the original CBA donor. Recipients of lymphoid cells reject skin homografts more promptly than animals that receive serum.

Additional evidence for the complicity of cells rather than soluble serum elements in the destruction of solid-tissue homografts was provided by Algire et al. (15–17). They demonstrated that homologous "target" tissues placed within the confines of diffusion chambers and inserted intraperitoneally into previously sensitized hosts were not destroyed unless the pore size of the diffusion chambers was sufficiently large to allow the passage of host leukocytes (Fig. 15-3).

These findings ended further attempts to classify homograft reactivity as a serum-antibody-mediated immediate hypersensitivity phenomenon. Transferability of an immune state by cells of the lymphoid series rather than immune serum is one of the cardinal features of hypersensitivity reactions of the delayed type. Thus the immunologic processes of the homograft reaction are considered similar to those involved in delayed sensitivities or allergies to drugs, microorganisms (particularly tubercule bacilli), and autoantigenic body constituents (7,18).

Genetic Aspects

The incompatibility of skin or of other tissue and cellular homografts transplanted from an alien donor and the consequent rejection of these foreign grafts represents an immunologic expression of genetically deter-

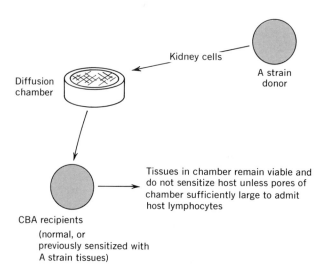

Kidney cells

Diffusion chamber

A strain donor

Tissues in chamber remain viable and do not sensitize host unless pores of chamber sufficiently large to admit host lymphocytes

CBA recipients
(normal, or previously sensitized with A strain tissues)

Fig. 15-3 Homologous tissues or cells enclosed within the confines of cell-impenetrable diffusion chambers when placed into the peritoneal cavities of recipient mice remain viable even if the hosts are sensitized and do not provoke a state of immunity in normal hosts.

mined differences between individuals. It is the outcome of an immune response directed against transplantation, or histocompatibility (H) antigens, present in the graft and absent in the host, determined by H genes with chromosomal locations designated as H loci. At some of these loci, one of an alternative series of genes is expressed. Others seem to be more complex, consisting of a very closely linked, or pseudoallelic series of genes, each of which probably determines a single antigenic specificity.

The genetic basis for the acceptance of grafted tissues or cells is simply that the complement of donor H genes must also be represented in the host so that, as with identical twins or individuals of a highly inbred, isogenic strain, no foreign transplantation antigens confront the immunologic apparatus of the host. Although tissues grafted between individuals of a single isogenic strain are not rejected, they are rejected if donor and host differ by even a single H gene. One other circumstance of donor and host tissue compatibility occurs when tissues from either of two unrelated parental isogenic strains are grafted to their F_1 hybrids. Whereas hybrid hosts accept parent grafts, tissues from F_1 donors on parental strain hosts are rejected. This demonstrates that H genes are codominant, that they express themselves in the heterozygous condition, and therefore, that each hybrid possesses all of the H antigens of both its parents (7).

The availability of numerous isogenic mouse strains has permitted detailed immunogenetic analyses of histocompatibility. By appropriate mating procedures mouse strains can be produced which differ with respect to their entire genotype by only a single H gene (coisogenic strains); grafts exchanged between individuals of two such strains will be rejected. The recent development of isogenic, and in some cases coisogenic, strains of other species (rats, guinea pigs, hamsters, and chickens) has permitted immunogenetic analyses of their H antigens, especially, (1) the establishment of the number of H loci and the number of different H alleles at each locus in different species; (2) the relative immunologic potency of the antigens determined by different loci and of individual genes in an allelic series of a specific locus; (3) identification of various H loci with specific linkage groups; and (4) an evaluation of the expressivity of the various H genes in different tissues and cells.

In the mouse, many histocompatibility systems have been defined (H-1 through H-13, H-Y, and H-X), although the total number probably exceeds 20 in both rats and mice (7,19). Grafting studies with coisogenic strains have shown that not all of the H antigens determined by the various loci are of equal strength. One in each species, the H-2 in mice, AgB in rats, and B in chickens, has proven to be a major locus (19a). The basis for designating a locus as being "major" or "minor" is that a difference between donor and host with respect to a single strong antigen determined by an allele at a major locus is sufficient to provoke a homograft reaction of such intensity as to destroy a skin homograft within 10 or 11 days. Weaker antigenic differences determined by minor loci may be compatible with the survival of skin grafts bearing them for 100 days or more before succumbing to the inevitable host reactivity. The existence of multiple weak H antigens between donor and host determined by several minor loci may lead to a synergistic effect and result in a more prompt tempo of graft rejection (20).

With the use of specific isoantisera it has been shown that the H-2 system in the mouse is a complex locus composed of at least 20 different alleles which determine at least 30 distinct antigenic specificities. Some of these specificities may be the product of a single allele and others of two or more alleles (7,19).

Studies with rodents have revealed the simplest conceivable histocompatibility situation which occurs within an isogenic strain. In some strains of rats and mice a weak histocompatibility locus on the Y chromosome, hence absent in females, determines the existence of a weak male associated transplantation antigen(s), with the result that male isografts to female recipients of these strains are rejected, whereas all other donor/host sex combinations are permanently accepted. This situation is of particular value, since female hosts and male donors differ by the presence or absence of a histocompatibility antigen rather than by the substitution of one or the other of an alternative pair of antigens as with grafts between isogenic or coisogenic strains (21).

Nature and Distribution of Transplantation Antigens

Sensitization of the host can be accomplished through the use of a wide variety of donor tissues or cellular homografts. The implication of this fact is that (1) the full spectrum of antigens determined by an individual's histocompatibility genes seems to be present in all of the living nucleated cells of its body, and (2) there is no tissue specificity to transplantation antigens, that is, no one tissue contains an H antigen not represented in other tissues. It is possible, however, that various tissues or cells may differ quantitatively in their content or the expression of their transplantation antigens. In spite of the anucleate character of blood platelets there is some suggestion that they contain transplantation antigens and are capable of eliciting a state of homograft sensitivity (22).

The relationship of the antigens contained on erythrocytes to those on other cells of the body has been difficult to decipher. There is no evidence that an effective immunity to test tissue homografts can be provoked by prior sensitization with red blood cells. Yet some of the serologically detectable erythrocyte antigens are determined by important histocompatibility genes. Possible explanations for this histoimmunogenic shortcoming of erythrocytes are that they are not capable of transporting antigen to immunologically reactive sites and their antigens may be inadequately expressed or inappropriately located (7). Another possibility is that antigens located on red cells give rise to serum-mediated immunities rather than an effective state of delayed hypersensitivity, and it is the latter that is primarily involved in the homograft reaction. In fact, some studies have suggested that the existence of a serum-mediated immunity can inhibit the development of delayed hypersensitivity against the same antigen(s) ("immune deviation") (22a).

One of the important objectives of studies of transplantation antigens is the identification of their chemical nature. To date, most of the information on this subject has been derived from studies of aqueous extracts prepared from lymphoid tissues of mice and relates specifically to the products of the H-2 locus (23). The most exacting test for the antigenicity of an extract is its ability to elicit a state of homograft immunity in animals against subsequent test skin homografts. Important ancillary assay procedures include the ability of extracts to elicit the formation of anti-H-2 hemagglutinins, to inhibit hemagglutinating activity of H-2 antisera, and to enhance the growth of test tumors in mice.

There is good evidence that the antigenic specificities determined by the H-2 locus in mice are associated with lipoproteins found in the microsomal fractions of homogenized cells (23). Suspensions of intact cells and fractions thereof, capable of provoking homograft sensitivity, are also effective in eliciting a humoral antibody response. However, these two modalities of sensitization are separable. Repeated freezing and thawing or lyophilization of cells apparently abolishes their capacity to elicit a homograft response but not a serological response. Although the same antigenic determinant is probably responsible for these two different responses, it is questionable whether they are located on the same carrier molecules within different cell types.

Graft-versus-Host Reactions

The concept that the lymphocyte was an essential participant in immunologic phenomena in general and a prime mover of the homograft reaction in particular was well established in the early 1950s. Therefore, it might have been predicted that the transfer of immunologically competent lymphoid cells into an antigenically alien environment, that is, a situation wherein the graft would respond immunologically against the host, would result in dramatic if not fatal consequences to the host. Though not the result of a conscious reasoning process, such a phenomenon was subsequently described. Dempster (24) and Simonsen (25) noted the presence of pyroninophilic cells of the plasma cell series in the cortices of canine renal homografts 3 to 4 days following transplantation and suggested that these cells were of donor origin and might be engaged in an immunologic reaction against the antigens of the host. Billingham and Brent (26) subsequently noticed that attempts to procure tolerance of homografts both in bird embryos and in young rodents by inoculating them with blood or suspensions of homologous lymphoid cells from adult donors were frequently complicated by a fatal wasting syndrome which exacted a heavy toll among the recipients. This condition was acute or chronic, sometimes of delayed onset, and characterized by a failure of normal development, hepatomegaly, splenomegaly, hypertrophy and then atrophy of the lymphoid tissues, and frequently striking abnormalities of the skin. They concluded that these pathologic effects, for which they coined the term "runt disease," were the outcome of an immunologic graft-versus-host (GVH) reaction (27).

Several lines of evidence indicated that the basis for GVH reactions involved an immunologic reaction directed against host transplantation antigens. The severity of the disease in afflicted recipients was directly related to the degree of immunogenetic disparity between donor and host, the dose of inoculated immunologically competent cells, and whether or not the transferred cells were obtained from normal or specifically pre-sensitized donors.

Subsequent studies established the following straightforward conditions under which a graft might be capable of reaction immunologically against its host: (1) the graft must contain immunologically competent cells; (2) the host must possess the important histocompatibility antigens not represented in the graft donor to stimulate a response on the part of the grafted cells; (3) the host itself must be naturally or artificially rendered incapable, at least temporarily, of developing and executing an immune response to the graft.

There are two experimental situations which provide "security of tenure" of immunologically competent grafted cells in an antigenic environment and where grafted cells are genetically qualified to react against their hosts. One instance occurs when lymphoid tissue from parental strain animals is transplanted to F_1 hybrid recipients derived from matings between the two parental strains. Another case occurs when homologous tissues from adult donors containing immunologically competent cells are transferred into immunologically immature hosts.

Use of the GVH reaction has provided much information and insight into the immunologic capabilities of the lymphocyte, and it has been suggested that GVH reactions may serve as a model for studies on auto-immune diseases. To date, the capacity to bring about a GVH reaction constitutes one of the easiest and most conclusive means of determining whether a tissue or a suspension of cells in question contains immunologically competent cells (27).

Several pathologic conditions symptomatic of systemic runt disease in adult animals arise as a result of various experimental manipulations involving the transfer of immunologically competent cells.

F₁ Hybrid Disease

This is a wasting syndrome in adult F_1 hybrid recipients following inoculation with parental lymphoid cells (28).

GVH Reactions in Adult Tolerant Animals

Animals previously made tolerant of transplantation antigens of an alien donor strain by neonatal inoculation with immunologically incompetent cells are fully susceptible to runt disease if grafted with competent cells from the original donor strain (29).

Parabiosis Intoxication

The parabiotic surgical union (30,31) of an animal to an unrelated partner, with the establishment of vascular anastomoses between them, may result in a wasting syndrome: parabiosis intoxication, characterized by severe anemia, loss of weight, and other pathological conditions, including death of one of the partners. Immunogenetic analyses with mice have shown that when both partners differ by a major histocompatibility locus, they reject each other, without overt parabiosis intoxication, with the result that the pedicle uniting the two parabionts becomes necrotic, leading to their separation. When partners differ by only minor loci, one or both may become tolerant of the other. In the instance where parabiosis involves the union of immunologically competent and nonresponsive partners, as for example, parental and F_1 hybrid individuals, the immunologically incompetent partner dies (32).

Secondary Disease

It has long been known that animals may be protected against the effects of otherwise lethal doses of x-radiation by grafting them with bone marrow cells from isologous or homologous donors (33). These grafted marrow cells become established in the host and replace radiation-depleted lymphoid and myeloid tissues. Long-term survival generally results when isologous cells are transferred. However, with the use of bone marrow cells of homologous or heterologous origin, the hosts recover from the primary effects of the irradiation only to succumb frequently to a secondary wasting disease culminating in death, due to the immunologic activities of competent cells in the marrow inoculum (34).

Besides the systemic forms of GVH reactions, several local manifestations of the GVH reaction have been described. These are essentially the outcome of immunologic reactions occurring locally at the site of inoculation of homologous, immunologically competent cells (27).

Intrarenal GVH Reactions

Elkins (35–37) has described the outcome of inoculating lymphoid cells from parental strain rats beneath the renal capsules of F_1 hybrid hosts. A local self-limiting invasive-destructive reaction develops which can destroy 25 percent of the renal parenchyma, leaving the contralateral kidney and other organs and tissues unaffected. This reaction is accompanied by marked proliferation on the part of the donor cells and occurs with approximately the same intensity and tempo whether the donor cells are derived from normal or previously sensitized donors. There is evidence that the destructive reaction does not involve only the simple confrontation of immunologically competent donor cells and antigen-bearing cells of the host renal parenchyma. Prior irradiation of the host, to the extent that the level of circulating host mononuclear leukocytes is severely depressed, inhibits the development of the renal lesion following implantation of the donor cells. Also, inoculation of lymphoid cells into an isologous kidney newly grafted into an F_1 hybrid recipient produces an invasive-destructive reaction. Elkins has interpreted these findings to indicate that the development of lesions in the host kidney requires the continuous interaction of the specifically reactive donor cells with a population of infiltrating mononuclear antigen-bearing host cells of hematogenous origin.

Intracutaneous GVH Reactions

When lymphoid cells from presensitized homologous donors are inoculated intradermally in hamsters and guinea pigs, a delayed inflammatory reaction develops. This immune lymphocyte transfer reaction (ILT reaction) reflects the outcome of an immunologic attack by the sensitized lymphoid cells against host antigenic constituents at the site of the inoculation (38). A similar local inflammatory reaction results when antigenic material, that is, cells or cell extracts, is transferred subcutaneously to previously sensitized recipients. This direct reaction, the outcome of the recognition of and response to locally implanted antigenic material, has the appearance, tempo, and histologic characteristics of tuberculin-type reactions and, although formal proof for this is lacking, it is one of the bases for considering that homograft reactivity, and delayed type hypersensitivity reactions are related phenomena. When cells from normal, unimmunized donors are transferred subcutaneously into homologous recipients, a similar local inflammatory reaction occurs, the normal lymphocyte transfer reaction (NLT reaction), which is initially less intense and develops more slowly than the ILT reaction. The reaction in this case reflects the development of reactivity to host isoantigens by donor cells prior to the development of a host response, and the intensity is related to the degree of immunogenetic disparity between donor and host (39,40).

Brent and Medawar (39,40) have recently analyzed the events which occur in the NLT reaction in irradiated, hence temporarily immunologically incompetent, guinea pigs. They have described an "initial inflammatory episode" which reaches its peak at 24 hours following transfer of the cells. This is considered the outcome of an immunologic recognition event and does not involve proliferation by the donor cells, since it is not inhibited by antiproliferative agents. This phase is succeeded on the third to fourth day by a "flare-up," which leads to a second and more violent inflammatory episode, and which depends on the proliferation of the donor cells. After the sixth day, the lesion quickly disappears because of the immunologic recovery of the host. Use of presensitized cells in this system results in a similar sequence of events, except that the first episode immediately achieves the intensity of the flare-up reaction.

Chorioallantoic Membrane Lesions

When a suspension of leukocytes derived from adult chickens is distributed over the chorioallantoic membrane (CAM) of a genetically unrelated chicken embryo, a number of white focal lesions develop within a few days (41). These "pocks" represent local GVH reactions of competent cells to histocompatibility antigens present in the membrane. Use of this system established that the small lymphocytes in fowl blood were the immunologically competent cell type (42,43), and that as few as 30 of these were capable of producing 1 pock (44).

In addition to the localized GVH reactions described above, one of the features of systemic runt disease, splenomegaly, has been of particular value in quantitative studies of the immunologic behavior of lymphocytes. This splenomegaly assay, introduced by Simonsen (45), is applicable to both chickens and mice and consists of weighing the enlarged spleen of an animal a few days after inoculation with immunologically competent lymphocytes (44).

THE ROLE OF LYMPHOCYTES AS EFFECTOR CELLS
IN HOMOGRAFT IMMUNITY

The early studies of Medawar (2–6), which established the immunologic nature of the homograft reaction, included a description of mononuclear cells and histiocytes which invaded the graft parenchyma. Although this infiltration of host cells preceded the onset of degenerative changes in the graft, a causal relationship between these cells and graft destruction could not be established, since some areas of skin homografts exhibited necrotic changes with only a sparse infiltration of host mononuclear cells (46).

That mediation of homograft immunity, and other types of delayed hypersensitivity, is the province of cells and not of circulating humoral factors and is based principally on the failure to transfer an effective state of homograft sensitivity to isologous recipients with sera and the unqualified success with lymphoid cells from immunized donors. This notion was reinforced by studies which demonstrated the survival in sensitized animals of sequestered target homografts in cell-impermeable diffusion chambers. There is, however, no evidence which contradicts the possibility that humoral antibodies may play an ancillary, supportive, but not an essential or exclusive role in the rejection of tissue homografts. In some situations serum antibody can lyse suspensions of dissociated homologous cells. In any case, knowledge of the effector mechanisms involved in the destruction of tissue homografts has been difficult to obtain, partly because of the failure to isolate an immunospecific product which could be associated with the destructive behavior of immunologically active lymphocytes.

In Vivo Studies

From histopathologic studies of the homograft reaction in rats, Waksman (47) concluded that contributory processes leading to the demise of a skin homograft included a local endo- and perivascular accumulation of host mononuclear cells followed by a direct cytopathic action by these cells on cells of the vascular wall as well as in the graft parenchyma. Vascular stasis and consequent ischemia of the graft were considered to be important factors in graft necrogenesis.

With the use of tritiated thymidine in autoradiographic procedures, Gowans (48) demonstrated that the majority of infiltrating cells in a skin homograft undergoing destruction were newly formed cells and not an accumulation of cells at random from the circulating lymphocyte pool. Prendergast (49) extended these findings with rabbits and showed that labeled cells, newly formed in the regional lymph nodes draining a homograft from donor A, had a marked tendency to infiltrate the distant site of a test homograft from A rather than remaining in the circulating pool. However, the invasive behavior of these newly formed cells was not immunologically specific, since they could be found with equal frequencies at the site of a third party B donor skin homograft as well as at a delayed hypersensitivity lesion provoked by a heterologous protein antigen.

Studies in which sensitivity of skin homografts is transferred adoptively with labeled cells to normal or tolerant isologous hosts have shown rather convincingly that of the cells which infiltrate a test homograft, very few are the committed cells of donor origin. It is supposed, therefore, that the vast majority of infiltrating cells in this situation are immunologically uncommitted cells of host origin (48). Apparently the presence of a very small number of sensitized, committed infiltrating cells is sufficient to bring about the termination of a graft. The possibility remains, however, that the uncommitted host cells are not irrelevant bystanders, but fulfill some participatory role, perhaps as the result of their recruitment and conversion to an immunologically committed status by agents released from the sensitized donor cells. Two such recruitment agents might be "transfer factor" and RNA (50,51). Transfer factor is an RNase-insensitive extract prepared from disrupted leukocytes of sensitized donors which is capable of transferring delayed hypersensitivity passively to normal recipients (50a).

The first convincing evidence that lymphocytes from sensitized animals possess direct destructive potentialities emerged from Winn's studies (52) with adoptive immunization to transplantable tumor cells in mice. He showed that if sensitized lymph node cells were mixed in the same inoculum with a suspension of homologous tumor cells, the subsequent growth of the latter was inhibited, even with ratios of lymphocytes to tumor cells as low as 1:10. Similar numbers of sensitized lymphocytes inoculated at a site distant from the tumor cells did not retard their growth. This suggested that the inhibition required close contact between the lymphocytes and "target" tumor cells. Studies using local manifestations of the GVHR, CAM assays, and the ILT reaction discussed above, showed that the immunologic effector activities of sensitized lymphoid cells in these systems required that they be live cells. Use of devitalized cell preparations or cell extracts had no effect (46).

On the basis of studies involving the NLT reaction in guinea pigs, Brent and Medawar (39,40) developed the hypothesis that the intensity of the immunologic activities of lymphocytes is directly related to the number of cells involved. Reactions of greater or lesser violence by various numbers of sensitized cells against stronger or weaker antigens differ only in amplitude, thereby reflecting the number of lymphocytes which take part in them. The violent response produced by a population of normal lymphoid cells at the peak of the flare-up phase in the NLT reaction is considered to be an arithmetic multiple of that produced at the outset of the recognition phase from an inoculum of sensitized cells in the ILT reaction. According to this view, the intrinsic differences between a population of lymphoid cells from normal or immunized donors reflect a higher proportion of immunologically competent activated cells among the latter.

It became evident that the manner in which the cytopathogenic effect of sensitized lymphocytes was mediated would be difficult to resolve in studies employing the intact animal. To provide a closed system where cells would not leave or enter the site of reaction and where the fate of the active cells could be scrutinized more easily, Dvorak et al. (53) incorporated normal rabbit lymphoid cells with homologous skin tissues into cell-impermeable millipore diffusion chambers and inserted these into the peritoneal cavities of neutral hosts. After a period of 4 days, a population of lymphoid cells could be recovered which had the capacity to incite intracutaneous ILT reactions in the epidermal tissue donors, thereby demonstrating the acquisition of a state of sensitivity by the lymphoid cells while in residence in the chambers. This test system would be useful in studying the involvement of other cell types, such as macrophages, and the interactions between various cell types (e.g., lymphocytes and macrophages) in the development of primary immunologic reactivity and the production of immunologic effector cells.

In Vitro Studies

Govaerts (54) and Rosenau and Moon (55) went one step further by studying the destructive activities of sensitized lymphoid cells in a tissue culture system. Govaerts demonstrated that thoracic duct lymphocytes obtained from dogs that had rejected renal homografts were capable of destroying cultures of target renal cells obtained from the donor of the organ graft. The cytocidal capabilities of lymphocytes and macrophages (56) from specifically immunized animals were quickly confirmed in a number of laboratories, and although as yet unconfirmed, isolates of nuclei from sensitized lymphocytes were claimed to be cytocidal (57).

Koprowski and Fernandes (58) found that within a few hours following the addition of lymphoid cells from the regional lymph nodes, spleen, or thoracic duct of animals immunized to monolayer cultures of target cells obtained from a donor against whose tissues the sensitivity is directed, many of the lymphocytes were clustered around and over the target cells, a phenomenon termed *contactual agglutination*. Within 10 hours of culture DNA synthesis in the dividing target cells ceased, the cells retracted their cytoplasmic processes, acquired a fragmented appearance, rounded up, and by the twentieth hour lysed or detached from the surface of the culture vessel (59).

The finding that cytocidally active cells can be obtained from the thoracic lymphatic duct of dogs that had rejected renal homografts (54) or from rats immunized with skin grafts is of particular importance (59). Here, the attacking cells are part of the circulating lymphocyte pool and, by the strictest criteria, immunization is provoked by transplantation iso-antigens. Use of target cells rendered incapable of division by x-radiation showed that immune lymphoid cells actually kill the target cells rather than merely inhibiting their growth (59).

The destructive interaction of sensitized lymphocytes and homologous target cells is the outcome of an immunologically specific event (54–64). Target cells are destroyed only if they bear the histocompatibility antigens to which the lymphocyte donors are immunized. Activated lymphocytes have no adverse effect on isologous target cells, and lymphocytes obtained from animals immunized to heterologous antigens or to transplantation antigens of a third party are completely ineffective against specific homol-ogous target cells. In some circumstances, however, the interaction be-tween an antigen in culture, such as tuberculin and lymphoid cells sensitized to that antigen, results in the destruction of innocent bystander cell mono-layers (65,65a).

Use of this immune lymphocyte–target cell culture system has pro-vided important information on the destructive capabilities of sensitized lymphocytes (66–68). The cytopathogenic activities of lymphocytes are developed approximately 1 week after immunization and apparently do not require the presence of complement (69) nor of serum antibodies. That cytophilic antibody might be involved has been ruled out on the basis of reconstruction experiments in which normal or immune sera were combined with normal or sensitized lymphocytes. Destructive activities are not acquired by otherwise normal cells in the presence of immune sera. Furthermore, immune sera, even in high concentrations, do not augment the cytopathogenic capabilities of sensitized lymphocytes; in fact, the de-structive reaction is inhibited (66).

Provisions for intimate cytoplasmic contact between the attacking lymphocytes and target cells are essential. Extracts prepared from sonically disrupted sensitized lymphoid cells were ineffective, and when separated from intact sensitized lymphocytes by a diffusion membrane, target cells were not destroyed. This indicates that if a cell-bound immunospecific agent is involved, it is not itself toxic nor can it be detached from the sensitized cells (66).

Quantitative studies in which the number of target cells surviving were determined after various times of incubation revealed a latent period of approximately 20 hours before demonstrable target cell destruction occurred (66). The duration of this latent period depends on the nature of the event being scored. Cell death occurs after 20 hours and is generally complete by 48 hours, while morphological alterations occur within a few hours (66,70). Lymphoid cells producing lytic antibody to sheep erythrocytes, when used as target cells, cease antibody synthesis following 5 hours of contact with specifically sensitized attacking lymphocytes (71). Injury to target fibroblasts, assessed by changes in their plating efficiency, begins shortly after contact with immune lymphocytes and is complete after 12 hours (72).

Increasing the ratio of attacking lymphocytes to target cells does not shorten the length of the latent period. However, the number of surviving target cells is inversely proportional to the number of attacking lymphoid cells added to the cultures. It can be shown that the percent surviving target cells versus the "dose" of lymphocytes follows an exponential relationship similar to a "single hit" inactivation curve. This indicates that a single lymphocyte, if immunologically active, is sufficient to destroy or have a detectably adverse effect on one target cell. From such a model, it can be computed that approximately 1 to 2 percent of a population of lymphocytes derived from the regional lymph nodes of a sensitized rat donor is immunologically active (66). Similar conclusions were subsequently derived from the experiments of Brunner et al. (72) where the target cell injury was assessed in terms of decreases in plating efficiency.

Drugs which have immunosuppressive effects in vivo have been shown to inhibit the cytotoxic properties of sensitized lymphocytes in vitro. Cortisone and Imuran do not prevent the clustering behavior of lymphocytes around target cells but do reduce subsequent cytotoxicity (67,73). Cultures conducted at room, rather than body, temperature also exhibit the clustering behavior, but not target cell destruction. These findings are consistent with the notion that destructive interaction between sensitized lymphoid cells and homologous target cells in vitro requires an intact metabolic capacity for protein synthesis on the part of the lymphocytes (60,74).

So far, the exact means by which sensitized attacking lymphocytes destroy homologous target cells has not been determined. The available evidence suggests that the cytopathogenic action of sensitized lymphocytes proceeds via a two-step process: (1) the attachment of attacking lymphocytes to target cells (contactual agglutination), and (2) lysis of the target cells as the result of some lymphocyte metabolic activity. Whether lysosomes and lysosomal enzymes are involved remains to be demonstrated. Close contact involving receptor sites or "cell-bound antibody" on sensitized lymphocytes may represent the only step which is immunologically specific although clustering itself is not destructive. The effectiveness of immunosuppressant drugs in inhibiting the destructive process, but not the viability of the attacking lymphocytes nor their clustering behavior, suggests that they act on the metabolism of the lymphocyte (60).

In applying the information derived from these culture systems concerning the destructive activities of sensitized lymphocytes in vitro to the question of how lymphocytes fulfill their effector role in vivo in the rejection of tissue homografts or in the various GVH reactions, the following premise deserves serious consideration. Antibody or immunoglobulin molecules are not the ultimate mediator of graft destruction. The role of surface-bound immunoglobulins is primarily that of recognition and of ensuring close contact between attacking and target cells. Following this recognition event, sensitized lymphocytes release or secrete and/or induce host target cells to release an immunologically nonspecific, perhaps pharmacologically active, agent, which is the ultimate effector. Supportive evidence for this premise is provided by the finding that extracts from sensitized cells or devitalized cell preparations routinely fail to incite ILT reactions or [with one exception, transfer factor in man (50)] to transfer an effective status of homograft immunity (46). Therefore, synthesis or release of effector agents is not initiated until lymphocytes interact with antigen. Willoughby (75) has described lymph node permeability factor, (LNPF), extractable from lymph node tissues and from the sites of a tuberculin reaction, where its level rises and falls in parallel with the local inflammatory response. When administered locally, LNPF causes increased vascular permeability to plasma proteins and a massive local leukocytic infiltration. This factor, which does not possess immunologic specificity, is currently under consideration as the mediator of delayed hypersensitivity reactions.

David (76) and Bloom and Bennett (77) have studied an in vitro phenomenon which may have great relevance to the destructive capabilities of lymphocytes. When lymphocytes obtained from an animal sensitized to natural antigens, such as tuberculin proteins, or to artificially synthesized haptenic antigen-carrier molecules are cultured in the presence of the specific antigens, they release a substance called migration inhibition factor (MIF) which inhibits the migratory behavior of macrophages. This substance has the following properties: (1) It is only released by lymphocytes from animals possessing a state of delayed hypersensitivity. Cells from animals immunized so as to produce only circulating antibodies do not release MIF. (2) It exhibits the characteristics of a newly synthesized, and not a previously existent, protein; its production is blocked by mitomycin C and puromycin, and it is nondialyzable. (3) It is produced by sensitized lymphocytes only in the presence of specific antigen, but it has no immunologic specificity of its own. It serves simply to inhibit the migratory behavior of an indicator population of macrophages. (4) It apparently does not kill the macrophages, but it may have an adverse effect on other cell types (65,76,77).

Recently, a toxic soluble material, of mol. wt 90,000 to 100,000, has been described. This material causes destruction of target cells and is produced by lymphocytes stimulated by a variety of procedures, all of which cause lymphocyte transformation. This material seems to act on membranes of target cells, thereby causing lysis (78a,78b).

The possibility that cells from normal, immunologically virgin animals may have cytocidal capabilities has recently received attention. It has been reported that normal, unsensitized lymphoid cells can destroy homologous target cells in culture systems if the lymphoid cells are artificially aggregated around the target cells with phytohemagglutinin (PHA) or heterologous antisera (78). This destructive effect, termed *allogeneic inhibition*, was not attributable to the aggregation process itself, since isologous lymphoid cells under similar circumstances were innocuous. A comparable in vivo phenomenon was described where parental strain tumors were shown to grow better in isologous recipients than in F_1 animals. Several findings ruled out the possibility that the in vitro destructive reaction and its related in vivo counterpart, syngeneic preference, involved conventional immunologic mechanisms. It was found that lymphoid cells previously exposed to 3000 r x-radiation were not inhibited in their capacity to kill target cells; cells from hybrid F_1 mice, when aggregated to parental target cells with PHA, exerted a marked cytotoxic effect; this contact cytotoxicity is not restricted to lymphoid cells, but is reported to be exhibited by various neoplastic cells; extracts of sonically disrupted homologous or F_1 hybrid tumor cells exert a growth inhibition effect on target tumor cells in culture. Hellström and Möller (78) suggested that these inhibition and destructive effects are the outcome of cell contacts involving structurally incompatible cell surfaces; however, no plausible mechanism has been proposed.

THE ROLE OF LYMPHATIC VASCULATURE

Whatever the mechanism of antigen recognition is, it is clear that an intact lymphatic and blood vasculature is required for the completion of subsequent steps leading to the production of an effective immune state. This can be inferred from recent studies on naturally occurring and artificially prepared immunologically privileged sites (79). Whereas in most instances, homografts of skin or other tissues orthotopically transplanted to potentially responsive recipients are rejected, when transplanted to certain other sites, they may be partially or completely exempt from destruction. The special dispensation afforded homografts at these immunologically privileged sites, such as the cornea, brain, hamster cheek pouch, and testis, may depend on the failure to respond to an existent state of immunity and/or the failure to excite an effective immune response.

Tissues transplanted into the corneal stroma will survive even in an immunized host only so long as the graft does not become vascularized. This status of absolute privilege is terminated only when the efferent arc of the immunologic reflex, the route by which effector cells would enter the graft, is established in the form of the blood vasculature.

Foreign tissues grafted into the brain of unsensitized animals are generally not rejected, in spite of the fact that they acquire vascular connections with the host. They fail to provoke an effective state of immunity because lymphatic drainage, the structural route of the afferent arc of the immune response, is absent in the brain. They are, however, fully vulnerable to a state of immunity previously or subsequently provoked. Studies with the hamster cheek pouch as a site for the implantation of homografts have shown that the survival time of such grafts is abnormally prolonged. This has been attributed to an absence of draining lymphatics and regional lymph nodes in this tissue.

Frey and Wenk (80) showed that when the lymphatics draining an area of skin were surgically interrupted, a state of delayed hypersensitivity to locally applied dinitrochlorobenzene (DNCB) could not be evoked in guinea pigs. These investigators demonstrated that an immunized animal would not display the conventional local lesions to DNCB expected of a state of delayed hypersensitivity if the blood supply to that area were not intact. Barker and Billingham (81) applied a modification of these surgical techniques to a study of privileged sites in homograft immunity. They showed that a flap of skin where the blood vasculature was maintained but the draining lymphatic vessels interrupted would support a test skin homograft indefinitely.

The lymphatic vessels draining the site of a homograft can thus be considered as playing an essential role in the evocation of homograft sensitivity. It has long been thought that these vessels serve as channels through which antigenic matter escapes from a graft and travels to the regional lymph nodes, the cells of which subsequently become activated (60).

More recently, Medawar (82) proposed that the inductive phase of the homograft reaction need not take place within the environment of the lymph node, but peripherally within the graft itself. According to this concept of peripheral sensitization, host lymphocytes contact and then interact with foreign antigens in the grafted tissues to become immunologically primed before returning to the lymphoid tissues, where they continue their differentiative processes to the status of effector cells. Evidence favoring the premise that circulating lymphocytes can engage in a peripheral recognition process is as follows:

1. Thoracic duct lymphocytes which have been perfused through a homologous kidney when returned to recipients of their strain of origin will produce an effective state of immunity against antigens of the kidney donor (83).

2. Peripheral blood lymphocytes have the capacity to respond to the presence of foreign antigens in the NLT reaction and in the mixed lymphocyte interaction (39,40,84–86).

3. Thoracic duct lymphocytes incorporated into cell-impermeable diffusion chambers with antigens undergo blastogenic changes, produce antibody, and provoke ILT reactions (52,87,88).

IMMUNOSPECIFIC PROLIFERATION AND ANTIGEN RECOGNITION

A large body of evidence has been accumulated from studies both in intact animals and in tissue culture systems that stresses the importance of cell proliferation, most notably by lymphoid cells, in the mechanism of the immunologic response. Blastoid transformation of lymphocytes in the lymph nodes and spleen has been seen to accompany the immunologic response to injections of soluble protein antigens (89) and the rejection of tissue homografts (90). Furthermore, lymphocytes transferred into an alien recipient, and thereby exposed to the homologous transplantation isoantigens of the host, undergo similar morphologic changes indicative of blastoid transformation during the course of a GVH reaction (91).

The significance of proliferation by cells in the peripheral lymphoid organs, the spleen and lymph nodes, during secondary responses has been stressed by Dutton (92). Autoradiographic studies with cells in tissue culture systems have shown that up to 4 or 5 percent of splenic or lymph node cells from previously immunized animals, boosted in vivo or in vitro with specific antigens, are engaged in the synthesis of DNA, and it is clear that increases in the rate of antibody synthesis by these cells depend on the extent of proliferation of antibody-forming cells or their precursors.

A small percentage of cells of the circulating lymphocyte pool obtained from the peripheral blood of human or other animal donors, in which a state of delayed hypersensitivity has been induced, undergo blastogenesis when cultured in the presence of the specific antigen (e.g., purified protein derivative of tuberculin-PPD). This mitogenic response is immunologically specific; it requires the use of lymphocytes from sensitized donors and the presence of the sensitizing antigen. Cells from normal, unsensitized individuals or from sensitized animals in the presence of no antigen or of an indifferent antigen do not respond. There is some indication that this proliferative activity of peripheral blood lymphocytes is the property of cells from donors with delayed rather than immediate hypersensitivities (93,94).

More recently, it has been shown that cultures consisting of cells derived from the peripheral blood of unrelated human donors, undergo blastoid transformation and proliferation; this can be measured quantitatively by the incorporation of tritiated thymidine (H^3-TdR) into newly synthesized DNA. Proliferation in these mixed cultures involves the lymphocyte fraction of the peripheral blood and occurs despite the fact that the donors have not been deliberately sensitized to one another (95). For the following reasons, it is considered that the proliferation in mixed lymphocyte interaction (MLI) results from the stimulation of immunologically competent lymphocytes which recognize and respond to histocompatability isoantigens (60):

1. Cells of the circulating lymphocyte pool obtained by cannulation of the thoracic lymphatic duct of rats, and consisting predominantly of thymus derived, long-lived small lymphocytes, the cell type acknowledged to be immunologically competent, undergo proliferation when exposed to cells of homologous origin (84).

2. The magnitude of the proliferative response is related to the degree of immunogenetic disparity of the two codonors; peripheral blood lymphocytes obtained from identical twins or from members of the same inbred strain show no reaction, while moderate reactions result in cultures from familially related human donors, and maximal proliferative activity occurs in cultures from unrelated donors (95).

3. In the first careful immunogenetic analysis of the MLI, Dutton (96) demonstrated that responses were obtained with splenic cells from murine donors that differed by a single histocompatibility gene at the H-2 locus. Differences involving multiple weak histocompatibility loci (non-H-2) resulted in some response but never with strain combinations differing by a single weak histocompatibility gene.

4. That the stimulatory factors in the MLI are, in fact, histocompatibility antigens was demonstrated in experiments employing cell donors from a genetically defined population of backcross and parental strain rats. Each member of the backcross population had been typed by serologic procedures for the presence or absence of segregating major histocompatibility antigens determined by the AgB locus. Only those individuals differing from parental strain donors with

respect to this antigen stimulated a proliferative reaction in mixed cell cultures (86). With the use of rat donors of two strains which possess the same AgB allele, no response occurs (84, 85). A similar dependency of the MLI on differences at a major histocompatibility locus has been described for human mixed cell cultures (97).

5. The extent to which cells proliferate in the MLI reflects the immunogenetic status of the cell donors. Responding cells in cultures from parental and F_1 hybrid rat donors of different sexes were shown by karyologic examination to be of parental origin. This finding is particularly important in view of the fact that F_1 hybrid hosts do not respond immunologically to tissues grafted from parental strain donors. Cells from immunologically tolerant donors are nonreactive to cells bearing the specific histocompatibility antigens to which they have been rendered tolerant but are fully responsive to cells from an indifferent third-party donor strain. Thymectomy of the cell donors at birth results in an inability to exhibit proliferative activity in the MLI without impairing the capacity of these cells to respond to a nonspecific mitogen such as PHA (85). A recent comparative study of the conditions required for positive responses in the MLI and local renal GVH reactions has found them markedly similar (98).

The nonreactivity of lymphocytes from (1) F_1 hybrid donors against parental strain cells even in a proliferating environment, (2) tolerant donors, against antigens to which they have been rendered unresponsive, and (3) thymectomized donors when confronted with antigen provide strong support for the premise that proliferation in the MLI represents an immunologically specific event engaged in by cells of an immunologically competent population. Any involvement of a nonspecific inducer of cell division, even one that might act following a specific triggering event, can be discounted; otherwise, mitoses would have been detected among F_1 cells in parental-F_1 mixed cell cultures. Furthermore, it is unlikely that mitogenesis in the MLI has any relationship to a nonspecific phenomenon based on structurally incompatible cell surfaces such as allogeneic inhibition (78).

The foregoing discussion highlights the immunologic relevance of the MLI, and from this it is clear that this culture system might serve as a useful experimental model for study of the inductive phases of the immune response involving primary contact between antigen and immunologically competent cells. The simplest or "minimal" hypothesis of the immune response mechanism (99,100) holds that antigen-sensitive cells (ASC) bear on their surfaces antigen-specific receptor sites which endow that cell with the capacity to recognize specific antigenic determinants. These receptor sites are considered to be immunoglobulin molecules which are a sample of what that cell can produce if stimulated. In the presence of antigenic determinants specific for these receptor sites, the ASC are stimulated to proliferate and to differentiate with the result that there is a clonal expansion of specific ASC which may act as immunologic effector cells. This hypothesis does not indicate whether a cell may possess receptor sites specific for two or more antigen determinants. However, the simplest scheme is provided by the clonal selection hypothesis: that of 1 antigenic determinant/1 receptor site/1 cell/1 antibody (99,100). In all likelihood, ASC are lymphocytes, and in view of the large number of antigens in the immunologic universe and the restrictions of the clonal selection hypothesis, the proportion of lymphocytes capable of recognizing a given antigenic determinant, by virtue of the specificity of their receptor sites, is small—of the order of 10^{-5} to 10^{-6}.

In view of the possible relationship between ASC and the cells which respond by proliferating in the MLI, closer examination of the MLI is warranted. Recent stathmokinetic studies (101) of the proliferative behavior of responding, parental strain cells in mixed cell cultures from parental and F_1 rats have shown that

1. After initiating the cultures there is a latent period of approximately 40 hours during which time no mitotic activity is detectable.

2. This is followed by a period of proliferation in which previously nondividing cells enter the mitotic cycle for the first time. Proliferative activity, detected by incorporation of radioactive thymidine and measured by autoradiography or scintillation spectrometry, increases exponentially with a doubling time (T_2) of approximately 9 to 10 hours.

3. During this exponential proliferative phase, which lasts approximately 100 hours, the dividing cells undergo a series of rapid sequential divisions with a generation time (Tc) of 8 hours. Few, if any, cells drop out of the mitotic cycle.

4. In addition to the cells which first entered mitosis at the beginning of the proliferative phase and then proceeded through multiple divisions, significant numbers of new, previously nondividing cells continue to enter the mitotic cycle during the entire exponential growth phase. The total number of these newly responsive, first division cells throughout the culture period amounts to 1 to 3 percent of the original parental cell inoculum.

The proportion of lymphocytes which recognize and are stimulated to proliferate by a particular histocompatibility antigen system is surprisingly high. It is at least three orders of magnitude in excess of the frequency of ASCs (10^{-5}) which respond to heterologous erythrocyte antigens (102–104), and therefore it is difficult to reconcile this large number with the clonal selection hypothesis, which predicts that the receptor sites possessed by a given antigen-sensitive lymphocyte would be of single or limited specificity. However, unlike the cellular reaction to histocompatibility antigens, immunities to heterologous red cells involve predominantly the serum antibody response, and the mechanisms involved in these two modalities of immune response may be quantitatively very different.

Simonsen (44) has reported that as few as 30 to 50 adult fowl lymphocytes from unimmunized donors inoculated into homologous embryos can produce a marked splenomegaly, symptomatic of a GVH reaction. He concluded that a minimum of 1 to 2 percent of the peripheral blood lymphocyte population of adult chickens can respond to a strong histocompatibility antigen in this species. Simonsen has also described the results of quantitative studies in mice on the comparative effectiveness of lymphocytes from normal or immunized donors to produce GVH reactions in F_1 hosts. When donor and host differ by a major histocompatibility antigen, deliberate sensitization of the cell donors did not substantially increase their capacity to produce GVH reactions over that of cells from unimmunized, normal donors. In this instance, the factor of immunization, the comparative effectiveness of sensitized cells, was in the range 1 to 3. With donor and recipient combinations differing by weak histocompatibility antigen systems, the factor of immunization was much greater. Sensitized cells were 10 to 100 times as effective as cells from normal donors. This finding has been interpreted to indicate that the size of the clone of reactive cells in a normal animal against strong histocompatibility antigens is already so large that deliberate immunization does not significantly increase its size (44). Along these same lines Simmons and Fowler (42), with another GVH system, have recently demonstrated that a large proportion, approximately 1 in 50, of adult fowl lymphocytes are capable of provoking a destructive focus or "pock" on the chorioallantoic membrane of homologous chick embryos.

If we accept the immunologic relevance of the mixed lymphocyte interaction and the fact that the responsive cells are ASCs there are several general possibilities which might account for what appears to be an inordinately large number of cells responsive to a particular antigen system.

The AgB histocompatibility antigen system of the rat may consist of a very large number of antigenic determinants. If ASC are restricted in their potentiality and can respond to only one determinant, then assuming their frequency to be as high as 10^{-4}, the observed number of responding cells in the MLI would indicate that 100 to 300 separate antigens are associated with the AgB differences of the two strains employed. This seems an unlikely possibility. By comparison, the H-2 antigenic system in mice consists of only about 30 different specificities, detectable by serologic procedures, and no two strains differ by more than 14 or less than 2 (19). It is probable that the various AgB alleles in the rat differ from one another with respect to multiple antigenic specificities (105). However, first estimates would not suggest that there is a sufficient number of them to account for the number of responding cells observed even if the frequency of ASC were as high as 10^{-4}.

Proliferation in the MLI might be initiated and conducted by cells which have had some prior experience with a ubiquitous cross-reacting antigen, and hence proliferation is a manifestation of a secondary response. Under these circumstances, "strong" histocompatibility antigen systems (the HLA in man, H-2 in mice, AgB in rats, and B in chickens, the first three of which have been demonstrated to be potent mitogens) could be defined as those antigens to which a native immunity exists in the intact animal. This might explain the apparently unique characteristic of strong histocompatibility antigens; in hosts with preexistent immunities, one might expect to find reactive cells in the frequency of 10^{-2}. Although in some respects this is an unattractive possibility, it is perhaps the most difficult one to deny. Studies with animals that have been raised under pathogen- and antigen-free conditions as cell donors or with cultures stimulated with unnatural, synthetic antigens might help to resolve this question.

The foregoing two possibilities assume that receptor sites of a given ASC have a limited specificity. This is a central issue and requires closer examination. There is some support for the possibility that a given cell can produce antibodies to two determinants if they are presented on the same carrier molecule (106,107). If valid, this would imply that ASC are pluripotential with respect to their capacity to respond to multiple antigenic configurations. In the MLI, where parental strain lymphocytes are exposed to a barrage of antigens, all of them are represented on each cell from the F_1 donor. The great majority of studies with single cell systems, however, have shown that antibody produced by a single cell has only one specificity.

The recent observations of Dutton and Mishell (108,109) also make the multipotentiality of responsive cells a difficult interpretation to accept. They showed that two populations of antigen-sensitive cells are involved in the production of antibodies to two unrelated antigens. When a heterologous antigen in the form of sheep erythrocytes is added to cultures of mouse splenic lymphocytes, the cells are stimulated to proliferate, and antibody-forming cells appear which are detectable with the Jerne plaque assay procedure. The development of these antibody-forming cells could be inhibited by allowing the proliferating cells to incorporate suicidal amounts of a radioactive DNA precursor, H^3-TdR, during the 24 to 48 hours after adding the antigen to the cultures. Under these conditions no antibody-forming cells were detectable on the fourth day. When, however, a suicidal H^3-TdR pulse and a second antigen (burro erythrocytes) is given to cultures of mouse lymphocytes to which the first antigen (sheep erythrocytes) had been added 24 hours earlier and a proliferative response had been induced, antibody production to the first, but not the second, antigen is selectively abolished.

Direct evidence which favors the unipotentiality of the responsive cells in the MLI is the following: (1) Responses in mixed cultures with parental strain cells provoked by the simultaneous presence of two different AgB histocompatibility antigen systems approximate the sum of the separate responses to these antigen systems; (2) Peripheral blood lymphocytes from a donor tolerant of one histocompatibility antigen system respond in culture to a second antigen system with the same magnitude as normal cells from nontolerant donors (110).

The best interpretation of this information is that different subpopulations of lymphocytes are stimulated by different antigen systems. The induction of immunologic tolerance is accompanied by the inactivation or destruction of a particular subpopulation of cells which would otherwise be responsive in the MLI. The disappearance of this subpopulation in no way affects the capacity of a different population to respond to a different antigen system.

Another obvious possibility, although it was dismissed earlier, is that of nonspecific recruitment of large numbers of cells into the mitotic cycle in the mixed lymphocyte interaction as the result of some activity on the part of a small minority of specifically responsive cells. Presumably, a large proportion of these recruitable cells observed in the response to one antigen could be coerced equally well to a second antigen system by a different subpopulation of specific cells. As mentioned earlier, there is some evidence that weighs against this possibility; namely, in mixed cultures of cells from parental and F_1 hybrid donors, the F_1 cells do not participate by entering the mitotic cycle in significant numbers (101). Nevertheless, there may be a requirement that the specific and recruited cells be genetically more similar in order for some interaction to occur between them.

Although cells from tolerant donors do not respond in mixed cultures with F_1 hybrid cells bearing the tolerance-inducing antigens, this nonreactivity may reflect the inability of these cells to initiate a proliferative reaction. Presumably, this would stem from the deficit induced with the tolerant state in the small subpopulation of specific triggering cells. This missing group of cells might therefore be replaced in a mixed culture system simply by supplying a population of lymphocytes from a normal, isologous donor.

This premise has been tested by exposing cells from normal and tolerant members of the same inbred strain in the same cultures to F_1 cells bearing the tolerance-inducing antigens. The normal and tolerant parental strain donors were, however, of different sexes so that responding cells could be identified by an examination of the sex chromosomes in the mitotic figures. Under these conditions, the vast majority of the responding cells were derived from the normal animal, suggesting that nonspecific recruitment is not the basis for the large number of responsive cells in the MLI (110). If it were, one would expect to find as many as 50 percent of the cells derived from the tolerant animal.

It must be concluded, therefore, that even though it is large—approximately 1 cell in 50—the fraction of cells which recognize and proliferate in response to a particular histocompatibility antigen system is specific. This implies that (1) "strong" antigens possess that property by virtue of the fact that a large number of lymphocytes can recognize them, and, conversely, "weak" antigens are those for which there are smaller numbers of reactive cells; and (2) that weak antigens, which ordinarily constitute a negligible proliferative stimulus, become effective mitogens in lymphocyte cultures derived from immunized donors that presumably possess an expanded clone of ASCs. Thus while cultures of lymphocytes from donors which have not been immunized with antigens such as tuberculin or penicillin are not stimulated by the presence of these antigens, mitotic activity is readily observed if cells are derived from previously immunized donors.

If the clone(s) of reactive cells to a particular histocompatibility antigen system is specific and, at the same time, it consists of a significant proportion of the total number of cells available, it follows that only a few antigen systems can stimulate proliferative responses of this magnitude. The number of strong histocompatibility antigens which can provoke significant mitogenic responses has not been determined; however, it can be predicted that 30 would be approaching an upper limit. The remainder of the circulating lymphocytes would consist of the numerous subpopulations of ASCs, each present in a frequency of 10^{-5} to 10^{-6}, which are specific for the rest of the antigens of the immunologic universe. It can therefore be predicted that the "strong" histocompatibility antigens of one species should not induce significant proliferation by lymphocytes from a different species unless these are derived from immunized donors.

Preliminary studies (110) with mixed cultures of human and rat lymphocytes indicate that this is indeed true. Lymphocytes from rats can be stimulated to proliferate by human leukocytes only if they have been obtained from a donor that has previously been immunized with human cells. Lafferty and Jones (110a) have shown that lymphocytes of one species are not capable of producing GVH reactions in another species unless the donors were previously immunized to the species antigens of the recipient.

The foregoing discussion, although somewhat speculative, is not altogether out of place in this chapter since it highlights certain aspects of the mechanism of the immune response which are under active investigation. Furthermore, it hints at the possible biological significance of histocompatibility isoantigens. It is more than a consequence that (where information is available) of the histocompatibility antigens possessed by each species, some are stronger than others, and the strong antigens are determined by alleles at a single genetic locus. The products of each of these major loci provoke an immunologically specific proliferative response by lymphocytes of other animals of the same species not possessing such antigens. For some reason the major histocompatibility antigens are more "foreign" and provoke a greater response involving more cells to individuals within the species than to members of different species.

One possibility is that the polymorphism of histocompatibility antigens and the genetic systems to produce them, as well as to react to them, were developed and retained in vertebrate evolution to provide the bearer with the capacity to react immunologically against (1) transmission of oncogenic viruses or (2) somatic mutations or other genetic mistakes which might otherwise give rise to neoplasia, especially when associated with the development of new antigens (110b).

One other possibility concerning the significance of histocompatibility antigens and the immunologic capacity to react promptly to them was recently presented by Jerne (110c). This hypothesis, an extremely powerful one because it is open to experimental verification, links the generation of immunologic diversity, i.e., the capacity to respond immunologically to the many antigens of the immunologic universe, with tolerance to "self" antigens. Jerne postulates that (1) the germ line contains structural genes which code for antibodies specifically directed against histocompatibility determinants of the species, (2) mutations occur among the v-cistrons, those coding for antibody specificity, and these mutations specify reactivity to antigens other than histocompatibility antigens, and (3) the survival of these mutant cell clones is favored by the suppression of nonmutant antecedents. The suppression of nonmutants takes the form of tolerance induced in ontogeny to self antigens. Since no one individual of a species possesses all the H antigens of his species, the v-genes of his germ line must code for antibodies to all his species' antigens in order to insure reactivity against those self antigens he does possess. Consequently, Jerne's hypothesis predicts that the portion of germ-line cells with v-genes determining antibodies against self antigens are suppressed, and the survival of mutants of this germ line is thereby favored. On the other hand, cells expressing the other set of v-genes which code for H antigens of the species that the individual does not possess are not suppressed and are therefore available in large numbers for reactivity against H antigens of other members of the species.

CONCLUDING REMARKS

It is perhaps pertinent to reconsider the cellular events which might be operative in the homograft reaction in the light of recent information, especially on the cooperation of lymphoid cells of different lineage involved in the development of immune reactivity to sheep erythrocyte antigens (111).

It is generally accepted that the homograft reaction operates via cellular mechanisms which (1) recognize that the grafted tissues are, in fact, foreign, and (2) produce immunologically activated effector lymphocytes which (3) bring about the destruction of the graft by some as yet ill-defined process. The initial recognition events following the application of a homograft to an immunologically virgin recipient entail the passage of antigenic cellular or subcellular material to the regional draining lymph nodes via the afferent lymphatics. In the nodal tissue, antigen-stimulated cells proliferate and bring about the production of immunologically activated effector cells. These cells exit the lymph node, travel to the graft via the bloodstream, infiltrate the graft, and effect the ultimate destruction of the foreign tissue.

The results of numerous studies suggest that this is an oversimplified view and that it may require modification along the following lines:

1. In the afferent stages of the homograft reaction, immunologically competent lymphocytes of hematogenous origin may be engaged locally in the graft itself and interact with graft antigens. These "peripherally sensitized" cells may then pass from the graft via afferent lymphatics in the graft bed to the draining lymph node and thence continue their proliferative and differentiative activities to produce a state of homograft immunity. To date, no evidence can be offered against the concept of peripheral sensitization. Lymphoid cells in a variety of circumstances outside the environment of a lymph node have the capacity to recognize and respond to the presence of antigens. Neither should this concept be considered as an exclusive alternative to the possibility that cells in the lymph node are sensitized directly by antigen which has escaped the graft tissues.

2. The recent studies of Elkins (37) and Steinmuller (112) have suggested that host leukocytes, transferred with the grafted tissues as passenger cells, may be an important, if not the exclusive, source of antigen in the graft.

3. Convincing evidence suggests that the initial recognition of antigen and the production of specific antibody involve lymphocytes of two distinctly different cell lineages, one derived from the thymus and one from the bone marrow. This requires that some form of interaction must occur between the two cell types. Perhaps one specifically concentrates antigen so that it can be recognized by, and can result in the effective stimulation of, antibody-forming cell precursors. Another possibility, although not an easy one to accept, is that some transfer of informational RNA is involved. Even though this cooperative involvement of two cell types has been shown only for sheep erythrocyte antigens thus far, and in an immune system involving a humoral response, the possibility that a similar mechanism may be operative in the homograft reaction must be considered. Thymus-derived lymphocytes may recognize the presence of antigen peripherally in the graft or within the draining lymph node tissue and then influence the production of specific effector cells from bone marrow–derived cells in the lymph node or even distally in the graft.

4. In terms of the effector arc of the homograft reaction, several facts seem incontrovertible. The majority of host cells infiltrating the site of a homograft reaction are proliferating and incorporate a label (H^3-TdR). However, labeled lymphoid cells obtained from the lymph nodes of immunized donors and transferred to isologous recipients bearing the homografts do not appear in the homograft under destruction in significant numbers. Instead, they migrate to the lymph nodes. It is thought that they may divide several times in the lymph nodes, diluting their label, and that it is the progeny of the inoculated cells which infiltrate the graft in large numbers. Cells which become labeled in a node stimulated by a homograft migrate via the bloodstream and appear, in preference to reside in the bloodstream, at the sites of rejection of test grafts, but they are still a minority of the infiltrating cells (10 to 20 percent) and appear with equal frequency also in nonspecific sites of delayed hypersensitivity lesions or at a skin homograft from a second, unrelated donor under destruction. In these experiments, it is a distinct possibility that the infiltrating cells were derived ultimately from sources other than the inoculum or the draining lymph nodes. It must be seriously considered that cells of host bone marrow origin serve as active participants in the infiltrate.

5. Finally, the actual mechanism of destruction of foreign cells and tissues by immunologically activated effector lymphocytes is far from clear. It is certain that it does not proceed by the same or similar mechanisms involved in complement- and antibody-mediated cytotoxicity and hemolysis reactions. However, there is a growing body of evidence to sustain the premise that sensitized lymphocytes can produce certain substances, such as MIF, which might mediate delayed hypersensitivity reactions in general in addition to the homograft reaction. These substances have no immunologic specificity themselves, i.e., they are nonspecific in their inhibitory or destructive action on target cells, however they are produced by lymphoid cells under conditions which are strictly specific immunologically. The cells must derive from immunized donors, and they must be maintained in the presence of specific antigen under conditions acceptable for their metabolic activity.

REFERENCES

1. Billingham, R. E.: *J. Invest. Dermatol.*, **41**:165, 1963.
2. Medawar, P. B.: *J. Anat.*, **78**:176, 1944.
3. Medawar, P. B.: *J. Anat.*, **79**:157, 1945.
4. Gibson, T., and Medawar, P. B.: *J. Anat.*, **77**:299, 1943.
5. Medawar, P. B.: in The Harvey Lectures, *Series* **52**:144, 1956–1957, Academic Press, Inc., 1958.
6. Medawar, P. B.: *Proc. Roy. Soc. (Biol.)*, **149**:145, 1958.
7. Billingham, R. E., and Silvers, W. K.: *Annu. Rev. Microbiol.*, **17**:531, 1963.
8. Snell, G. D.: in "Conceptual Advances in Immunology and Oncology," Harper & Row, New York, 1962.
9. Brent, L., and Medawar, P. B.: *Proc. Roy. Soc. (Biol.)*, **155**:392, 1961.
10. Kaliss, N.: *Ann. N.Y. Acad. Sci.*, **101**:64, 1962.
11. Winn, H. J.: *Nat. Cancer Inst., Monogr.*, No. **2**:113, 1960.
12. Mitchison, N. A.: *Proc. Roy. Soc. (Biol.)*, **142**:72, 1954.
13. Mitchison, N. A.: *J. Exp. Med.*, **102**:157, 1955.
14. Billingham, R. E., Brent, L., and Medawar, P. B.: *Proc. Roy. Soc. (Biol.)*, **143**:58, 1954.
15. Algire, G. H., Weaver, J. M., and Prehn, R. T.: *J. Nat. Cancer Inst.*, **15**:493, 1954.
16. Weaver, J. M., Algire, G. H., and Prehn, R. T.: *J. Nat. Cancer Inst.*, **15**:1737, 1955.
17. Algire, G. H., Weaver, J. M., and Prehn, R. T.: *Ann. N.Y. Acad. Sci.*, **64**:1009, 1957.
18. Medawar, P. B.: in "Cellular and Humoral Aspects of the Hypersensitive State," Harper & Row, New York, 1959.
19. Snell, G. D., and Stimpfling, J. H.: in "Biology of the Laboratory Mouse," E. C. Green (ed.), 2d ed., McGraw-Hill, New York, 1966.
20. Graff, R. J., Silvers, W. K., Billingham, R. E., Hildemann, W. H., and Snell, G. D.: *Transplantation*, **4**:605, 1966.
21. Billingham, R. E., and Silvers, W. K.: *J. Immunol.*, **85**:14, 1960.
22. Wilson, D. B.: *Transplantation*, **1**:318, 1963.
22a. Stone, S. H.: *Ann. Rev. Microbiol.*, **21**:181, 1967.
23. Manson, L. A., Foschi, G. V., and Palm, J.: *Proc. Nat. Acad. Sci. U.S.*, **48**:1816, 1962.
24. Dempster, W. J.: *Brit. J. Surg.*, **40**:447, 1953.
25. Simonsen, M.: *Acta Pathol. Microbiol. Scand.*, **32**:36, 1953.

26. Billingham, R. E., and Brent, L.: *Trans. Bull.*, **4**:67, 1957.
27. Billingham, R. E.: *The Harvey Lectures, Series* **62**:21, 1966–1967.
28. Oliner, H., Schwartz, R., and Dameshek, W.: *Blood*, **17**:20, 1961.
29. Billingham, R. E., and Silvers, W. K.: *Trans. Bull.*, **28**:113, 1961.
30. Bert, P.: *J. Anat. Physiol.*, **1**:69, 1862.
31. Sauerbruch, F., and Heyde, M.: *Munchen. Med. Wochschr.*, **55**:153, 1908.
32. Eichwald, E. J., Lustgraaf, E. C., and Strainer, M.: *J. Nat. Cancer Inst.*, **23**:1193, 1959.
33. Micklem, H. S., and Loutit, J. F.: "Tissue Grafting and Radiation," Academic Press, Inc. New York, 1966.
34. Trentin, J. J.: *Proc. Soc. Exp. Biol. Med.*, **92**:688, 1956.
35. Elkins, W. L.: *J. Exp. Med.*, **120**:329, 1964.
36. Elkins, W. L.: *J. Exp. Med.*, **123**:103, 1966.
37. Elkins, W. L., and Guttmann, R. D.: *Science*, **159**:1250, 1968.
38. Brent, L., and Medawar, P. B.: *Brit. Med. J.*, **II**:269, 1963.
39. Brent, L., and Medawar, P. B.: *Proc. Roy. Soc. (Biol.)*, **165**:281, 1966.
40. Brent, L., and Medawar, P. B.: *Proc. Roy. Soc. (Biol.)*, **165**:413, 1966.
41. Burnet, F. M., and Boyer, G. S.: *J. Pathol. Bacteriol.*, **81**:141, 1961.
42. Simons, M. J., and Fowler, R.: *Nature (London)*, **209**:588, 1966.
43. Szenberg, A., Warner, N. L.: *Brit. J. Exp. Pathol.*, **43**:123, 1962.
44. Simonsen, M.: *Cold Spring Harbor Symp. Quant. Biol.*, **32**:517, 1967.
45. Simonsen, M.: *Acta Pathol. Microbiol. Scand.*, **40**:480, 1957.
46. Billingham, R. E.: *Transplantation*, **5**:976, 1967.
47. Waksman, B. H.: *Lab. Invest.*, **12**:46, 1963.
48. Gowans, J. L.: *Brit. Med. Bull.*, **21**:106, 1965.
49. Prendergast, R. A.: *J. Exp. Med.*, **119**:377, 1964.
50. Lawrence, H. S., Al-Askari, S., David, J., Franklin, E. C., Zweiman, B.: *Trans. Assoc. Amer. Physicians*, **76**:84, 1963.
50a. Lawrence, H. S.: *Advan. Immunol.*, 1969. In press.
51. Mannick, J. A., and Egdahl, R. H.: *J. Clin. Invest.*, **43**:2166, 1964.
52. Winn, H. J.: *J. Immunol.*, **86**:228, 1961.
53. Dvorak, H. F., Kosunen, T. U., and Waksman, B. H.: *Lab. Invest.*, **12**:58, 1963.
54. Govaerts, A.: *J. Immunol.*, **85**:516, 1960.
55. Rosenau, W., and Moon, H. D.: *J. Nat. Cancer Inst.*, **27**:471, 1961.
56. Granger, G. A., Weiser, R. S.: *Science*, **145**:1428, 1964.
57. Svet-Moldavsky, G. J., and Chernyakhovskaya, I. J.: *Nature (London)*, **204**:799, 1964.
58. Koprowski, H., and Fernandes, M. V.: *J. Exp. Med.*, **116**:467, 1962.
59. Wilson, D. B.: *J. Cell. Comp. Physiol.*, **62**:273, 1963.
60. Wilson, D. B., and Billingham, R. E.: *Advan. Immunol.*, **7**:189, 1967.
61. Wilson, D. B., and Wecker, E. E.: *J. Immunol.*, **97**:512, 1966.
62. Brondz, B. D., Folia Biol. (Praha): **10**:164, 1964.
63. Vainio, T., Koskimies, O., Perlmann, P., Perlmann, H., and Klein, G.: *Nature (London)*, **204**:453, 1964.

64. Old, L. J., Boyse, E. A., Bennett, B., and Lilly, F.: in "Cell-bound Antibodies," B. Amos and H. Koprowski (eds.), Wistar Institute Press, Philadelphia, 1963.
65. Ruddle, N. H., and Waksman, B. H.: *Science*, **157**:1060, 1967.
65a. Ruddle, N. H., and Waksman, B. H.: *J. Exp. Med.*, **128**:1237, 1968.
66. Wilson, D. B.: *J. Exp. Med.*, **122**:143, 1965.
67. Wilson, D. B.: *J. Exp. Med.*, **122**:167, 1965.
68. Rosenau, W.: *Federation Proc.*, **27**:34, 1968.
69. Taylor, H. E., and Culling, C. F. A.: *Nature (London)*, **220**:506, 1968.
70. Taylor, H. E., and Culling, C. F. A.: *Lab. Invest.*, **12**:884, 1963.
71. Friedman, H.: *Science*, **145**:607, 1964.
72. Brunner, K. T., Mauel, J., Schindler, R.: *Immunology*, **11**:499, 1966.
73. Rosenau, W., and Moon, H. D.: *J. Immunol.*, **89**:422, 1962.
74. Wilson, D. B.: *Transplantation*, **5**:986, 1967.
75. Willoughby, D. A.: *J. Pathol. Bacteriol.*, **92**:139, 1966.
76. David, J. R.: *Proc. Nat. Acad. Sci. U.S.*, **56**:72, 1966.
77. Bloom, B. R., and Bennett, B.: *Science*, **153**:80, 1966.
78. Hellström, K. E., and Möller, G.: *Progr. Allergy*, **9**:158, 1965.
78a. Granger, G. A., and Kolb, W. B.: *J. Immunol.*, **101**:111, 1968.
78b. Williams, T. W., and Granger, G. A.: *J. Immunol.*, **102**:911, 1969.
79. Barker, C. F., and Billingham, R. E.: in "Advance in Transplantation," J. Dausset, J. Hamburger, and G. Mathé (eds), Munksgaard, Copenhagen, 1968.
80. Frey, J. R., and Wenk, P.: *Int. Arch. Allergy*, **11**:81, 1957.
81. Barker, C. F., and Billingham, R. E.: *Transplantation*, **5**:962, 1967.
82. Medawar, P. B.: *Proc. Roy. Soc. (Biol.)*, **B149**:145, 1958.
83. Strober, S., and Gowans, J. L.: *J. Exp. Med.*, **122**:347, 1965.
84. Wilson, D. B.: *J. Exp. Med.*, **126**:625, 1967.
85. Wilson, D. B., Silvers, W. K., and Nowell, P. C.: *J. Exp. Med.*, **126**:655, 1967.
86. Silvers, W. K., Wilson, D. B., and Palm, J.: *Science*, **155**:703, 1967.
87. Holub, M.: in "Mechanisms of Antibody Formation," M. Holub and L. Jaroskova (eds.), Czechoslovak Academy Science, Prague, 1960.
88. Holub, M.: *Ann. N.Y. Acad. Sci.*, **99**:477, 1962.
89. Leduc, E. H., Coons, A. H., and Connolly, J. M.: *J. Exp. Med.*, **102**:61, 1955.
90. Scothorne, R. J.: *Ann. N.Y. Acad. Sci.*, **64**:1028, 1957.
91. Gowans, J. L.: *Ann. N.Y. Acad. Sci.*, **99**:432, 1962.
92. Dutton, R. W.: *Advan. Immunol.*, **6**:253, 1967.
93. Pearmain, G., Lycette, R. R., and Fitzgerald, P. H.: *Lancet*, **II**:816, 1965.
94. Mills, J. A.: *J. Immunol.*, **97**:239, 1966.
95. Bain, B., Vas, M. R., and Lowenstein, L.: *Blood*, **23**:108, 1964.
96. Dutton, R. W.: *J. Exp. Med.*, **123**:665, 1966.
97. Bach, F. H., and Voynow, N. K.: *Science*, **153**:545, 1966.
98. Wilson, D. B., and Elkins, W. L.: in "3rd Lymphocyte Conference," Iowa City, Iowa, 1969.

99. Mitchison, N. A.: *Cold Spring Harbor Symp. Quant. Biol.*, **32**:431, 1967.
100. Lennox, E. S., and Cohn, M.: *Annu. Rev. Biochem.*, **36**:365, 1967.
101. Wilson, D. B., Blyth, J. L., and Nowell, P. C.: *J. Exp. Med.*, **128**:1157, 1968.
102. Albright, J. F., and Makinodan, T.: *J. Cell. Physiol.*, **67**(Suppl. 1):185, 1966.
103. Kennedy, J. C., Till, J. E., Siminovitch, L., and McCulloch, E. A.: *J. Immunol.*, **94**:715, 1965.
104. Kennedy, J. C., Till, J. E., Siminovitch, L., and McCulloch, E. A.: *J. Immunol.*, **96**:973, 1966.
105. Štark, O., Frenzl, B., and Křen, V.: *Folia Biol. (Prague)*, **14**:169, 1968.
106. Hiramoto, R. N., and Hamlin, M.: *J. Immunol.*, **95**:214, 1965.
107. Attardi, G., Cohn, M., Horibata, K., and Lennox, E. S.: *J. Immunol.*, **93**:94, 1964.
108. Dutton, R. W., and Mishell, R. I.: *J. Exp. Med.*, **126**:443, 1967.
109. Dutton, R. W., and Mishell, R. I.: *Cold Spring Harbor Symp. Quant. Biol.*, **32**:407, 1967.
110. Wilson, D. B., and Nowell, P. C.: Submitted to *J. Exp. Med.*
110a. Lafferty, K. J., and Jones, M. A. S.: *Australian J. Exp. Biol. Med. Sci.*, **47**:17, 1969.
110b. Snell, G. D.: *Folia Biol.*, **14**:335, 1968.
110c. Jerne, N. K.: *Proc. Nat. Acad. Sci. U.S.* In press.
111. Mitchell, G. F., and Miller, J. F. A. P.: *Proc. Nat. Acad. Sci. U.S.*, **59**:296, 1968.
112. Steinmuller, D.: *Science*, **158**:127, 1967.

Name Index

Subject Index

Page references in bold indicate tables or figures.

Toxin:
  in acquired immunity, 9–10
  anti-, 376–377, 382–383
  endo-, 21, 376, 377, 381, 382
  exo-, 376, 377
  inactivation of, 376–377
  in innate immunity, 5
  natural antibodies to, 7
  vaccination and, 383
  as virulence factor, 381
Toxoid, 10
Transplantation of tissues:
  antigens in, 388, 437–440, 447
  autografts, 246, 432
  effect of antilymphocyte serum on, 280
  graft versus host reaction and, 439–443
  homograft reaction and, 432–439, 444–463
  homotransplantation, 250, 298
  in invertebrates, 94–95
  isograft, 246, 437
  second set reaction, 244–245, 433
  in vertebrates, Cyclostomata, 98
Tuberculosis, 383
Tumor immunity, 387–389, 445
Two-cell theory of antibody production, 252

Ultracentrifugal analysis of antigen-antibody complexes, 343

Vaccination, 1, 383–384
  intrauterine, 126, 127
  of invertebrates, 95
  smallpox, 130
Vaccines, 9
  adjuvants in, 261, 266
  against viruses, 383–384

Valence of antibodies, 79–80
Vertebrates, evolution of immunity in, 96–115
  amphibians, 113
  birds, 113–114
  chondrosteans, 107–110
  Cyclostomata, 96–103
  elasmobranchs, 104–106
  holosteans, 110–112
  major steps in, **97**
  mammals, 113–114
  reptiles, 113
  teleosteans, 110–112
Virulence:
  bacterial capsules and, 374, 376, 380–381
  factors in, 380–381
  reduction of, 9
Virus:
  adeno-, 386
  incubation period of, 384, 386
  induced tumors, 387–389
  neutralization, 378
  protection against, 384–387

Waldenstrom macroglobulin, 36, 43, 46
  antigenic determinants and, 38–39
  dissociation of, 58, 62
  structure of, 60, 62
Wax D of tubercle bacillus, 264–265

X-radiation:
  colchicine and, 289
  effect on immune response, 284–291
    in primary and secondary response, **285, 287, 322**
    restoration, **289**
  protection against, 287–291
X-ray scattering, shape of IgG molecule, 55